Survival:
A Medical Memoir

FROM DRUG DISCOVERY TO
CLINICAL CANCER TRIALS

Lorne J. Brandes, MD

◆ FriesenPress

Suite 300 - 990 Fort St
Victoria, BC, V8V 3K2
Canada

www.friesenpress.com

ISBN
978-1-4602-8506-0 (Hardcover)
978-1-4602-8507-7 (Paperback)
978-1-4602-8508-4 (eBook)

1. MEDICAL, ONCOLOGY

Distributed to the trade by The Ingram Book Company

ACKNOWLEDGEMENT

I thank numerous participants in this story for their recollections and insights. I am grateful to several colleagues and friends for taking the time to read the manuscript as well as for their comments and encouragement. A very special tip of the hat to my wife, Jill, herself a writer extraordinaire, for suggesting the title and helping me to make the story "flow".

This book is dedicated to Jill, Jason and Carolyn for always believing in me, and to the memory of four other very special people: my parents, Lorraine and Bill Brandes; Dr. David B. Meltzer who, by his example, inspired me to become an oncologist; and Dr. Lyonel G. Israels, who shaped my career, gave me wings and let me fly.

LJB

FOREWORD

It is my great pleasure to write a few introductory words to Dr. Lorne Brandes' book. I first came across Lorne when he embarked on the adventure in drug development he so well describes in this book.

To say that I saw him, from the start, as a "unique character" is an understatement. He was passionate and persistent about his findings on DPPE, his basic and clinical research, as well as his practice of oncology. This passion likely came from his calling, but also from the Jewish dictum: "Tikun Olam" (saving the world). This phrase is viewed by many in their own way, but the concept of "doing good" is embedded in all their interpretations. All of this comes out so clearly in this book.

This view and his passion made Lorne some rivals, but also friends along his journey. I am happy to count myself amongst his friends.

The story he writes is a good read after all the years that have passed. It is a story that was worthwhile writing to have researchers understand that many endeavours do not end successfully. This is true, especially, in the realm of drug development.

Solid and confirmed clinical studies, with at least two convergent outcomes are needed to have a drug product become viable. I have often noted that regulators require certainty to be able to make solid decisions. However, achieving certainty does not necessarily ensure uptake by the health care system. In addition to clinical benefit, pharmacoeconomic factors also must be shown convincingly for that product to become a standard in therapy.

Then, there is the issue of what the scientific world demands, increasingly, for credibility: declaration of financial or other competing interests, registry of the trials, and fully independent peer review, among others. In parallel, the regulatory bar continues to be raised. Finally, conducting clinical trials with adequate rigor is difficult, while the expectations of the public keep increasing, an added complexity. All of these factors make it increasingly costly and difficult to bring a drug to market and common use.

Decades ago, basic and clinical scientists, as well as regulators, estimated that 1:10,000 substances reach the viable and marketable drug product stage. That ratio has not decreased with time: indeed, over the last 40 years the ratio of success to failure is still approximately the same. Hence, it was a bit surprising, but not shocking that, despite its initial success, DPPE failed at a point in its development where most failures occur, namely at the stage of clinical trials aimed at confirming its therapeutic activity.

Nonetheless, the dedicated work and effort as well as the years Lorne spent on DPPE were, most likely, not wasted as a significant body of knowledge on "targeted therapies" may have emerged and could be considered one of the heralds of "personalised" medicine.

The story of DPPE, as described by Lorne, is accurate as much as memory can reproduce. While not present at some of the conversations between other parties, the essence and feel of each episode is accurate in terms of tone and direction of the conversations. The "feel" for what went on had been described to me by Lorne in much the terms reflected in the book. I believe the book deserves to be published to remind researchers, physicians, other health care professionals and even a regulator like me, that the road to a successful drug is paved with pitfalls, despite all good intentions, and that while many active substances never "make it", much new knowledge can be acquired along the way.

So, my friend Lorne, do not despair. Your work was not in vain.

Agnes V. Klein, MD
Director, Centre for Evaluation of
Radiopharmaceuticals and Biotherapeutics
Biologics and Genetic Therapies Directorate
Health Canada
November, 2015

PREFACE

This is the amazing true story of medical research, far outside the box, that led to a promising cancer drug discovery. The word *Survival* in the title refers not only to the life and death struggle of DPPE (tesmilifene), a drug that was prematurely declared inactive in an aborted international breast cancer trial only to rise from the ashes and win a second chance, but also to the surprising survival advantage that DPPE appeared to confer in an analysis performed 18 months after the trial was stopped. Ultimately, *Survival* is a story about the resilience of the human spirit amid rejection and failure.

The saga chronicles the roller-coaster ride of a novel cancer treatment with potentially enormous benefit to patients; the unprecedented facilitation of its development by university and government bureaucrats; the premature decision of a U.S. pharmaceutical giant that stopped it in its tracks for five years; and its dramatic rescue by a small Canadian biotech company that, with a combination of luck, private venture capital and the FDA's blessing, took it back into a pivotal trial needed for its approval. Intertwined with the human drama is an account of the politics and science behind the story, including an unanticipated research finding with implications that shook the public, drug companies and regulatory agencies.

In the absence of a diary, telling the story of a journey that took place over more than twenty years has involved, to a large degree, vivid recollections long ingrained in my memory, aided by reams of correspondence, public records and discussions with many of those who took part.

Given the long interval over which events unfolded, there may be inadvertent omissions, or minor errors in timelines. Also, with the exception of interview transcripts, quoted conversations are my reconstruction of what was said. At the end of the day, this is my version of what happened. While others may have a different perspective, I stand by the overall accuracy of my recounting of history. As in any story, there are those who deserve praise or, in some cases, less than praise; I have tried to give each person their correct due.

With notable exceptions, such as James D. Watson's remarkable and entertaining account of the discovery of the structure of DNA in *The Double Helix* (never out of print since its publication in 1968!), and Eric Kandel's *In Search of Memory*, a unique blend of personal memoir and Nobel Prize-winning research into the biological basis of memory, books about science can make dull reading at best, or miss the mark at worst. Who will be interested in reading the story if the passion behind the discovery is lost behind dry prose, or complexity in the telling causes bafflement in the reader, even among colleagues who attempt to understand research that may be unrelated to their own?

Mindful of these pitfalls, I have tried to write this story in such a way as to engage the reader, while explaining important scientific concepts as simply as possible, and only when necessary, to help both laypersons and experts understand the "whys and wherefores" of the bigger picture as I saw it.

Sadly, many of the key players in this book are no longer alive, including those incredibly brave patients who allowed me to test

DPPE on them in the early stages of its development. Without their help, it would have never gone into clinical trials.

Over those tumultuous years, my dear wife and family, as well as many close friends and colleagues, accompanied me down the long and uncertain road that I chose to follow. To say that it was not always easy is an understatement of vast proportion. To them I say, "Thank you for your love, support and, most of all, your understanding."

LJB

WHO'S WHO, AND WHERE

1. *Manitoba Cancer Treatment and Research Foundation (CancerCare Manitoba)*

   Asher Begleiter, Professor of Pharmacology, Manitoba Institute of Cell Biology

   David Bowman, Medical Oncologist

   Susan Bracken, Chemotherapy Nurse

   Julia DeFehr, Head, Donations and Media Relations

   Linda Friesen, Clinic Nurse

   Jon Gerrard, Professor of Pediatrics, Manitoba Institute of Cell Biology

   Arnold Greenberg, Director, Manitoba Institute of Cell Biology

   Lyonel Israels, CEO, Manitoba Cancer Treatment and Research Foundation

   Kerry McDonald, Nurse Practitioner

   Frixos Paraskevas, Professor of Immunology, Manitoba Institute of Cell Biology

   Arnold Portigal, Chairman of the Board

Brent Schacter, President and CEO (successor to
Lyonel Israels)

2. *University of Manitoba*

Wayne Beecroft, Assistant Professor, Department of Surgery

Ranjan Bose, Research Associate, Department
of Pharmacology

Ratna Bose, Senior Scholar, Department of Pharmacology

Gary Breit, Executive Director, Technology Transfer Office
(successor to Janet Scholz)

Harvey Chochinov, Professor, Department of Psychiatry

Henry Friesen, Professor and Head, Department
of Physiology

Gary Glavin, Associate Professor, Department
of Pharmacology

Gordon Grahame, Chairman, Ethics Committee (successor
to John Maclean)

Clive Greenway, Professor and Head, Department
of Pharmacology

Landis Henry, Assistant Manager, Technology Transfer Office
(successor to Morris Silver)

Terry Hogan, Vice-President, Research (successor to
Marion Vaisey-Genser)

Georgina Hogg, Professor Emeritus, Department of
Pathology (retired)

Joanne Keselman, Vice-President, Research (successor to
Terry Hogan)

Ed Kroeger, Professor, Department of Physiology

Frank LaBella, Professor, Department of Pharmacology

John Maclean, Chairman, Ethics Committee

Leigh Murphy, Post-doctoral Fellow, Department of Physiology

Carl Pinsky, Professor, Department of Pharmacology

Ernest Ramsey, Professor and Head, Section of Urology

Janet Scholz, Manager, Technology Transfer Office

Morris Silver, Assistant Manager, Technology Transfer Office

Keith Simons, Professor, Faculty of Pharmacy

Marion Vaisey-Genser, Vice-President, Research

3. *Sim and McBurney*

Michael Stewart, Patent Agent

4. *University of Saskatchewan*

Robert Warrington, Professor, Department of Biochemistry

5. *University of Southern California (USC), Los Angeles*

Derek Raghavan, Professor, Chief, Division of Oncology

6. *Health Protection Branch (Health Canada), Ottawa*

Ivo Hynie, Assessment Officer, Clinical Trials

Agnes Klein, Head, Division of Hematology/Oncology/Gastroenterology

7. *Food and Drug Administration (FDA), Bethesda, MD*

Gregory Burke, Director, Division of Oncologic and Pulmonary Drug Products

Charles Grieshaber, Director, Office of Testing and Research

Robert Temple, Director, Office of Drug Evaluation

8. *National Cancer Institute of Canada Clinical Trials Group (NCIC-CTG)*

   Elizabeth Eisenhauer, Director, Investigational New Drug (IND) Program

   Kong Khoo, Member, IND Committee

   Kathy Pritchard, Chair, Breast Cancer Site Group

   Len Reyno, Chairman, MA.19 Trial

   Lesley Seymour, Co-Director, IND Program

9. *Burroughs Wellcome*

   Pedro Cuatrecasas, Vice-President, Research and Development

   Gertrude Elion, Head, Department of Experimental Therapy

   Indu Parikh, Associate Head, Molecular Biology

   Howard Schaeffer, Vice-President, Research

10. *Eli Lilly*

    Bernie Abbott, Manager, Technology Acquisition

    Stan Marshall, Senior Chemist and Vice-President

    Patrick Roffey, Senior Vice-President

11. *Schering-Plough*

    Allen Barnett, Vice-President, Technology Acquisition

12. *Sparta Pharmaceuticals*

    Bill McCulloch, Medical Director

Bill Sullivan, CEO

13. *Pharmacia*

Langdon Miller, Vice-President, Oncology

Hooshmand Sheshberadaran, Director, Licensing

Franzanne Vreeland, Oncology Group

14. *Bristol-Myers Squibb*

Renzo Canetta, Vice-President, Oncology

Robert Kramer, Head, Oncology Discovery Group

David Lebwohl, DPPE Project Manager (successor to Bill Slichenmyer)

Alice Leung, Vice-President, Licensing

Ana Menendez, Researcher, Oncology Discovery Group

Sol Rajfer, Vice-President, Worldwide Clinical Research and Development

Bill Rose, Head, Experimental Therapeutics

Lee Schacter, Director, Clinical Cancer Research

Bill Slichenmyer, DPPE Project Manager

Jeff Usakewicz, Clinical Research Manager, Oncology

15. *YM BioSciences*

David Allan, CEO

Craig Binnie, Director, Clinical Product Development

David Harper, Director, Licensing

Paul Keane, Medical Director

Vincent Salvatori, Executive Vice-President (successor to Nic Stiernholm)

Gail Schulze, CEO, YM BioSciences USA

Jennifer Seibert, Director, Intellectual Property

Igor Sherman, Director, Clinical Research and Scientific Affairs

Nic Stiernholm, Executive Vice-President and Chief Scientific Officer

Mark Vincent, Medical Consultant

16. *Pharm-Olam*

Bruce Ross, Manager, North American YM Trial Recruitment

17. *European Histamine Research Society (EHRS)*

Michel Dy, Institute Nêcker, Paris, FR

Wilfried Lorenz, Professor, Department of Anaesthesiology, Marburg, DE

Pier Mannaioni, Professor, Department of Pharmacology, Florence, IT

Henk Timmerman, Professor and Head, Department of Pharmacology, Amsterdam, NL

Börje Uvnäs, Emeritus Professor of Pharmacology, Stockholm, SE

Takehiko Watanabe, Professor, Department of Pharmacology, Sendai JP

CHAPTERS

PROLOGUE

On a Monday morning in early May, 2001, I unlocked the door to my office, turned on the light and proceeded to open some mail. I had no reason to believe that this Monday would be different from any other of recent memory. I was quickly proven wrong. David Bowman, an oncologist and longtime colleague, poked his head in the door. He was just back from the spring meeting of the National Cancer Institute of Canada (NCIC) Clinical Trials Group. "Lorne, did Kathy Pritchard call you?" he asked. Kathy chaired the organization's Breast Cancer Site Group. From the blank look on my face, he quickly realized she had not. "So you haven't heard?" he tried again.

"Heard what?" I replied, unsure of what would follow.

"I think you had better sit down," David suggested. I followed his instruction.

"The MA.19 survival data have just been analyzed and presented at the meeting. Are you ready for this?" he asked, now clearly savoring what he was about to tell me.

"David....enough of the suspense," I implored.

"Follow-up after the trial ended showed a highly significant, fifty percent increase in survival in the one hundred and fifty patients who received DPPE. It's been analyzed every way possible and they can't make the result disappear. It caught absolutely everyone off guard. It was the talk of the meeting. You should have been there."

MA.19 was a major international breast cancer study testing DPPE, a drug that I had developed over a fifteen year span. Given in combination with chemotherapy drugs, DPPE was intended to make them more effective as cancer-fighters. The trial had been abruptly stopped eighteen months previously, when what is called an "interim analysis" failed to show any evidence of an early benefit from adding DPPE to a breast cancer drug called doxorubicin. Without waiting for the survival outcome, a much more meaningful endpoint that would take many additional months of observation to measure, Bristol-Myers Squibb, the drug company to which DPPE was licensed, immediately pulled the plug. However, the NCIC continued to follow the patients' survival as part of the original study plan.

A fifty percent increase in survival, that most elusive of all endpoints? Unheard of! No drug had ever achieved such a result in this group of patients. I just sat there, thunderstruck, shaking my head, not knowing whether to be happy or sad, to laugh or cry. David well understood my reaction. "I think you should be elated by this news. Congratulations. You deserve it," he said, shaking my hand, a wide grin evident on his face.

I was totally unprepared for this momentous news. After my drug was very publicly declared a failure, I mourned the loss and then got on with my life. Now, as in a bad Hollywood movie, the "baby" I thought was buried had just reached up from the grave and grabbed me by the neck. What had I done to deserve such cruel and unusual punishment?

So begins the amazing story of DPPE....

PART 1

"Nothing great was ever achieved
without enthusiasm."

Ralph Waldo Emerson

CHAPTER ONE:

Eureka!

According to my late parents, when I was very young they would take me for a walk down our street on warm summer nights. I would invariably look up to the sky, raise my stubby little finger and point to the moon or myriad of tiny stars twinkling overhead. "Whaddat?" I would ask them. They marveled at the inquisitiveness of their not yet two-year-old son. But then again, they were biased in my favor. Aren't are all mothers and fathers? Of course, I have no recollection of doing this, but if they told me it happened, it was so. They always told the truth.

As I grew, so did my "whaddat?" curiosity. Unfortunately, I, and it, were often synonymous with trouble. Although there were attempts to distract me with chemistry, Erector and even crystal sets (remember those?), I just could not resist taking apart household items, including windup clocks and everything that plugged into the wall. After all, I needed to understand how they worked. For example, the small table radio in the bedroom forever squeaked and squawked after I ignored the printed warning about electrocution on the back cover, removed it, pulled out some wires attached to strange-looking objects in its innards, and then tried unsuccessfully to put them back. My younger brothers looked on, promising to rat on me. In turn, I threatened the two of them with bad things if they squealed. They didn't have to. My parents soon figured out who and what.

Approaching puberty, I fancied myself an inventor, a budding Thomas Edison. At the age of twelve, excited by Sputnik, I sent the U.S. Defense Department a drawing of four diamond-shaped vanes, black on one side, white on the other, similar to the ones that sunlight caused to rotate on a spindle in a vacuum bulb in my science class. I suggested that, in the sunlit vacuum of space, the vanes could turn a small built-in generator to make electricity for satellites. In those early days, they ran on regular batteries that soon wore down. Several months went by without a reply. Finally, an official-looking envelope arrived from Washington, addressed to a Mr. L. Braneles. *Brainless?* Undaunted by the embarrassing misspelling of my last name, I excitedly ripped it open to find a short, polite letter of rejection. Unfortunately, my invention did not fit the needs of the Department of Defense. However, my suggestion would be kept on file "for future reference".

Closer to the ground, a friend and I kept trying to improve on the "two tin cans attached by a string" concept, making fancy hollow cone-like receptacles to amplify the sound, and laboriously waxing long pieces of string to improve the vibration that transmitted our voices from one cone to the other. Once I had the bright idea that if we connected a small battery to an aerial made from a wire coat hanger, the electricity would power our voices through the cone into the air without the need for any string! Unfortunately, it was a bust. But didn't it come close to today's cell phones? Okay, so it didn't. Why do I tell you all of this? To give you some insight into the mind of a precocious kid who grew up to be a scientist.

Thirty years later, in 1984, slightly less precocious but still curious, I was now a medical doctor with post-graduate training in oncology. Keenly interested in research, I had given up taking

apart radios and, instead, took apart cells. My lab in the Institute
of Cell Biology at the University of Manitoba was conducting
research on tamoxifen, a drug widely used to shrink estrogen-
driven breast cancer. As usual, I was trying to figure out how
it worked.

It was well established that tamoxifen hones in on an important cell component called an estrogen receptor. A receptor can be
thought of as a lock into which a specific key must fit. When the
female hormone, estrogen, inserts itself into the receptor in breast
cancer cells, a series of events are set into motion that include cell
division. This results in tumor growth. Tamoxifen is called an
"antiestrogen" because it too fits the receptor, thereby blocking the
entry of estrogen and preventing it from fueling the cancer. But
was that the whole story?

I had become intrigued by a second potential tamoxifen target,
described in a 1980 paper in *Nature* by Robert Sutherland's group[1]
at the Ludwig Institute in Sydney. It was called the "antiestrogen
binding site (AEBS)", simply a descriptive term to denote the
ability of tamoxifen to latch on to it. While its exact nature was
a mystery, the AEBS had been found to reside in what are called
"microsomes", derived from thin-walled canal-like membranes
inside cells that are involved in metabolism and in making important substances such as proteins. Unlike the estrogen receptor,
which is mainly present in the breast and uterus, the AEBS is
found in all body tissues, especially in the liver, an easy organ to
obtain from rodents.

Thus, the question: although blocking the attachment of
estrogen to its receptor in breast cancer cells appeared vital to the
clinical activity of tamoxifen, could binding to the AEBS also con-
tribute to its ability to shrink tumors? To answer that question, we

---

1   One member of the group, Dr. Leigh Murphy, who moved to the
     University of Manitoba in 1985, laughingly reminded me of the time I
     phoned Rob Sutherland to ask him some naïve questions about the
     methodology of his AEBS experiments. "I just got the strangest call from
     a guy in Canada," he told her.

needed to find a substance that, unlike tamoxifen, would bind only to this newly-discovered entity, and not to the estrogen receptor. At a breast cancer research conference earlier in the year, I had met Benita Katzenellenbogen, a prominent investigator from the University of Illinois. She told me that she was also interested in pursuing this approach. From this encounter, it became clear that the race was on to find a selective agent for the AEBS.

I had some idea of what was needed to succeed. In very basic terms, a great many common drugs, including tamoxifen, are small molecules. Their chemical structures consist of two main elements: rings and chains. There are innumerable permutations and combinations, based on the number, shape and size of each component, and how they relate to each other in space (i.e. in three dimensions). This determines the overall shape of the drug. In turn, the shape of the drug, like a piece of a jigsaw puzzle, determines its target in the cell. Only the right piece, with the proper dimensions, will fit into position in a receptor of specific size and configuration.

In the case of tamoxifen (Figure 1), there are three rings, each having six sides. A special "stilbene" bridge[2] links one of the rings to the other two. In addition, a side chain, made up of various atoms joined one to the other, dangles like a tail from one of the rings.

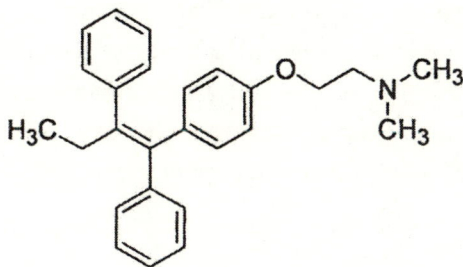

Fig. 1 Structure of tamoxifen

---

2   The stilbene bridge consists of two carbon atoms joined together by a double bond: -C==C-

Recent studies had shown that tamoxifen's side chain was essential, but not sufficient in itself, to bind to the AEBS. Therefore, I hypothesized that a selective drug for the AEBS must include that vital side chain, but any rings attached to it could not have the specific configuration to fit the estrogen receptor. This likely meant that we would have to exclude at least one of them from any molecule we would make.

The first attempt would be kept simple: one ring attached to the side chain. Dr. Asher Begleiter, a colleague at the Institute who had a background in chemistry, gave instructions on how to put it together. Luckily, it would be quite easy to do, requiring some heat and alkali to fuse together two chemicals purchased from a laboratory supply house. This was followed by some "cleanup" steps with common solvents to remove impurities. The product was dried overnight on filter paper to form a white crystalline powder.

The new compound was then tested in what is called a radioligand binding assay.[3]

In this case, we would see if it prevented the binding of two radioligands: tamoxifen to the AEBS and estrogen to its receptor. In this way we could determine the selectivity of our newly-made molecule for one site or the other. By using a machine similar to a Geiger counter, the energy emitted when the radioactive substance binds to a receptor in cells or tissue can be measured. If the non-radioactive compound we just made could prevent the binding (i.e., compete for the attachment) of either, or both, radioligands, the amount of measured radioactivity would decrease.

The answer in the assay was clear: our first compound did not prevent the binding of radioactive estrogen to its receptor (good!). However, there was only the slightest hint of interference with the

---

3   The prefix "radio-" means radioactive. The term "ligand" means a substance or molecule. Therefore, a "radioligand" is "a radioactive substance". "Binding" means "to attach to something". "Assay" is just another word for "test". Taken together, it is "a test to detect the attachment of a radioactive substance". In this case, the radioligands were estrogen (estradiol) and tamoxifen, obtained from a company that added a radioactive hydrogen atom to each molecule.

binding of radioactive tamoxifen to the AEBS (not good!). Hardly close and definitely no cigar. Yet I thought we might be on the right track.

The next logical step was to make a molecule containing two of tamoxifen's rings. To avoid mimicking the structure of estrogen, I chose the two not joined by the stilbene bridge (Figure 2). One of the rings was then attached to the side chain….again, surprisingly easy to do with two purchased precursor chemicals, followed by the same type of cleanup and drying procedures that were used to formulate the first compound. That Asher…what a genius!

The resulting creamy-white powder was ready to test within a couple of days. It showed no interference with estrogen binding to its receptor (again, good!). However, it proved to be as strong as tamoxifen in its ability to bind to the AEBS. We appeared to have synthesized exactly what we had wanted, and on only the second try! Sometimes you get lucky. We called our promising new find "DPPE", an acronym for its long chemical name, N,N-diethyl-2-[4-(phenylmethyl) phenoxy] ethanamine.

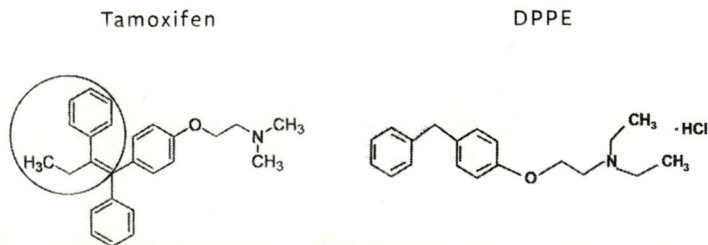

Tamoxifen   DPPE

Figure 2: Removing the top left ring, stilbene bridge and ethyl (CH$_2$CH$_3$) group from tamoxifen (left) leaves a two-ring structure attached to the side chain. The resulting molecule is DPPE.HCl (right), an easily-dissolved hydrochloride salt.

Could DPPE stop the growth, or even kill breast cancer cells in tissue culture? For these experiments, we used estrogen-driven cells called "MCF-7", isolated many years earlier at Detroit's Michigan Cancer Foundation (hence the designation) from the tumor of a woman with advanced breast cancer. Long after her death, these cells continued to grow in culture dishes around the world and were widely employed in laboratories conducting breast cancer research. The results were unequivocal: DPPE did not block the estrogen-stimulated growth of the MCF-7 cells[4] but, nonetheless, slowed them considerably. Higher concentrations of DPPE killed the breast cancer cells, just like tamoxifen. The findings supported the hypothesis that the AEBS might be important to the growth-slowing and cell-killing action of both DPPE and tamoxifen. This story was getting exciting!

Now it became even more important to establish the identity of the AEBS. The first question that came to mind was, "What kind of a substance is DPPE?" Thumbing through a chemical dictionary called the *Merck Index*, revealed that its structure most closely resembled certain antihistamine drugs, such as diphenhydramine (Benadryl), dimenhydrinate (Gravol) and hydroxyzine (Atarax), used for years to treat hay fever, nausea and itching. What could this mean, apart from the obvious inference that DPPE itself might treat these symptoms? Did histamine have any hidden properties that might be relevant to the killing action of tamoxifen and DPPE? I was not aware of any.

Down the hall to the Institute library I went! As luck would have it, on the shelf was a copy of *Goodman and Gilman's The Phamacological Basis of Therapeutics*, the "bible" of pharmacology. I signed it out. The next afternoon, when I did not have to see patients in my clinic, I went to my office, closed the door, picked up the heavy reference textbook and turned to the chapter on histamine.

---

4   Tamoxifen's growth-inhibitory action at the lowest concentrations can be reversed by adding excess estrogen to the cell culture, meaning that low-dose tamoxifen slows growth by blocking the estrogen receptor in these MCF-7 cells, a site that DPPE does not bind. In contrast, the slowing and killing at higher concentrations by tamoxifen and DPPE is not reversed by added estrogen, suggesting that higher concentrations of each slow or kill the cells by a different mechanism, possibly implicating the AEBS.

The preamble went like this: histamine, like many of the body's important small chemicals, acts by binding to specific cell receptors. But while many receptors, such as those for estrogen, reside inside the cell, others, like those for histamine, reside outside the cell, on its membrane, or outer "skin". Two distinct types of histamine receptors had been identified at that time: the H_1 receptor, which was linked to allergic symptoms, and the H_2 receptor, which was linked to the stimulation of acid secretion in the stomach. Specific antihistamines had been developed to counteract the effects of histamine at each of these receptors.

That said, since its discovery almost a century earlier by British physiologist Sir Henry Dale, many questions still surrounded histamine. The mystery deepened in the 1930s, when histamine was identified in "mast cells" that make and store it in dense, blue-staining granules, and release it in the presence of many substances to which a person may be allergic.[5] Mast cells are abundant in the body, especially the skin, liver, gut, heart and bone marrow. Why are they there and what do they do? No one was sure.

On and on the text droned....past the usual stuff about histamine and mast cells; H_1 receptors and allergy; H_2 receptors and acid secretion in the stomach; the pharmacology of H_1 and H_2 antihistamines. As the chapter wound down, it seemed that I would not find any new revelations.

And then I saw it...right near the very end....a sentence, in smaller print than all of the preceding, that would literally change my life: "*A conspicuously high histamine-forming capacity is present*

---

5   I once heard a lecturer estimate the total weight of mast cells in the adult human body to be about two kilograms! If true, that's an awful lot of mast cells containing an awful lot of histamine. Are mast cells simply there to burst open, release their granules of histamine and cause a severe reaction that might kill you if you are allergic to shrimp or peanuts? That notion always seemed nonsensical to me because it represents abnormal pathology rather than normal physiology. So what is the real function of all that stored histamine in our tissues? the great unanswered question, then and now.

in many tissues undergoing rapid growth or repair, such as embry-onic tissue, regenerating liver, bone marrow, wound and granula-tion tissue, and malignant..." Rapid growth? Malignant? Eureka!

CHAPTER TWO:

Audrey's Special Loan

A book reference had been given: *Kahlson, G. and Rosengren, E. In: Biogenesis and Physiology of Histamine. Edward Arnold Ltd., London, 1971.* Where would I ever locate such an arcane source? I immediately walked across the medical school campus to the main library, hoping against all odds that a copy of this must-have tome could be found there.

On entering the cluttered main room, I looked for Audrey Kerr, our head librarian. She was in her office. "Audrey, is there any chance that we might have this book somewhere?" I asked, thrusting into her hand (the one not holding the ever-present cigarette) a paper on which I had written the reference. Audrey, always kind and helpful, immediately went over to the main cardex (computer inventories were in their infancy) and started the ritual flip of the cards to search by author, title, and category.

"It looks like we have it," she reported a few minutes later. My heart skipped a beat. I followed her like a little puppy up and down the stacks that housed the decades-old collection of materia medica as she looked for that magic Dewey decimal combination indicated on the card.

Halfway down the second-last row, Audrey stopped. "Well, Lorne, here it is," she said triumphantly, plucking a small black-covered book from in between two others and handing it to me. I still couldn't believe my good luck. I blew off an accumulation of dust as I opened it. Inside, the pages were pristine; the spine was stiff. The library stamp on the inside back cover indicated that it had been signed out only once before in the preceding twelve years! The preface indicated that this was a special monograph, commissioned by the British Physiological Society in 1971. In it, Kahlson summarized his life's work on "nascent" histamine, which he defined as *"intracellular histamine formed at very high rates in some tissues and circumstances....seemingly involved in certain kinds of rapid tissue growth...."* That did it. I had to read this book!!!

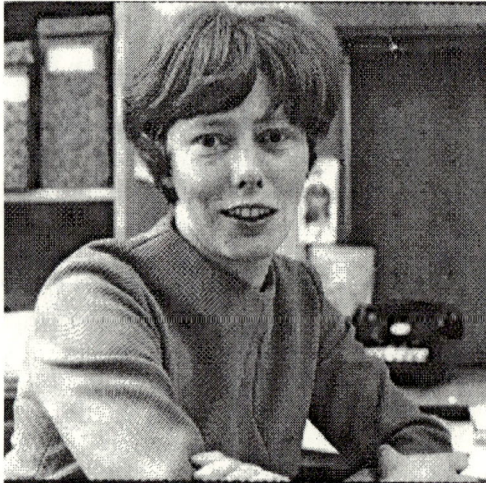

Audrey Kerr, circa. 1965 (Photo courtesy of Audrey Kerr)

"Keep it for two weeks, rather than the usual one," Audrey immediately offered, a twinkle in her eye. I eagerly accepted. After two weeks, I renewed the book at the library. I kept reading and rereading its two hundred and eighty-nine pages over the next three months.

Again and again I renewed the book. After about the sixth time, Audrey decided I should keep it "on special loan", as she euphemistically called it, and filled out the requisite form for her records. Ever since that time, the book has remained on my shelf. I will always love Audrey for that.

The essence of the book was this: Professor Georg Kahlson, assisted by his colleague, Elsa Rosengren, and other members of his group in the Department of Physiology at the University of Lund, Sweden, had carried out a series of experiments that he believed linked histamine, made directly inside the cell (which he termed "nascent", or newly-formed, histamine), to growth and other vital cell functions. These experiments were centered on the newly-discovered ability to measure the activity of an enzyme, called histidine decarboxylase, that specifically converts a precursor amino acid, called L-histidine, into histamine.

An enzyme is a cell chemical that removes or adds molecules to an existing substance, thus making a new substance. The term "decarboxylase" means a specific enzyme that removes a molecule of carbon dioxide. *Histidine decarboxylase removes a molecule of carbon dioxide from histidine to form histamine.*

By tracking the activity of the enzyme, Kahlson and Rosengren were able to show a marked increase in new histamine formation under a variety of circumstances, including the rapid growth of plants, embryos and malignant tumors. Interestingly, even though this "nascent" histamine was being formed rapidly, its actual level *decreased* in the growing tissue, much of it leaving the cells. Why? There was no good explanation. All Kahlson knew was that the histamine apparently was consumed as fast as it was being made.

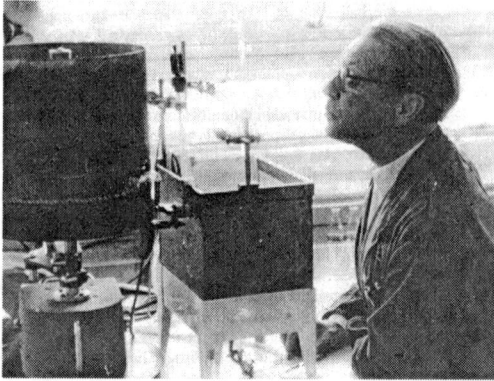

Georg Kahlson in his laboratory in Lund, Sweden, circa. 1950s. (Photo courtesy of Prof. Lo Persson)

To what purpose? "It sounds like a car engine going full-tilt, the gas gauge heading for empty," I concluded. Was histamine fueling cell division? Based on the high activity of the histidine decarboxylase enzyme in growing tissues, I assumed that Professor Kahlson thought this to be the case.[6]

That was quite a revelation. Now there appeared to be something altogether new for me to consider: in addition to mast cells, histamine apparently could also be made inside other cells and tissues, especially those that undergo rapid cell division...as in cancer cells! *Histamine and growth...histamine and growth... histamine and growth....*it was becoming my mantra. Here I had

---

6   In later years, at a meeting of the European Histamine Research Society, I gained "insider knowledge" about Professor Kahlson from my beloved octogenarian friend and colleague, Professor Börje Uvnäs, Emeritus Chairman of the Department of Pharmacology at the Karolinska Institute in Stockholm, and former Chairman of the Nobel Prize Committee for Medicine or Physiology. As a young man, Börje had worked in Kahlson's lab in Lund. He believed that the real credit for any success of Kahlson's research on nascent histamine must go to an American, Dr. Richard Schayer, who had laboriously developed the histidine decarboxylase assay. He said that Kahlson "was a difficult fellow" who "never gave Dick Schayer the credit he deserved". As will be told, I later corresponded with Dr. Schayer.

DPPE....some sort of an antihistamine structure....the AF tamoxifen....slowing and killing breast cancer cells in the test tube.....

Suddenly, on the second-last page of the book, it all came together for me in the following admonition from Dr. Kahlson: "Students of the physiology of histamine are denied the guidance that would be provided if specific antagonistic compounds were available. The principal actions of the [hist]amine, in the ranking as we see them at present, namely the part played in..... tissue growth and protein synthesis, are not obviated by antihistaminics.[7] This is presumably because in these functions histamine is not engaging receptors of the conventional sort." It was at that precise point that I had my epiphany: *Maybe the AEBS was Kahlson's unconventional histamine receptor inside the cell that mediates growth! Maybe DPPE was a unique type of antihistamine with which we could unravel that mystery! Was tamoxifen also an antihistamine???* Eureka (again!).

---

7   At least not by any recognized antihistamine at that time.

C H A P T E R   T H R E E :

Patent Or Perish

Although the researcher in me wanted to publish my findings as quickly as possible, the oncologist in me considered that DPPE might have a unique potential in treating cancer. However, this very possibility conflicted with publication because to have any chance of developing a potentially promising new drug, a patent must be filed *prior to* any public disclosure such as publication in a journal.[8] But before I could worry about that, I first had to know whether DPPE had been synthesized previously by someone else. If so, was it already patented?

To my disappointment, I discovered that, indeed, a "composition" patent on DPPE and at least twenty other antihistamine-like compounds had been granted in 1954 to the Bristol-Myers laboratories by the United States Patent Office (USPO). This was at the time when antihistamines had just been demonstrated to be effective in treating allergic symptoms associated with hay fever. As a result, all

---

8   There are no exceptions to this rule

the drug companies were rushing to develop their own version of this new type of blockbuster drug.[9]

One of the compounds covered in the patent was phenyltoloxamine. Very similar in structure to DPPE, apparently it proved in tests to be the best Bristol-Myers candidate to treat allergy and was eventually marketed under the trade name "Bristamine". It appears that DPPE and the rest of the "also-rans" were left to sit, undisturbed, on a laboratory shelf for the next twenty years. Then, by law, the original composition patent expired in 1974, a full ten years before DPPE was rediscovered in my laboratory! Was the "new" DPPE compound dead in the water as a potential commercial entity?

I sought advice from Janet Scholz, the University of Manitoba's expert on patents. She told me that a second type of patent can be obtained when a new use is discovered for a previously-patented drug, old or new. From the point of view of a pharmaceutical company, a "use patent", as it is called, is much more likely to be of value if the drug in question is not already marketed for another indication. However, this is not always the case, especially if the pharmaceutical company already holds the composition patent on the marketed drug and it is still on-patent. But, if the composition patent for DPPE had already expired, and the drug was not marketed by anyone else, a new use for it should be far more attractive to a drug company. I told her that from my investigation of its status, this latter scenario would seem to be the case.

Then came more good news from Janet. Pending a formal patent filing, there was a simple means of establishing priority with the USPO. This involved sending a letter to the Commissioner for Patents, describing the invention and requesting priority. Upon receipt in Washington, the letter would be date-stamped and filed in

---

9   Pyrilamine was the first, patented in 1950 and subsequently marketed by Rhône-Poulenc, now part of Aventis. H_1 and H_2 antihistamines (to treat allergy and ulcers, respectively) are perennial "billion dollar drugs" for pharmaceutical companies. Long before the patent on one runs out, drug companies usually make sure that a "tweaked" molecule, covered by a new composition patent, is ready and waiting to hit the market.

the USPO; I would receive a copy along with the reference number. This rather simple procedure allowed a grace period of one year from the official date of receipt to formally filing a patent. It would also allow me to publish our work on DPPE without prejudicing the subsequent patent application, the perfect solution to my dilemma.

At that moment, the University was just dipping its toe into the waters of protecting intellectual property. It appeared that my timing in contacting Janet was right. She called back a short time later to tell me that Vice-President of Research, Marion Vaisey-Genser, wanted to know more about my discovery. Marion, who had earned a doctorate in nutritional sciences, brought to her position impeccable credentials. A handsome woman noted for her silver hair pulled back into a bun, a quick laugh and warm demeanor, she was internationally recognized for pioneering studies on canola that led to its acceptance as an important edible oil.

I submitted a summary of my findings for her review, explaining in the report that we had only cell-culture evidence that DPPE could slow or kill breast cancer cells. However, the linkage of this finding to the demonstration that DPPE selectively bound to the AEBS, a recently-discovered site that was also a target for the proven anti-breast cancer drug, tamoxifen, appeared to sway her in my direction.

That accomplished, Marion concluded that the University had to start somewhere in its protection of health-related intellectual property. That was it. The decision was made. I was soon informed that, despite uncertainty about any potential clinical benefit of DPPE, the University would indeed undertake a patent filing on my behalf… the first they had ever done for a pharmaceutical discovery![10]

The disclosure issue solved, I decided to submit the findings in two separate papers to *Biochemical and Biophysical Research Communications (BBRC)* a widely-read, rapid-publication, basic

---

10 That first use patent, claiming DPPE to have activity, alone or with tamoxifen, in the treatment of breast cancer, was ultimately granted. However, as will become apparent, it was not a claim that we could ever utilize. Further research resulted in the multiple other use patents needed to commercialize DPPE.

science journal popular with investigators who believe they have made novel observations and hope to have them disseminated as quickly as possible (a forerunner to today's online publication of "rapid communication" papers by many reputable medical and scientific journals). Manuscripts were to be sent to one of six editors, all scientists, named on the inside cover of the Journal. I did not know any and randomly chose Dr. William D. McElroy[11] at the University of California, San Diego.

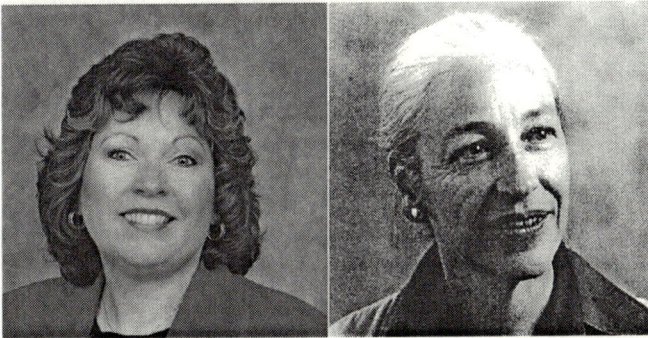

Janet Scholz (L) and Professor Marion Vaisey-Genser (R), circa 1985 (Photos courtesy of Janet Scholz and Marion Vaisey-Genser)

The first paper reported the structure of DPPE and described its binding to the AEBS, but not to the estrogen receptor. The second showed the correlation between the ability of DPPE and tamoxifen to bind to the AEBS, and to inhibit or kill MCF-7 breast cancer cells. I concluded the second paper with the suggestion that the AEBS was biologically important to the action of tamoxifen and that DPPE might have clinical potential as an anticancer agent. To my delight, both papers were accepted by the prescient Dr. McElroy and published within a few months of the rebirth of DPPE.

---

11   I later found out that Dr. McElroy was a previous president of the prestigious American Association for the Advancement of Science and also the National Science Foundation. He was famous for having discovered luciferase, the enzyme responsible for "chemoluminescence" that causes the firefly's flash of light. On learning this, I was humbled that my papers were accepted for publication by such an eminent scientist.

CHAPTER FOUR:

Waiting For Pedro

Those were heady days…a new discovery published in two papers; trumping Benita's lab in synthesizing a potent and selective ligand for the AEBS[12]; a patent in the works; an exciting new lead about histamine; great prospects for continuing research funding. It was mid-1985. Was I doing great, or what? (As this story proceeds, "or what?" becomes the more operative phrase.)

I went to see my boss, Dr. Lyonel Israels, CEO of the Manitoba Cancer Treatment and Research Foundation (now known as CancerCare Manitoba); the Manitoba Institute of Cell Biology, established by him in 1973, was, and remains, its productive and prestigious laboratory research arm. Lyonel was recognized across Canada, and internationally, as a great teacher, clinician and scientist. To me he was an icon, my mentor, singly responsible for my

---

12 Benita's group subsequently developed a somewhat complex compound and published the finding in 1985 in the journal, *Cancer Research*. Predictably, from its single-ring structure, it was significantly weaker than DPPE to bind AEBS and, also as predicted by our findings, did not show much activity. The data suggested to the authors that AEBS may not be of biological relevance, a conclusion not shared by me.

coming to Winnipeg in 1971 to complete postgraduate training in hematology/oncology. The program included a two-year stint in the laboratory, where I discovered I loved research.

Although I had a longstanding offer to return to my alma mater, the University of Western Ontario in London, Ontario, Lyonel wanted me to join his growing cadre of clinician-scientists in Winnipeg. He recommended to Reuben Cherniack, the distinguished respirologist who chaired the Department of Medicine, that I be given a full-time University appointment with my office and laboratory at the Cancer Foundation. I eagerly accepted the offer. With the exception of marrying my college sweetheart, Jill, this was the best decision I ever made.

Lyonel closely followed the progress of all his protégés and loved nothing more than to discuss science, so on the morning I went to see him, we talked at length about DPPE and its possible clinical application as a novel anticancer agent. Lyonel had been exposed to the excitement of new drug discovery during his own training. Each of us had spent a year, he in 1953, I in 1971, at the Royal Marsden Hospital in the real London. The "Marsden" has long been affiliated with the Chester Beatty Research Institute (now The Institute of Cancer Research), located just down the Fulham Road, next to an old walled Jewish cemetery beyond the Brompton Chest Hospital.

Lyonel had been there at a particularly fertile time in the history of the "Chester Beatty"; Professor David Galton (with whom I also trained) was instrumental in the early clinical development and testing of a group of anticancer drugs, called alkylating agents, that had been synthesized by chemists working under the Institute's director, Sir Alexander Haddow. One, called chlorambucil, was found to be effective in the treatment of chronic lymphocytic leukemia and later, in slow-growing forms of non-Hodgkin's lymphoma. Along with Galton and his colleagues, Lyonel played an important role in assessing the efficacy and safety of chlorambucil in patients at the Marsden; subsequently he co-authored one of the first published clinical papers on the drug.

Amazingly, even now, despite being succeeded by newer drugs, chlorambucil still has a role in the treatment of these diseases.

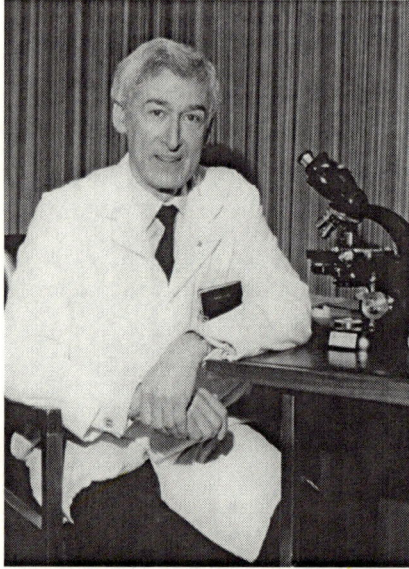

Dr. Lyonel Israels (CancerCare Manitoba Archive)

Remembering that Burroughs Wellcome, the U.K.-based pharmaceutical company, had funded the breakthrough work on alkylating drugs at the Chester Beatty laboratory, Lyonel suggested that we contact its U.S. head office to see if they might be interested in looking at DPPE. Excited by this prospect, I eagerly agreed. Within hours he had spoken with Dr. Howard J. Schaeffer, a career chemist with the company who was now a senior vice-president at their Research Triangle Park, North Carolina facility. I have no doubt that Lyonel quickly established his credentials with Dr. Schaeffer and then probably wowed him with the revelation about the role he had played in the early development of chlorambucil. Whatever was said, it seemed to catch the executive's attention.

Dr. Schaeffer called me the next day. When I started to tell him about DPPE, he cautioned me not to divulge anything until we signed a confidentiality agreement (the first, but far from last, time I was to sign such a document over the next few years). When it arrived shortly after, Janet Scholz' office suggested some minor modifications which were agreeable to both sides. Within a few days of his initial call to Howard Schaeffer, Lyonel and I were on a plane to Research Triangle Park.

Landing at the Raleigh-Durham airport in the late afternoon, we were met by Dr. Indu Parikh, BW's associate head of molecular biology, whose research interests included estrogen and other hormone receptors. He worked under Dr. Pedro Cuatrecasas, research VP, who had made his name in the discovery of the insulin receptor and in the development of a widely-adopted method for separating proteins and other substances. Indu, a very modest and accommodating individual, gave us a tour of the area as we drove to our lodging at the historic Carolina Inn in nearby Chapel Hill, a small college town that is home to the University of North Carolina.

"Oh yes, gentlemen. I have you sharing a room with a queen-size bed, is that correct?" cooed the desk clerk. Lyonel and I quickly looked at one another like two deer caught in the headlights. We were close, but not that close. Indu immediately apologized for the mistake and had him correct the reservation. We each were given a beautiful colonial-style room decorated with period furniture, including a four-poster bed with canopy. I slept well that night. I'm sure that Lyonel did too.

The next morning Indu met us for breakfast. Over corn muffins, and bacon and eggs washed down with copious amounts of black coffee, he reviewed our itinerary: my lecture to the BW scientists later that morning, an all-important lunch meeting with Pedro Cuatrecasas after the talk, a tour of the company research laboratory that afternoon and dinner with several BW executives at a Chapel Hill restaurant that evening. Except for my talk, it sounded great.

We then drove to Research Triangle Park, an impressive industrial development a few miles down the highway, where

Burroughs Wellcome had their corporate offices and laboratories. Frank Lloyd Wright had designed the rather unusual-appearing building, with its backward slanting windows. It wasn't my cup of tea.

On arrival, we were immediately escorted to Howard Schaeffer's office for a short but pleasant introduction, then taken to a large conference room where I was to present my data. I looked around nervously as the room filled up with at least fifty people, almost all with notepad and pen in hand. Someone closed the shades and switched on the overhead projector for my transparencies. This was it! Lyonel's eyes met mine. "Stay calm," they said. I tried.

Indu introduced me to the crowd and within a minute I had launched into a summary of my findings, starting with a short background on the action of tamoxifen, the recent discovery of the AEBS, our synthesis of the AEBS-selective agent DPPE, and its effect to kill breast cancer cells, unimpeded by the presence of estrogen, at the same concentration as tamoxifen. About ten minutes into the talk, my eye caught the blur of the late-arriving Pedro Cuatrecasas, whom I recognized from a picture hanging on the wall in Howard Schaeffer's office. At the end, there were quite a few questions from those in attendance, but none from Cuatrecasas, who soon ducked out as surreptitiously as he had appeared.

It was now noon, the meeting was over, and everyone had filed out of the room. Lyonel and I waited in the hall for Indu, who had temporarily excused himself to finalize our lunch meeting with his boss, Pedro. He returned a few minutes later, obviously embarrassed, to extend Cuatrecasas' regrets that something important would prevent him from joining us. Lyonel and I exchanged glances...we knew the score...my findings were apparently of little or no interest to the research director. We were out of luck.

Our lunch, now switched to the BW cafeteria, was a bit muted; however, talking very sincerely, Indu told me that he believed I could be on to something important. He had recently published a paper showing strong estrogen binding in microsomes. In view of my data, he suggested that something of biological relevance might be going on between the estrogen receptor and the AEBS. This was a novel piece of information, the more so because it was dogma that the estrogen receptor simply shuttled back and forth, carrying its cargo of estrogen from the cytoplasm (the semi-liquid cell sap) to the DNA-containing nucleus, with no stops in-between. He promised to send me a reprint.

For the rest of the afternoon we somewhat dejectedly went through the motions of touring the research laboratories where we were introduced to various and sundry scientists, all of whom kindly took a few moments out of their busy schedule to give us a synopsis of their research programs. That completed, Indu had one more thing he wanted to show us: a history of discovery at the BW laboratories. It took the form of a wall display that was, in large part, a photographic tribute to the careers of Dr. George Hitchings, the company's scientific director, and his longtime colleague, Gertrude B. Elion.

Over the years, these two scientists led a group of chemists responsible for the discovery of many important drugs, including 6-mercaptopurine and thioguanine for the treatment of acute leukemia; allopurinol (Zyloprim) for the treatment of gout; aza-thioprine (Imuran), a mainstay immunosuppressive drug used to prevent organ rejection; acyclovir (Zovirax), the first effective drug to treat the herpes virus; and trimethoprim, a component of the antibiotic Septra. "Amazing," I thought to myself.

Just then, a short, well-coiffed woman in a white coat appeared. She looked to me to be in her mid-sixties. From some of the black and white pictures in the display montage that showed someone much younger, I realized it was Gertrude Elion as I and the others shook her hand. "Call me Trudy," she requested. Her accent suggested northern, east coast roots. I must admit that, up to that minute, I had known nothing of her or her outstanding career. It was altogether different for Lyonel, who was soon sharing stories with Trudy and discussing colleagues they had in common. "I was asked by Howard to join you for dinner tonight," she announced.

I thought that was great news. By his smiling nod, I knew that Lyonel was equally delighted.

Now firmly in the role of protective "grandmother", Trudy insisted on driving Lyonel and me back to Chapel Hill in her snappy new Buick Regal coupe, complete with landau leather top and all the trimmings. Along the way, she proudly pointed out her well-kept older home along a lovely tree-lined street near the centre of this small southern town. Looking through the car window at the many large colonial-style homes, I could not help but be reminded of the pre-Civil War days of the Confederacy. Dropping us off to walk the grounds of the beautiful UNC campus near our hotel, she offered to return at seven to drive us to our dinner date. We gladly accepted.

That night at the restaurant we had a wonderful meal over wine with Trudy, Howard Schaeffer and an engaging young female oncologist they invited along. Trudy sat directly across the table, giving me the opportunity to tell her about my excitement over my current research findings with DPPE and their possible implications in cancer therapy. She could not have appeared more interested or supportive, sharing with me her own experiences in drug discovery and taking the opportunity to point out the many disappointments along the way. "The majority of drugs never make it into the clinic because they have unexpected toxicities or just don't pass muster in humans," she cautioned. That said, she wished me all the luck in the world with DPPE and told me to leave no stone unturned in my quest to help my patients. Her own decision to become a scientist was influenced by the death of her grandfather from cancer. "Given what you have accomplished, your grandfather would be proud of you," I opined. Trudy did not answer, but her eyes said it all. Yes he would.

At the end of the evening, Howard Schaeffer wished us a safe trip home, telling Lyonel that he would get back to us as soon as possible with a company decision on DPPE. We heard nothing for weeks. Finally, Lyonel contacted Howard, who apologized for the delay, saying there had been much discussion but, so far, no decision. Give him a couple of more weeks. Lyonel filled me in on this latest non-development and we again agreed that the failure of Dr. Cuatrecasas to meet with us after my talk was a bad omen. The two weeks came and went.

Finally, after another month without any news, I sat on the sofa in his office while Lyonel again called Howard Schaeffer. "Howard, a simple 'yes' or 'no' will suffice. There will be no hard feelings on our side. We would just like an answer either way," said Lyonel, always the smooth diplomat. On the other end, Howard apologized but regretted having to report that, although there was some potential interest in my "novel finding", the company just didn't have enough information on which to proceed. Please call him in the future if and when we had more data. Lyonel thanked him for his time and effort. We did not know it then, but there was not to be a future for us with Howard Schaeffer. For the first, but not last, time in this story, a drug company with whom we were dealing would exit the stage….Burroughs Wellcome was taken over a few years later by a rival company, Glaxo.

That aside, there is a wonderful followup to the BW story. Three years later, Gertrude "Trudy" Belle Elion was named co-recipient of the 1988 Nobel Prize in Medicine,[13] which she shared with her partner George Hitchings, and Sir James Black[14] "for their discoveries of important principles for drug treatment". I got to congratulate her myself soon after her award, when we again crossed paths at the 1989 meeting of the American Association for Cancer Research in New Orleans; she was a past-president of the organization.

---

13   Amazingly, Gertrude Elion was one of the only Nobel laureates who held neither an MD or PhD. After graduating at the top of her class with BA and Masters degrees, she worked for many years as a chemist in industry. Although she subsequently completed 2 years of a doctoral course at Brooklyn Polytechnic while working as a research chemist at Burroughs Wellcome, she was forced to withdraw when given the choice of devoting full time to her studies or quitting her job.

14   Black was cited, in part, for his discovery of the histamine H_2 receptor.

Gertrude Elion remained active and involved until her death ten years later at the all-too-young age of 81. On hearing the sad news of her passing, my immediate thought was, "Gone too soon". I then reflected on those precious few hours when I had been privileged to be in the presence of, and receive encouragement and advice from, a great human being. As a pioneering woman in science, I am sure she faced many personal and professional hurdles. Her example of stick-to-itiveness would remain firmly etched in my memory as I traveled the long road ahead.

CHAPTER FIVE:

Proving The Case...Sort Of

Following our return from North Carolina, I again immersed myself in my research. The next question to tackle: how to prove whether the AEBS was some sort of growth-promoting histamine receptor. I must admit that my knowledge of receptors and pharmacology in those days was, to put it kindly, primitive, and based mainly on what I had learned in medical school or read for myself in books and journals. I certainly did not know all the "ins and outs" of the area I was about to enter. The irony is that, very occasionally, "not being confused by the facts" can work in your favor. As it turned out, this may have been one of those rare times.

As simplistic as it now appears, my thinking was as follows: If the AEBS is a histamine receptor, both histamine and antihistamines (the H_1 anti-allergy types, including phenyltoloxamine that Bristol-Myers had developed for treating allergies all those years ago, and/or the H_2 anti-ulcer types) should compete for the binding of radioactive tamoxifen to the AEBS in liver tissue. Patricia Bogdanovic and Linda Macdonald, my two new enthusiastic lab assistants, quickly got to work.

So what did we find? The allergy-fighting H_1 antihistamines did indeed compete for radioactive tamoxifen binding to the AEBS! However, there were wide differences among the drugs: some were as strong, or almost as strong, as DPPE, while others, including pyrilamine (the "prototype" H_1 antihistamine), and phenyltoloxamine (Bristamine) were substantially weaker. The ulcer-fighting H_2 antihistamines, cimetidine (Tagamet) and ranitidine (Zantac), did not compete for the AEBS at all. Nor did histamine. *Oh, oh!*

This negative finding with histamine both surprised and disappointed me. The hypothesis must be wrong! However, on scouring the scientific literature, I learned that the liver extracts we were using contain a high concentration of metabolizing enzymes that can quickly and specifically break down natural substances such as histamine. "Perhaps not much histamine survived to bind the AEBS," I thought, grasping for straws. "Not good enough," my better sense told me.

Then I came across a 1969 publication that saved the day. Professor M. Rocha e Silva, a noted pharmacologist, pointed out that antihistamines interfere with histamine binding to the H_1 receptor *but not vice versa* because the molecules bind to different sites on the structure. Apparently because of its small size, the histamine molecule can bind to its own "nook" in the receptor without interfering with the binding of the antihistamines. However, mainly because of their larger size and dangling side chains, the antihistamine molecules can block the entry of histamine into the receptor[15], like a goalie extending his stick to deflect the puck from the net. "Thank you, Professor," I said to myself with a considerable measure of relief. If that could be true for histamine at the H_1 receptor, why could it not be true for histamine at the AEBS? My hypothesis appeared to be coming back from the dead.

---

15   The scientific term for the ability of a substance to block the binding of another ligand without actually attaching to the same site on the receptor is "steric hindrance".

With the results of the binding tests in hand, we then compared each antihistamine to DPPE and tamoxifen for their ability to slow or kill breast cancer cells. This time, in addition to the estrogen-driven MCF-7 cells (which contain estrogen receptors), we employed human breast cancer cells that did not contain estrogen receptors (and therefore were not estrogen-fueled). We were excited to find that the ability of the various antihistamines to slow or kill both types of breast cancer cells correlated almost perfectly with how strongly they bound to the AEBS.

Of one thing I was now certain: the AEBS appeared to be implicated in the ability of drugs to inhibit or kill breast cancer cells. Furthermore, with the inability of histamine to compete for tamoxifen binding to the AEBS possibly explained, I again believed that it could be Kahlson's growth-promoting histamine receptor, different from the H_1 and H_2 types.

Why? The H_2 receptor was out of the running because the H_2 blockers did not bind to the AEBS or slow the growth of our cells. The H_1 receptor was also on shaky ground because, while all of the H_1 antihistamine drugs we tested were equally strong allergy-fighters (i.e. equally strong as "H_1 blockers"), only two were as strong as DPPE to interfere with the binding of tamoxifen to the AEBS and to slow or kill the breast cancer cells, while three others, including DPPE's "cousin", phenyltoloxamine, were substantially weaker on both counts. I reasoned that, if the AEBS were an H_1 receptor, all the allergy drugs should show approximately the same ability to bind to it and kill the cells.

Then there was the question of location: the AEBS was located *inside* the cell, in the microsomes, whereas the H_1 and H_2 receptors were on the *outside* of the cell, on the membrane. Whatever I was dealing with, it was definitely a different "animal", both intriguing and worth pursuing.

I decided that these latest findings were "hot" and should be published as rapidly as possible (what researcher doesn't?). *BBRC* had been very obliging with the first two papers. Should I go back to Dr. McElroy? Why not? Even if he were to say no, the turn-around time was very short, normally just one or two weeks. I made the decision to try and chose a provocative title: "*Evidence that the antiestrogen binding site is a histamine or histamine-like receptor*". (I added "histamine-like" because it is always best to be at least somewhat tentative in case you turn out to be wrong.)

When the letter of acceptance arrived two weeks later, I was ecstatic. It was now early 1985 and I was on a roll: two published papers, with another accepted…a bases-loaded triple! Moreover, I was getting a lot of reprint requests for the first two, a sign that others were interested in my findings. Again I asked myself, "Was I doing great, or what?" (The "or what?" was coming closer.)

It was just about that time that Leigh Murphy and her husband, Liam, moved to Winnipeg from Sydney, Australia. Leigh had her PhD while Liam had both an MD and PhD. The couple had been recruited as post-doctoral fellows by Professor Henry Friesen, who had gained international prominence at McGill University following his discovery of an important hormone called pro-lactin. Henry, a Manitoba native and medical school alumnus, had since come back to his alma mater to chair the Department of Physiology and was looking to build up his area with top-notch people.

Leigh had been part of Rob Sutherland's team at the Ludwig Institute, where she co-authored several of the early papers on the AEBS, including the original paper in *Nature* that reported the discovery in 1980. I was bursting to meet her so that I could discuss my results. I quickly walked over to Henry's lab in the new Basic Medical Sciences building. One of the techs pointed her out to me (Leigh was hard to miss: tall, athletic-looking, red hair, blue eyes, pleasant smile) and I introduced myself. To my relief, we hit it off. She had read my first two papers in Australia. As we talked, I told her that I had now tentatively identified the nature of the AEBS. Her eyes widened at the news. Could we meet in my office so that I could show her the data? Absolutely. When? What about right now? Out the door I led her, across the medical campus to my laboratory on the second floor of the Cancer Foundation.

I quickly showed her around the lab, introduced my staff and ushered her into the cramped quarters that I called my office. As she sat down in a chair opposite me, I blurted out much too quickly, "The AEBS appears to be a novel histamine receptor." A moment's pause. Other than a slight nod, no reaction of "Aha!!" from Leigh. Sensing her bewilderment, I quickly launched into "the Kahlson story" (she was unfamiliar with it, but then again, who beside me had recently obsessed over his book?) and then summarized our binding studies with DPPE, tamoxifen and the antihistamines. Finally, I sat quietly, now with some trepidation, as she read a preprint of my just-accepted manuscript.

"Very interesting," she said, after what appeared like an eternity, "but I don't think you have definitely proven the case." I agreed that much work remained, but argued that histamine might be a good bet, given the binding results and Kahlson's implication of its role in growth. "True, but why don't you clone the receptor? That might give you the proof you need," she suggested. By this she meant using what was then an emerging technology to isolate and purify the genes that serve as the precise blueprint for the cell to make proteins such as receptors. In this way, the identity of the AEBS might be ascertained. I thanked her and said I would think about it. We agreed to keep in close touch.

After she left, I did think about it....for at least five minutes before deciding on a different approach to finding the answer. Not that Leigh's advice wasn't good. It was. However, from a practical point of view, I did not have the background to do this type of molecular research. I knew from my search of the journals that the genes for the H_1 and H_2 receptor had not yet been cloned, or at least not published, although it was only a matter of time before that would occur.[16] I decided on a different approach. I would continue to test DPPE and tamoxifen using proven "low-tech" methods that might inch me forward to the proof I sought.

---

16 Even if by some miracle I had cloned the gene for AEBS, I would not have been able to compare the sequence to the H_2 and H_1 receptors at that time. They were cloned in 1991 and 1993, respectively.

CHAPTER SIX:

Oldies But Goodies

There was a somewhat ancient test for H$_1$ antihistamine activity
that I remembered from my university days in the physiology
lab. A strip of muscle cut from the trachea (windpipe) of a rabbit
or other anesthetized animal is kept alive in a warm water bath
containing saline and other vital nutrients into which oxygen is
bubbled. One end of the muscle is connected by a fine wire to a
stylus that traces a line on moving graph paper (in medical school
we used charcoal-smoked paper, taped around a rotating drum…
in principle, not much different than Thomas Edison's first talking
machine where voice vibrations were traced on a roll of tinfoil).

When histamine is added to the nutrient solution, it attaches to
H$_1$ receptors present in the tracheal muscle cells and causes them
to contract. This results in a rapid sustained downward movement
of the stylus on the paper. Substances can be tested for H$_1$ antihistamine activity by their ability to prevent the muscle contractions,
and hence the downward movement of the stylus, when histamine
is added. By this method, I thought we should be able to find out
whether DPPE and tamoxifen were antihistamines and, more

importantly, how they stacked up against drugs like pyrilamine, a powerful H$_1$ blocker.

I needed someone with the expertise and lab setup to help me. Henry Friesen told me about Dr. Edwin Kroeger, a member of his department who conducted laboratory research on asthma. I quickly located his laboratory just down the hall. As luck would have it, inside the open doorway stood a tall dapper fellow, formally dressed in white shirt and tie and wearing a freshly-starched lab coat. He and a smiling middle-aged blond assistant were both intently gazing at a series of tracings on polygraph paper. At the epicenter of all this attention was a strip of muscle tissue in an organ bath bubbling with oxygen. They were clearly in the middle of an experiment …the very type of "oldie but goodie" test that I had remembered from medical school! "I'll come by later when you are finished," I said, not wanting to interrupt them at this delicate moment. Dr. Kroeger smiled and nodded.

The following afternoon, I returned and introduced myself to Ed Kroeger. As he ushered me into his office beside the lab, I could see that all the equipment from the previous day's experiment had been meticulously cleaned and laid out in an orderly fashion on stainless steel trays covered with white toweling. Various bottles of chemicals were sitting on the lab counter. "Coffee?" he offered as he poured three cups worth, giving the first to his assistant whom he introduced as Blanka Kucera. She had a very kind, motherly smile. Taking full advantage of the moment, I summarized my binding studies with DPPE, tamoxifen and the antihistamines, and gave him a copy of the *BBRC* papers. Then I told him what I would like to do next.

He was a quick study. "We should easily be able to test all your drugs as soon as I get a fresh muscle preparation."[17] He was set up and ready to proceed two weeks later. I brought over the samples of DPPE, tamoxifen and pyrilamine while Ed provided

---

17   Ed's lab used tracheal muscle strips from stray dogs that were going to be put to sleep anyway.

the histamine. He and Blanka quickly got to work as I watched over their shoulders.

Within a couple of hours we had our tracings: if enough DPPE or tamoxifen was added to the solution containing the muscle, they blocked the contractions caused by histamine. By definition they were antihistamines of the allergy type! That said, both were about one thousand times weaker than pyrilamine in this test. This contrasted starkly with the markedly weaker ability of pyrilamine to bind to the AEBS and to slow or kill breast cancer cells. Ed and I were in full agreement on the interpretation of our combined data: *If the AEBS was a histamine receptor, it was definitely distinct from the H_1. Put another way, while DPPE and tamoxifen were able to bind to the H_1 receptor, they bound to the microsomal AEBS/?novel histamine receptor with much greater strength.*[18]

Once again I thought we were sitting on hot data that deserved rapid publication. What did Ed think of (yet again) submitting a paper to my "pal", Dr. McElroy, at *BBRC*? "Given your track record with him so far, what have we got to lose?" was his sage reply. We wrote it together, and at the end, acknowledged Blanka's invaluable technical assistance. The title? *"Evidence that tamoxifen is a histamine antagonist"*. Two weeks after submission, a letter appeared in my mail box. With somewhat trembling hands I opened it to learn that this made four for four! I immediately called Ed, who was tickled pink. We had a good chuckle over my suggestion that perhaps *BBRC* should now stand for *Brandes Breakthrough Research Communications.*

My enthusiasm for the "low-tech" approach now firmly entrenched, I prepared to undertake a new series of animal experiments to assess whether, like tamoxifen, DPPE was an

---

18   The finding that drugs like DPPE and tamoxifen are active at more than one target is very common. In truth, no drug is absolutely selective for one site, only more active at one (or some) sites than at others. Activity at multiple sites in cells or tissues accounts in large measure for why most drugs have many side effects or can be used for more than one indication.

antiestrogen. But before proceeding, I went over to Henry Friesen's office to thank him for putting me onto Ed and to update him on the progress we had made on the histamine front. I had taken to visiting Henry often because he had a notoriously keen mind and his opinions were important to me.[19]

As I had done previously with Lyonel and Leigh Murphy, I enthusiastically recapped for Henry my hypothesis that the AEBS in some way might be linked to the growth function that Kahlson had envisioned for histamine. I showed him the graphs of the published binding experiments and the new data from Ed's lab, which he examined quietly for several minutes. Then, cocking his head toward me and squinting slightly through his glasses, Henry asked, "Have you considered radiolabeling DPPE?"

Pause

"No."

"Well I think you should." By this, Henry meant that we should have DPPE tagged with a radioactive label so that, like radiolabeled tamoxifen, we could assess how other non-radioactive substances compete for its binding to the AEBS.

"But why do that when I already have commercially-available radioactive tamoxifen?"

"Because," he explained, "you may learn more by using radiolabeled DPPE. It also may bind somewhat differently than tamoxifen to the AEBS. It will also allow you to do other types of studies that can concentrate on labeled DPPE."

I was quiet for a moment and then asked the sixty-four thousand dollar question. "If you were me, with only so much money in your grant, would you do this?"

"If at all possible, I would," he replied unequivocally.

"Then I will consider your suggestion very seriously," I said, shaking hands and thanking him as I went out the door.

---

19   Years later, Henry told me that his overly-protective secretary, Miss McDonald, would go into his office to warn him that I was outside, wanting to see him. "It's Dr. Brandes again. Do you want to clear out?" (He had a private exit door to the hallway from the back of his office.)

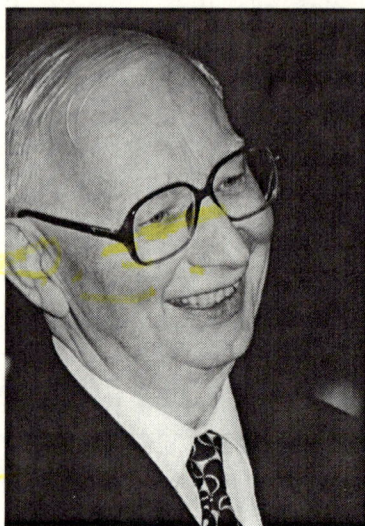

Professor Henry Friesen (Photo courtesy of Henry Friesen)

This time I sat in my office for a long while, considering Henry's unexpected advice. The more I thought about it, the more I knew he was right. I also knew it would be costly because the project would have to be farmed out to a nuclear isotope laboratory that did custom synthesis work. One of the two major isotope suppliers at that time was New England Nuclear in Boston. I called one of their technical people who explained that if I could provide them with a 200 milligram quantity of pure DPPE, they should be able to radiolabel my compound.

The cost would depend on where the radioactive tag was inserted (on the ring or side chain) and what radioactive tag was employed (hydrogen, carbon or phosphorus are the common atoms that can be labeled). With radiolabeled tamoxifen as a guide, I settled on labeling one of the ring hydrogens (the radioactive hydrogen is called tritium, denoted by the symbol ^{3}H). On hearing the quote of approximately $8,500, I audibly gasped. "Are you okay?" asked the voice at the other end. "Yes," I lied.

Before blowing my budget altogether, I discussed the matter with Lyonel, explaining the reasons behind Henry's suggestion and then told him the cost. Lyonel mulled it over for about a minute and then nodded in agreement. "I think that would be the way to go." That was good enough for me. I went to the office and filled out a purchase order.

Two months later, New England Nuclear shipped me three small vials of radiolabeled DPPE. "It's liquid gold. Guard it with your life," I instructed Pat. As she nervously took the small package from my hand to dilute the contents and store them in the freezer, she smiled, assuring me that she would. I really hoped I had done the right thing.[20]

---

20 Henry's suggestion would prove to be the best advice I could have received.

CHAPTER SEVEN:

Why Not Histamine?

At the very time the labeled DPPE arrived, we were planning an experiment to see whether, like tamoxifen, DPPE could block the effect of estrogen on the rat uterus. In other words, was DPPE an antiestrogen? Tamoxifen's actions on that organ are complex. In young female rats, whose ovaries have been surgically removed to render them estrogen-deficient, the uterus is very small and immature. When a type of estrogen, called estradiol, is injected into these rats for three days, the uterus is rapidly stimulated to grow. However, if the rats are first given tamoxifen, the effect of injected estrogen to enlarge the uterus is significantly blunted.

But the story does not end there. Although tamoxifen blocks estrogen, the drug itself behaves as a weak form of that hormone. As a result, when administered alone, tamoxifen also stimulates the immature uterus to grow, although to a significantly lesser extent than estradiol. This very property has been an albatross around the neck of an otherwise remarkable and effective breast cancer-fighting drug because, in some women, long-term use of tamoxifen, like estrogen itself, can lead to an abnormal degree of stimulation of glandular cells in the lining of the uterus, resulting in cancer.[21]

Dogma dictated that the antiestrogenic effects of tamoxifen resulted entirely from blocking the uterine estrogen receptors. But no one ever considered whether the AEBS might play a role here. Now, with DPPE, we might be able to determine the answer by comparing its ability with that of tamoxifen and placebo (saline) to block the stimulating effect of injected estradiol on the uterus. We could also test the effect of DPPE alone on the uterus to determine whether, like tamoxifen alone, DPPE made the uterus grow. Since the ability to stimulate uterine growth was linked to tamoxifen's weak estrogen action, I was betting that DPPE itself would have no effect on the size of the uterus.

None of these experiments would have been possible without Patricia, who was superb in her ability to handle the rats, inject them on a daily basis and then humanely kill them. I was her assistant as she rapidly removed each uterus through an incision, trimmed off all the excess tissue and recorded the uterine weights on a laboratory scale. Marveling at her surgical technique, I told her she missed her calling. She should have been a veterinarian, or, for less income, a surgeon (the human kind).

After repeated experiments to ensure they were correct, I was stunned by the findings. Like tamoxifen, DPPE also significantly blunted uterine growth in the estrogen-treated rats. In comparison, and as expected, saline did not prevent estradiol from stimulating the uterus to grow. More remarkably, whereas tamoxifen alone increased uterine weight (although, predictably, less than estradiol), the uteruses in rats given DPPE were actually *smaller*

---

21   The incidence of uterine cancer increases from about one case per thousand in the general population to six cases per thousand in women receiving tamoxifen for five or more years, still a very low risk to benefit ratio, considering that tamoxifen is estimated to save twelve lives per one hundred women who receive the drug to prevent the recurrence of breast cancer. Nonetheless, the increased risk of uterine cancer is significant and causes some women to refuse the drug. Newer drugs, called aromatase inhibitors, avoid this risk.

than in rats given the saline placebo. It now appeared to me that we were about to challenge the dogma on how tamoxifen works!! I just could not contain my excitement as I gave Patty a big hug. In my mind, the AEBS now loomed even larger as a candidate for the unconventional growth-promoting histamine receptor envisioned by Professor Kahlson.

There was just one piece of unfinished business before writing up the results ....we had to repeat those binding studies using our new radioactive DPPE. Although we had performed them on multiple occasions using radioactive tamoxifen, there was a palpable nervousness as we carried out our first test using our "liquid gold". We needn't have worried. DPPE bound to the AEBS, strong and true. Tamoxifen competed powerfully for DPPE. The H_1 antihistamines were weaker and the H_2 blockers did not compete at all. It was exactly what we had seen in our original experiments using radioactive tamoxifen.

Back to Dr. McElroy I went with a manuscript boldly entitled, *"New evidence that the antiestrogen binding site may be a novel growth-promoting histamine receptor (?H_3) which mediates the antiestrogenic and antiproliferative effects of tamoxifen"*.[22] "Accepted," replied Dr. McElroy after only three weeks. Five for five with *"Brandes Breakthrough" Research Communications!*

There is a charming anecdote associated with this part of the story. In researching the literature for that fifth paper, I came across a reference to work by Dr. Clara (Claire) Szego and her group at UCLA. These researchers, prominent in the field of how cells respond to hormones and other substances, reported that estrogen treatment causes histamine to be released into uterine tissue.

---

22   Receptors are numbered in order of discovery. I was later to be sorry that I had jumped the gun in the title because, unknown to me at the time, a new unrelated H_3 receptor had recently been discovered in the brain by J.-C. Schwartz and colleagues in Paris. Moreover, as I will soon tell, Frank LaBella chastised me for using the word "receptor" rather than "binding site". A receptor denotes a specific protein that mediates a proven function when it is bound by its ligand. I had not yet proven either. He was right.

I contacted Dr. Szego and we had several pleasurable telephone discussions about our mutual findings. Like me, she was intrigued by a possible role for histamine in growth. We exchanged reprints by mail over the next few months.

One day, a bulging manila envelope arrived on my desk. It was from Claire. She had sent me a rubber stamp on which the words "*Why Not Histamine?*" were embossed. An enclosed letter read as follows: "Dear Lorne. I may have told you about this little gadget that one of my classes gave me during the period when we were actively pursuing the histamine 'clue'. In view of your current vigorous contributions that have so advanced the 'plot', I hereby bequeath the contents to you. It was used so effectively by my students to poke gentle fun at my enthusiasm! All the best. Claire." The torch had been passed.

CHAPTER EIGHT:

Carl, Frank And The Lumpy Red Couch

Enthused by the exciting findings and encouraged by the flurry of publications, I was optimistic that my research monies would continue to be approved. It was the autumn of 1985 and my grant, funded by the National Cancer Institute of Canada (NCIC), was coming up for renewal. One of the real hardships for scientists involves the countless hours spent researching and writing grants, knowing all the while that the percentage of successful applications has always been one-third or less. But what was the alternative? Everyone grumbled and prepared their grant application.

Because there were multiple investigators at the Institute of Cell Biology who held NCIC grants, we received "block funding", meaning a global budget from NCIC to cover the various approved research programs. At renewal time, a site visit was made to the Institute so that the grants panel could meet personally with each researcher, grilling him or her in person. The outcome of that encounter would determine funding for a three-year period.

The members of the evaluation team, all scientists, were provided with a copy of our written proposals well ahead of time. I wrote up my grant with a flourish, pointing to the progress we had made after the synthesis of DPPE, the identification of a potential role for the AEBS in tamoxifen action, and the identification of a novel histamine site/receptor, related to the AEBS, that appeared to be involved in growth. I mapped out an ambitious plan for further experiments and budgeted for costs over the three years.

On the late October morning I was to appear before the panel, I stood outside the closed door of the Cancer Foundation boardroom, making mental notes of all the points I wanted to cover in my presentation, especially the histamine connection about which I was so excited. I was sure the examiners would share my enthusiasm. At the allotted time, the door opened and the chairman, Dr. Robert Phillips, an immunologist, bade me come in. I sat at the end of the long table and was introduced to the site visit team. Smiling to put me at ease, the chairman asked me to begin.

Within a few minutes of starting, any further smiles vanished. I had the distinct impression that those at the table were less enthusiastic than I about the proposed direction of my research. It was suggested that I was contradicting the dogma about the well-established role of the estrogen receptor in tamoxifen action. I had not established the structure of the AEBS. My hands started to sweat. The histamine connection was interesting but unproven and possibly a red herring. *Now they were really sweating!* It went from bad to worse as I was peppered with more and more questions, each less sympathetic than the previous. I could read this room only too well. I was in major trouble. When the inquisition finally ended, I felt totally beat up and dejected.

The next morning, the "word" came down from on high. The reviewers' written conclusion about my research was as follows: "In summary, although the importance of this new compound [DPPE] could be recognized and the potential seen for an understanding of the AEBS, Dr. Brandes' single-minded pursuit of the new histamine receptor was seen as a negative influence on his setting of priorities. Approval is therefore recommended but with low to medium priority." Translation: I received what was called a terminal award, meaning one year of reduced funding with the need to reapply as a new grantee. I was now off the block grant. Moreover, my chances for approval had just gone down a big notch since new grants had a significantly lower chance of funding than renewals. With the one year extension, I would have just enough money to carry me into the fall of 1987.

Discouraged, I discussed the situation with Lyonel. "Grants and grantsmanship," he sighed, shaking his head. He had been there many times himself, both as a reviewer and as an applicant. "Just keep working. You are making good progress but when you write a grant you have to keep it simple and focused on the facts. Reviewers do not respond well to speculation. We'll go over your next grant proposal together before you submit." I felt better. Maybe this had just been a small bump in the road. My enthusiasm soon picked up again. I believed in what I was doing. "History has been replete with skeptics and nay-sayers," I told myself.

During this time, I regularly visited and talked at length with Dr. Carl Pinsky, a senior member of the Department of Pharmacology. Carl was a most wonderful colleague; his appearance and kind demeanor reminded me of actor Edmund Gwenn's Kris Kringle character in *Miracle on 34th Street*. He was an eager and interested sounding board for my thoughts and ideas. Although mainly an expert in the science of neuropharmacology (the study of how nerve cell function is affected by chemicals and drugs), Carl's knowledge cut a wide swath. He was very familiar with Kahlson's work on "nascent" histamine and was highly complimentary about the studies that I had carried out to test my hypothesis about the AEBS.

After one of our many long discussions, Carl suggested that I speak with Frank LaBella, a fellow member in the department, whom he felt was the supreme expert on binding assays. "If anyone can help you with your studies and get you back on track with funding agencies, it's Frank," Carl advised optimistically. To his surprise, there was no immediate affirmative response to this suggestion. I did not know Frank personally, only his reputation as someone who did not suffer fools gladly. I had once heard him give a seminar. His monotone presentation resulted in one of the more boring hours I had spent in a lecture theatre.

Nonetheless, there was absolutely no doubt that Frank LaBella was a most accomplished scientist. Born into an immigrant Sicilian family in Connecticut, Frank received his PhD from Emory University in Atlanta. He had been lured to Winnipeg in 1958 by fellow American and former pharmacology head, Mark Nickerson, discoverer of a type of adrenalin receptor that is important in blood pressure regulation.

Within a few years, Frank established himself as one of the country's foremost investigators, one of only a select few to become a Career Scientist of the Medical Research Council of Canada. Along with Lyonel and Henry Friesen, he had recently been awarded the prestigious St. Boniface Hospital Research Award[23] for his long and distinguished research career.

"Okay, Carl, you win," I finally said after his further coaxing wore down my reticence. Victorious in his perseverance, he immediately called Frank's office. "He's there right now," proclaimed the exultant Dr. Pinsky. We took the stairs, two at a time, to the fourth floor. Entering his office, we found Frank sitting at his desk.

Plunking ourselves down on an old faded lumpy red couch facing the stone-faced Frank, Carl began speaking rapidly. "Frank, this is Lorne Brandes. He has done some absolutely fabulous research on histamine and growth that I truly believe represents a landmark discovery." Carl continued on in this somewhat overinflated way for what seemed like an eternity, telling Frank all about

---

23 St. Boniface Hospital is one of the two major Winnipeg teaching hospitals associated with the University of Manitoba Faculty of Medicine. Other recipients of the Saint Boniface award include D discovered the first successful polio vaccine, Danny Th ing St. Jude's Hospital and Mother Theresa, for her with the sick and indigent. All of these illustrious peopl awards in person.

Kahlson, my binding studies and DPPE. The more he talked, the more Frank's pained expression seemed to say, "Why are these two idiots wasting my time?"

Spotting his incredulous reaction, I grew more uncomfortable by the second. But when Carl finally came to the end of his spiel, Frank surprised me by saying, "I doubt you are correct, but we can probably help you find the real answer." Thus shakily began a collaboration that was to enrich us both for the next fifteen years. Frank LaBella's opinion about my binding studies and hypothesis would come to change, as would my first impression of him. Behind that stone face lurked a nice man who was a real softy.

C H A P T E R   N I N E :

Never Turn Down A Free Lunch

A few days later, Frank introduced me to Mark Hnatowich, his PhD student. Frank and Mark believed that DPPE most likely belonged to a group of chemicals called "calcium channel blockers". Examples are verapamil (Isoptin) and nifedipine (Adalat), valuable drugs in the treatment of angina and high blood pressure. Calcium is known to be an important cell "messenger". Its concentration increases dramatically inside cells when ligands, including estrogen, adrenalin, and even histamine, bind to their receptors.

By attaching themselves to specific sites on the small porous openings, or channels, that transport calcium through the cell membrane, verapamil and nifedipine block its entry into the cell, with the result that many important processes, such as cell division, are inhibited. Despite any interaction of DPPE with the AEBS, according to Frank and Mark it was probably also blocking calcium channels. I had not considered that possibility.

Mark's calcium channel studies involved the same radioligand binding assay that we had employed. However, rather than microsomes from rat liver cells, he used rat brain membranes, a cruder preparation containing both the outer cell membranes where the calcium channels reside, and the microsomes where the AEBS is located. Frank suggested that we compare the ability of DPPE to compete for radioactively-labeled verapamil and nifedipine binding to the calcium channels in the rat brain membrane preparation.

"We should have this thing sorted out in a few days," said Frank, sitting contentedly behind his desk, hands clasped behind his head.

"And what, exactly, are you predicting?" I questioned.

Looking pained for a second, Frank barely missed a beat as he replied, "I thought I had made it clear. DPPE should compete for the attachment of verapamil and nifedipine to the calcium channels. If that happens, DPPE is binding to calcium channels and that interaction may explain your other observations." For the second time since I had come across Dr. Kahlson's book, I was having some self-doubts about the viability of the histamine hypothesis.

A few days later, after "crunching the numbers", Mark proclaimed DPPE to be a potent inhibitor of verapamil and nifedipine binding to the calcium channel.[24] The results appeared unarguable. DPPE was a calcium channel blocker. Given the importance of calcium to cell function, I could no longer be sure that the AEBS was linked to the effects we saw in our various binding and functional assays. I must admit that I was feeling less than wonderful at that moment. But science is about truth, not fantasy. If I was wrong, I was wrong. That is not a sin. The sin is to ignore the facts and continue to proclaim that wrong is right. Suddenly I had a thought. "Let's have Mark test verapamil against radioactive DPPE."

---

24   As Frank and I would later discover, Mark had actually overestimated, by at least ten times, the ability of DPPE to interfere with verapamil binding. In truth, as we proved in subsequent binding assays, and in other, more direct, experiments, DPPE was very weak to block calcium channels. Mark's error caused us to constantly compare DPPE and verapamil in the various experiments we carried out over the next three years.

"Fine. But what do you expect that will change?" Frank asked.

"Maybe verapamil does not compete for DPPE," I answered.

Since the first test indicated that both substances were apparently binding to the same site on the calcium channel, Frank felt that the odds of that happening were extremely remote, but he had no objection to checking it out.

"Do you want to wager on the outcome?" I was upping the ante.

Silence from Frank; his expression suggested growing exasperation with this Luddite.

"Whoever is wrong takes the other to lunch," I continued.

Finally, he nodded in agreement. Frank never turned down a free lunch.

That Friday, I was Frank's guest at the noon buffet at the India Gardens.[25] Over a bottle of Kingfisher beer I silently toasted Henry Friesen as we discussed the surprising results. I had won the bet. Verapamil was a dud against DPPE. Based on Mark's initial findings, Frank had expected it to easily displace radioactive DPPE from the calcium channel. That had not occurred, casting some doubt on the mechanism of action of DPPE envisaged by Frank and his wünderkind, Mark. "I guess we now have to look further at the AEBS," he acknowledged. With those words, I enjoyed my beer and ate the delicious food.

As the place emptied we continued to sit, plotting strategy for further experiments. I would compare verapamil to DPPE in the cell growth and rat uterus experiments, while Frank would direct new binding experiments using radioactive histamine. *Now we were talking!* Once again, at least in my mind, a resurrection had occurred. The AEBS/histamine hypothesis was back from the dead.

---

25   This establishment, run by the Mehra family, was right across the street from the building housing Frank's lab. It boasted the best Indian cuisine in Winnipeg and was decorated with remarkable artifacts that Mr. Mehra brought over from India. The place was a perennial favorite with the medical school faculty and students, who jammed its two rooms for the noon buffet.

What I thought would be accomplished in a few weeks took longer to complete...much longer. Every time we finished one group of experiments, new questions arose for us to test. If I sound unhappy at this sudden snail's pace, that is not the case. I was now fully engaged with Frank on this project, so much so that Patricia had moved over to his lab, where she was working part time on the binding studies with Gary Queen and Doug Stein, Frank's highly experienced laboratory assistants.

The new work involved testing DPPE, verapamil and the various H_1 and H_2 antihistamines for their ability to inhibit radio-active histamine binding in the brain. We expected that radioactive histamine would bind to the brain membranes because H_1 receptors had long been known to exist there. Histamine is among the so-called "neuroamines", chemicals that mediate the complex functioning of the cells in our nervous system. However, its role in brain function has been less well defined than other amines, such as serotonin and dopamine, the major targets of antidepressant, antipsychotic and anti-Parkinson's drugs.

However, using a sophisticated computer software program, appropriately called "LIGAND", we were able to determine that the radioactive histamine was binding in huge amounts, and with a strength that was not compatible with binding to the much smaller numbers of H_1 receptors in the brain. Moreover, the number of these histamine sites was equal to the number of AEBS detected by radioactive DPPE (thanks again, Henry). I was not surprised. After all, if, as I believed, the AEBS was, in whole or in part, a novel histamine receptor, their numbers should match.

Equally noteworthy, DPPE was the most active of the drugs to block histamine binding in the brain; the "prototype" allergy (H_1) antihistamine, pyrilamine, was much weaker, as was verapamil, while the two ulcer-treating (H_2) antihistamine drugs, cimetidine and ranitidine, were virtually inactive. In other words, wherever most of that histamine was binding in the brain membranes, it was not, apparently, to the H_1 or H_2 receptors and not to a calcium channel! The results mimicked what we had seen when we had tested the various drugs to interfere with radioactive DPPE and tamoxifen binding to the AEBS in the liver microsomes.

The calcium channel theory put forward by Frank and Mark was dealt a further blow when Patricia compared the effects of DPPE and verapamil in the ovary-deficient rats. Unlike DPPE, verapamil had absolutely no ability to prevent uterine growth when the rats were injected with estradiol for three days. The coup de grâce came when we compared the effects of DPPE and verapamil on the growth of the MCF-7 breast cancer cells in tissue culture. The more DPPE that was added to the culture, the less the cells grew. Not so for verapamil. It did not affect growth but was toxic to the cells at high concentrations.

To add icing to the cake, we discovered that adding large quantities of L-histidine to the culture medium significantly decreased the ability of DPPE and tamoxifen to inhibit or kill the MCF-7 cells. Since histidine can cross the outer wall and get inside the cell, we believed that some was converted by the histidine decarboxylase enzyme to histamine, allowing the cells to overcome the blockade caused by DPPE and tamoxifen at the AEBS.

So it went. As the results accumulated test by test, Frank was becoming a believer. The AEBS had won out over the calcium channel. Moreover, Dr. Kahlson's concept of histamine as a major player in regulating cell growth was alive and well!

CHAPTER TEN:

If Only We Knew What
It Was Good For

In the midst of all of this, in late March of 1986, I received an unexpected phone call from New York. On the line was Dr. Julius Vida of Bristol-Myers, who introduced himself as vice-president of licensing for the company's Science and Technology Group. Our DPPE use patent had been filed with the USPO and he had seen the listing. He was interested and wondered whether he could come on short notice to meet with me in Winnipeg. I was both pleased and amused; although I did not allude to it on the phone, I wondered whether he knew that the original composition patent, now long-expired, had been awarded to his company.

A confidentiality agreement needed to be signed before we could talk. Dr. Vida offered to fax us one. Morris Silver, a very affable and enthusiastic PhD, had been hired to run the University's "satellite" technology transfer office at the medical school campus. He and Janet Scholz went over the document and, within a day or so, an agreement acceptable to both sides was ready to sign. The following week, Dr. Vida flew to Winnipeg, arriving early in the morning of April 9th. We met at Morris' office where, after the obligatory introductions, we all put our signatures on the document.

Julius Vida was an easy man to like. I was immediately struck by his immaculate appearance, cigarette holder and suave, sophisticated manner…a true European aristocrat. He told me that he had immigrated to the United States in the late 1950s, at the time of the Hungarian Revolution. Relatively nonplussed by my revelation that DPPE had been originally patented by Bristol-Myers, he allowed that he was not a stranger to drug "rediscovery" and use patents. If the drug was deemed valuable, Bristol-Myers would have no problem in reacquiring it through a licensing agreement.

We spent all morning discussing the experimental results. I then took him to Frank's office so that my colleague could fill him in as well. Frank was very supportive in his comments and by now I could see that Dr. Vida was both interested and enjoying himself. Noontime came quickly and Dr. Vida (by this time, it was "call me Julius") wanted to take me to lunch. I phoned Victor's, a wonderful continental restaurant, for a table. The place was always busy, but obtaining a last-minute reservation was never a problem, as the owner, Johanna Kattenfeld, always seemed partial to me. She wasn't bad herself.

The restaurant was located inside a renovated heritage building in Osborne Village, a tony part of town popular for its boutiques. Its name was derived from Osborne Street, a busy thoroughfare that runs through it and then passes by the well-manicured grounds of the Manitoba Legislature,[26] considered by many as la crème de la crème of Canada's provincial houses of parliament. I pointed out the restaurant to Julius, just across the street from where we were standing at a busy intersection. Before I knew what was happening, he started to cross against the red light. Out of the corner of my left eye, I saw a city transit bus barreling towards him. Time stood still for a split second as I grabbed the oblivious

---

26   Winnipeg is the capital of the Province of Manitoba.

Dr. Vida from behind by his expensive silk suit, almost ripping it as I yanked him back onto the curb. At literally the same time, the side of the bus passed three inches in front of us, the brakes screeching it to a halt just beyond a now very pale Julius Vida. As the front door opened for boarding, the bus driver's eyes met mine and a silent "That was close!" was exchanged.

"I did not have you come all this way to be flattened on Osborne Street," I said, trying to smooth out the maze of creases I had put on the back of his suit. Realizing that he had come within a second of being "toast", Julius just shook his head in disbelief, then quickly recovered from the shock of the moment as we crossed the now-clear street on the green light. Several glasses of red wine and a delicious meal soon put the harrowing experience behind us. The service was superb as a result of Johanna's attention, both to detail and to her favorite "Dr. Brandes", a point not lost on the ever-observant Julius.

Hot poppy seed cake for dessert was followed by more shop talk. "Your drug is w-e-e-e-ry interesting. Now if only vee knew vat it vas good for," he mused in his mellifluous Hungarian accent. I reiterated my hope that it might prove valuable in cancer treatment. "Ov courze, ov courze, zat vould be vunderful," he agreed. Clinking our glasses of Cabernet Sauvignon, we toasted the potential success of DPPE.

Lunch concluded, I took Julius back to my office for some final discussion. He told me he was very impressed by what he had learned and would take DPPE forward with the company. At his request, I provided him with a sample of the drug for general screening at the Bristol-Myers facility in Wallingford, CT and then drove him back to the airport. As we retrieved his valise from the trunk of my car, we shook hands and he promised that I would soon hear back from him.

About a month later he sent me a letter thanking me for arranging to see him on such short notice and suggesting that he would soon arrange for me to visit the company's Park Avenue headquarters in New York. Despite multiple efforts by Morris to contact him subsequently, that was the last we heard from the frequently-traveling Julius Vida for over two years! I was quickly learning about drug companies and how they work. A Brenda Lee tune, *Sweet Nothin's*, eventually became my theme song when dealing with them.

CHAPTER ELEVEN:

....Or What?

Bristol-Myers' "interest", now in limbo, quickly took a back seat to our research. After more than a year's work, Frank and I were finally ready to submit a paper. We decided to quit while ahead with *BBRC*. I suggested we submit to *Cancer Research*, a high-impact journal. Frank concurred. The review and revision process took several months but finally our paper was accepted and published. The title was, "*Histamine and growth: Interaction of antiestrogen binding site ligands with novel histamine sites that may be associated with calcium channels*".

The last seven words of the title were my idea, based on a lingering concern that Mark's binding studies might yet prove relevant. Frank did not think we needed to include them, since he fully accepted the evidence that the AEBS was distinct from the calcium channel. My argument prevailed and we left them in. As was also implicit in the title, Frank concurred with the notion that histamine plays a role in growth. "Now the NCIC will believe me," I told myself, as I eagerly dedicated the paper to Dr. Kahlson in an acknowledgement at the end of the manuscript.

By now, grant time had rolled around. Once again I spent weeks writing up my proposal to further assess the role of the AEBS and histamine in cell proliferation. Frank and Lyonel proof-read it and suggested revisions which I made. I confidently submitted the application to the NCIC. Appended to the grant were reprints of my five papers, including the one just published with Frank. As a backup, I also applied to the Medical Research Council. Three months later I received not one, but two rejections! How could this be happening? Was this how they rewarded innovative research?

Devastated, I went home early that afternoon. Jill and I took one of our innumerable walks up and down the majestic tree-lined streets of our River Heights neighborhood. My dear wife was both a good sport and a good listener. I often talked to her about the gobbledygook that was my research. Her expertise was in literature and theatre arts, not in science and medicine. Back when we were courting at the University of Western Ontario, with some degree of bravado I told her I wanted to find a cure for cancer. That statement won her heart. Her own mother had died a young woman of this disease. In December, 1966, I became the lucky guy who married the very popular and pretty Jill Leslie Colman.

"What if all of this work has been for nothing?" I agonized as we walked. That definitely would be the worst of all worlds, we both agreed. Nonetheless, if I wanted to succeed in my research, it had to be at the expense of other things, like a musician who must give up many of life's pleasures to practice for hours every day. Jill's unconditional love and support made my task easier, but great sacrifices were made along the way.

She and our two children had all too often come second to my career. On more than one occasion during those all-important years of raising a family, I had been guilty of self-absorption with my work. I even missed important events such as our son Jason's graduations from high school and the University of Manitoba. On both occasions I had busy clinics and believed that my cancer patients took priority. Jason later told me how hurt he was by my

absences. He was absolutely right to be upset with his dad. I had
been a fool. The past can never be recaptured. Chastened, I thereafter made it my business to attend all family milestones such as
Jason's receipt of his MBA from McGill and daughter Carolyn's
graduations with two degrees from the University of Winnipeg.

The next day I went to see my mentor in his office. Lyonel felt
for me, believing that I got a raw deal. Frank concurred. After
all, he, like Lyonel, had approved the contents of the application.
Lyonel immediately suggested that I submit my grant proposal
to the Manitoba Medical Services Foundation, a local funding
agency. He was one of their scientific advisors. The board was
due to meet in two months and the deadline for that year's applications was fast approaching. I filled out all the required forms
and rejigged the budget to cover one year of funding, all that was
allowed from this source.

Shortly after submission, I received a letter informing me that,
as one of three successful applicants, I was invited downtown to
present a short synopsis of my proposal to the board. "Now these
guys know good science when they hear it. They should be on the
NCIC panel," I said to myself as three retired family practitioners,
a businessman and an accountant nodded wisely and smiled with
approval during my fifteen-minute presentation. Joking aside,
they and Lyonel had saved my hide. I was safe for another year.
Nonetheless, the "…or what?" part of my rhetorical question had
now definitely descended on me for a second year in a row.

A few months later, Dr. Peter Scholefield, executive director of
the NCIC visited our Institute. I asked to meet with him to discuss
my research. During our private get-together, I tried to impress
upon him the potential scientific and clinical importance of my
findings. Listening courteously, he appeared sympathetic, but all
he could do was promise to send me the committee's commentary
outlining the perceived deficiencies of my research proposal. In
those days the critiques were not sent automatically and had to be
requested. True to his word, it arrived not long after.

Reading the report gave me heartburn. In their remarks, the NCIC panel of reviewers were now somewhat more positive about histamine, but once again the big "negative" was that we had not proposed to purify the AEBS. My grant had actually been approved, but with only "medium priority" and, therefore, not funded. I felt compelled to send Peter my commentary on their commentary. He soon replied with the following letter:

"Dear Lorne.

"This will acknowledge receipt of your letter of 31 March 1988. It prompts me to submit the following:

"There was a young medic called Lorne

"Who heaped on reviewers much scorn

"He'd debate and discuss

"And cause such a fuss

"They wished they'd never been born.

"My best regards.

"Yours sincerely, Peter."

I must admit I laughed at Peter's clever limerick, but at the same time I vowed to myself that, whether or not others saw value in my approach, I would continue on the same path. Shakespeare's admonition, "To thine own self be true" had long been ingrained in me. One advantage of being an MD/oncologist was that I was not dependent on research for my livelihood. In a perverse sense, if the lab program folded, it actually would be financially advantageous, since I would substantially increase my income by seeing more patients in the clinic one floor below. However, my research was a labor of love, and I was determined that it must, and would, survive. Besides, with Frank as my "partner in crime", things would work out eventually.

CHAPTER TWELVE:

Two Volatile Ethnics

Almost every day during our long collaboration, I would take the five-minute walk from my office to Frank's lab, crossing the hospital parking lot when the weather was warm or, during those months when the climate was less pleasant (Winnipeg has four seasons: winter, winter, winter and road construction), traversing the maze of underground tunnels that connected the various buildings. Frank usually could be found sitting at his desk, glasses hanging by a lanyard down the front of his open-collared shirt, pencil and pad nearby, perusing the latest issues of *Science* or *Nature*.

We would go over the latest experimental data or, if there wasn't anything "hot off the press", we would talk shop. During those discussions, certain of my buzzwords or phrases, especially "intracellular histamine receptor", were guaranteed to evoke an animated response. Based on our experiments, Frank now agreed with the possibility that the AEBS and histamine binding sites (which he distinguished from receptors) could be related but, until we had more data, that was as far as he was willing to go. I remained convinced that what we were looking at here was Kahlson's "unconventional" histamine receptor.

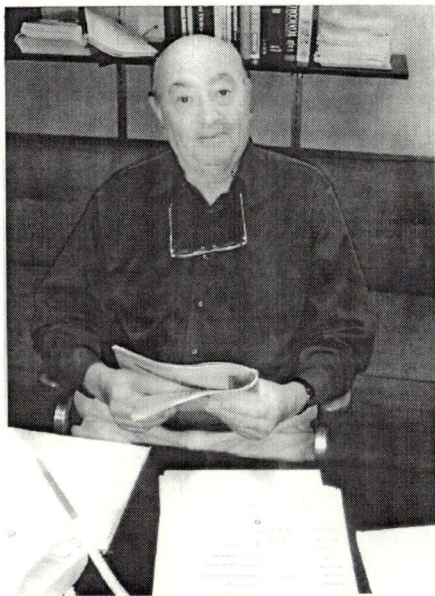

Frank LaBella (Personal photo collection)

"A receptor has a defined structure, with seven finger-like domains that go through the cell membrane," he would argue. "Moreover, a receptor has a proven function; for example when histamine binds to the H_1 receptor on a smooth muscle cell membrane it causes muscle contraction and when it binds to the H_2 receptor on a parietal cell membrane it causes hydrochloric acid to be secreted.[27] We just don't have enough information or evidence to call this new histamine binding site a receptor."

"We are talking about an unconventional histamine receptor inside the cell and it may have a totally different structure than the 'classical' receptors you describe on the cell membrane. There

27   Smooth muscles line the respiratory tract. They constrict when histamine binds to the H_1 receptor. Parietal cells line the inside of the stomach. They manufacture hydrochloric acid, important in the digestion of food, when histamine binds to the H_2 receptor.

is precedent for that in the estrogen receptor. Except in this case, it's a histamine receptor, probably part of the AEBS. I believe it has a function, which is the mediation of growth, and it can be inhibited by drugs such as DPPE and tamoxifen," I countered.

I also buttressed my argument by showing him a 1984 paper in *Cancer Research*. Rats with liver tumors were treated by Belgian researchers using a specific inhibitor of the histidine decarboxylase enzyme that makes histamine. The tumors shrank. "What further proof does one need for the existence of a growth-promoting intracellular histamine receptor?" I asked my colleague.

"Fine. That is your hypothesis," Frank retorted. "You may turn out to be correct. The work is definitely progressing and the findings are intriguing. Histamine appears to be a player here, but until you have definite proof, don't call it a receptor. It will just get in the way and antagonize both grant reviewers and experts in the field." I believed the proof was already there and couldn't see his point. We agreed to disagree. Then he hit me with a bombshell out of left field. Rather than a receptor, histamine and DPPE were probably binding to a type of metabolizing enzyme called "P450". I just looked at him incredulously, shaking my head, not appreciating the importance of this brilliant insight. That would come later.

Frank and I often argued like that... two volatile ethnics: a Sicilian and a Jew. At times the volume of our discourse permeated the hallway outside his office. Once, during a particularly enthusiastic exchange of opinion, Gary and Doug, Frank's two assistants, knocked on the closed office door to inquire whether all was well within. We assured them it was, notwithstanding the tell-tale white ring of antacid tablet residue visible around Frank's mouth. His consumption of Rolaids always increased noticeably when my visits lasted more than five minutes. I thought of writing to the company that made them to see if I could be their spokesman. Lyonel had once joked on the square that I was a carrier.... giving ulcers and grey hair to others.

Despite any differences of opinion, I can truthfully say that our frequent scientific disagreements never affected our friendship. Frank clearly respected me and I truly thought the world of him. Rarely before had he encountered a clinician who could argue science with him and, except for Lyonel, rarely had I known a colleague with the patience of Job to put up with a guy like me. Even if some of my ideas were hard for him to accept, Frank admired my verve and tenacity. He allowed that he was in it with me for the long haul, or until the money or life ran out, whichever came first. "Ditto for me," I agreed.

CHAPTER THIRTEEN:

New Colleagues, New Clues

Like sports, research sometimes requires you to play defense. A new finding suddenly forced me to undertake a study that, up to that point, was not on my radar screen. Ironically, it came from Peter Lam, one of my colleagues at the Institute, who published a paper showing that tamoxifen strongly inhibited a major calcium-regulating protein, called calmodulin. At the time, this molecule was a hot new topic among researchers interested in growth. If it was a target for tamoxifen, maybe DPPE would interact there as well. I had to find out, but had no procedure to assess this possibility. Even worse, I didn't have the money. Luckily, another colleague, Ratna Bose, had both. She was one of a triad of Boses in the pharmacology department. Her husband, Deepak, did cardiovascular research, while Deepak's brother, Ranjan, worked with Carl Pinsky in neuropharmacology.

Ratna had developed a specific calmodulin assay using muscle tissue. Despite her busy lab program, she was kind enough to test DPPE. Within a few weeks she reported that it was definitely not a calmodulin inhibitor. The AEBS was still the top contender.

We wrote up the findings and submitted them to a well-regarded journal called *Cancer Chemotherapy and Pharmacology*. The paper was accepted with no revision required. *Man alive*. Despite my problems with major funding agencies, I was still on a roll with the journals.

One never knows when experiments will prove to be "seminal". Collaboration with a third colleague in the pharmacology department resulted in findings that greatly contributed to the decision to test DPPE in patients with cancer. It grew out of my desire to determine whether there might be another role for histamine in the gut, unrelated to stimulating acid secretion in the stomach. Professor Kahlson showed that, in addition to copious numbers of mast cells that store histamine, gastrointestinal tissue had a high activity of the histamine-forming enzyme, histidine decarboxylase, suggesting that much of the histamine was newly-formed (nascent). He believed it to be involved in the rapid cell turnover and growth of new lining cells which have a short life and are constantly replenished; if not, ulcers will form. "Would DPPE have any effect on such cells?" was a logical question.

I brought up this question with Clive Greenway, pharmacology department chairman. Clive and I had both come to Winnipeg from the U.K. in the early 1970s. He was born and trained there, while I had just completed my year at the Royal Marsden. Coincidentally, in those early years, we lived a few doors from one another in a row of townhouses on Winnipeg's scenic Assiniboine River. Clive, who had just joined the medical faculty, kindly offered me a ride to work. However, after the first week I opted for alternate transportation because he was hopelessly addicted to nicotine and I just could not stand the heavy cigarette fumes. Sensitive to my plight, he even rolled down the windows of his well-worn Volvo station wagon. The incoming blast of wintry prairie cold made a bad environment even worse! That aside, we remained friends and colleagues through the years.

Like Carl, Clive was very supportive from the get-go. He had read Kahlson's book while a lecturer at Cambridge and, for that reason, was both interested in, and impressed by, my work. Clive's primary interest was in the control of the portal circulation (the all-important blood flow from the bowel and spleen through the veins into the liver). Where Ed Kroeger used dogs in his research, Clive used cats. What I always liked about Clive was that he was totally forthright in his appraisal of people and things. If he thought your work was worthwhile, he would tell you. If he thought your work was less than sensational, he would also tell you. Thus, his encouragement was heartening.[28]

On the particular day I posed the question about DPPE and its possible effect in the gut, he asked, "Do you know Gary Glavin?" When I replied in the negative, Clive told me that he had just recruited Gary, a PhD, to the department from the University of Winnipeg.[29]

His research focused on the mechanism of ulcer formation in the stomach and duodenum in rodents. "Sounds like I should see him," I suggested. Clive nodded, telling me that Gary's lab was at the end of the hall on the second floor. Down the stairs I went. As luck would have it, Gary was there. Lanky, bearded and athletic-looking, at well over six feet tall he was hard to miss.

We spent the better part of an hour talking about our mutual research. He could easily measure stomach acid in rats. In addition, he used two widely-employed methods to produce large stomach ulcers in rodents. The first, called "cold-restraint"[30] does not mimic the usual hyperacidity model in humans, but is definitely a counterpart of the "stress-ulcer syndrome", an acute type of stomach ulceration that can affect post-trauma and post-surgical patients, often with devastating results. The second, ethanol,

---

28 Clive later offered me a cross-appointment as adjunct Professor of Pharmacology. I was honored to accept.

29 The University of Winnipeg and the University of Manitoba are autonomous institutions, both located in Winnipeg. A healthy rivalry exists between them.

30 This procedure involved tying down a rat on its back in a cold room for one hour to produce stress ulcers. It would not be allowed today, but was ethically-approved in the 1980s.

the type of alcohol consumed by humans, is a direct irritan
stomach lining.

Using these two models, Gary could test various drug
their ability to protect against ulcer formation. His interest piqued
by my enthusiastic description of Kahlson's findings, he was more
than happy to test DPPE, especially because of its novel antihista-
minic properties that seemed to exclude blocking the H_2 receptor.
His assays would also provide a further opportunity to compare
DPPE and our calcium channel-blocking nemesis, verapamil.

Surprisingly, DPPE was a very potent drug to prevent stomach
acid production and prevented stomach ulcers induced by both
stress and ethanol. Verapamil, on the other hand, was weak to
block acid secretion and made ethanol-induced ulcers worse.
Clearly, DPPE was doing something very different from verapamil.
Perhaps the most interesting finding was that the ulcer-protective
effects of DPPE could be abolished by aspirin-like drugs. This
indicated that DPPE was not protecting the stomach at the H_2
receptor, but rather by stimulating the formation of certain cell
chemicals called prostaglandins.[31]

The prostaglandins are a fascinating lot: some are protective to
our tissues while others are injurious and cause fever, pain and
inflammation. It took scientists over a century to discover that the
wonder drug, aspirin, reduces pain and fever by blocking a family
of enzymes called "cyclooxygenases" (now commonly referred
to as COX-1 and COX-2) that make prostaglandins. However,
because aspirin also prevents the formation of a protective prostaglandin called prostacyclin, it can cause stomach irritation and
ulcers. As a result of Gary's experiments, we now knew that, in
the gut, DPPE worked in the opposite direction of aspirin: it was
stimulating the cells to make almost ten times as much prostacyclin as usual. It was not apparent then, but this highly important
finding influenced the design of future clinical trials in patients
with cancer.

---

31 The term "prostaglandins" derives from "prostate gland", the tissue in
which they were first identified.

Another paper was written, submitted and accepted! Again I marveled at the disconnect between getting papers published and getting grants funded. Both require critical peer review. "Where is the consistency here?" I wondered. It would not be the last time I asked that question. With just enough money to carry on for another twelve months, I now desperately needed to see whether DPPE had a future in cancer therapy.

CHAPTER FOURTEEN:

And The Winner Is.....

A year previously, I had sent a sample of DPPE to the U.S. National Cancer Institute in Bethesda. For decades, the government agency had offered a free screening program[32] to test substances for anti-cancer activity against a variety of tumor cell lines obtained from humans and rodents. Designated by the NCI as D-600011, DPPE was tested against forty tumor types in tissue culture. Although there were differences in its potency from tumor to tumor, in every case DPPE inhibited the growth or killed the cancer cells. From the actual test values provided by the NCI, I estimated that at least half of the cancers might be inhibited by DPPE at doses that could be achieved in the body.

In addition to the tissue culture experiments, the NCI also tested DPPE against several experimental tumors in rodents. Somewhat surprisingly, no tumor shrinkage was seen when DPPE was administered to the live animals. Indeed, I was puzzled by the results in two instances where, as compared to control animals that were injected with placebo (saline), DPPE appeared to cause

---

32   This valuable service was finally discontinued by NCI several years later.

a doubling or tripling of the growth of colon and breast cancer tumors. Since the number of animals tested was small, the results had to be interpreted cautiously. However, we ourselves had not actually administered DPPE to rodents to assess its toxicity or its effects on tumor growth. It was time we did.

There is a well-established breast cancer model in rats in which tamoxifen had been proven highly effective. A potent chemical carcinogen, called dimethylbenzanthracine ("DMBA"), is administered to young female rats. Within three months they develop multiple breast cancer tumors along the milk line on each side of their bellies. These tumors are usually fed by estrogen and can be significantly prevented or decreased in number by administering tamoxifen prior to, or just after, they start to form. Given our previous finding that DPPE, like tamoxifen, was active to block estrogen stimulation in the rat uterus, I thought we should put DPPE to the test against these chemically-induced breast cancers.

Once again Patricia was entrusted with the task. Linda helped with the administration of the DMBA. It was instilled using a syringe attached to a small rubber tube inserted directly from the mouth into the stomach, a procedure not particularly pleasant for the rats or my two brave assistants. But they got the job done. Once weekly, Pat and Linda, hands covered with thick gloves, examined the cages of rats for any developments. At the sixty-day mark none had yet developed tumors, but it was time to start treating them.

We randomly assigned seven rats to receive DPPE and seven to receive saline (placebo). Every Monday to Friday, Pat and Linda took the rats from their cages, injected them one by one with the designated treatment solution and checked for tumors, all the while trying to avoid bites and scratches imparted by their "patients". Within two weeks, lumps started to appear, slowly at first, then at a more rapid pace. The date of first occurrence of each tumor was recorded and the size was measured with calipers every week. By the time ten weeks had gone by there was a clear winner: *the placebo!!!*

Not only did DPPE not prevent or inhibit tumors from growing in the rats, it actually caused tumors to grow three times the size of those seen in rats receiving the saline. This was no tamoxifen. Maybe those NCI experiments were right!

There is a dictum in science that experiments must be repeated to verify a result. We had to determine whether what we had just seen was reproducible. Maybe it was an aberration or maybe it was true. We needed to know either way. However, although they understood the need for repetition, I could see that my two assistants were less than enthusiastic about another long encounter with a bunch of aggressive rats. Who could blame them? Moreover, Linda was getting married and was soon to move away. Pat was already overextended helping out with the binding studies in Frank's laboratory.

Reluctantly, I put the repeat experiment on hold until Max Cawker, a recent science graduate of the University, joined the lab to replace Linda. I had thought about strategy for some time and had a new idea. We could easily obtain mouse leukemia cells, called "L5178Y", from the lab down the hall. When as little as two hundred of these vicious tumor cells are injected under the shaved skin on the backside of genetically-identical mice, they rapidly grow to form tumors within a week. Max could retest DPPE versus saline all by himself using this second, simpler rodent model. We would have the added benefit of a rapid answer.

"In this experiment, inject two hundred leukemia cells and wait two days for them to take hold. Then separate the mice into two groups and inject DPPE or saline (placebo) once a day for just three days, I instructed." Max followed these directions to a tee. Thereafter, once a week he measured the growing tumors with his trusty calipers. And after four weeks, the winner was……
the placebo! Once again DPPE had stimulated tumor growth by almost two and one-half times compared to the mice treated with the saline. *DPPE, the great killer of cancer cells in the test tube was DPPE, the great stimulator of cancer cells in rats and mice!!!* The NCI had seen it and now we had, too.

I was now faced with two dilemmas. The first was a research issue: there was no disputing what had been found twice in a row. The decision to test a second tumor model, rather than repeat the DMBA experiment in the rats, greatly strengthened the case that DPPE was making malignant tumors grow faster in mice and rats. In other words, this was not a phenomenon limited to one type of tumor. Why the paradox between the inhibitory/killing effect against all sorts of cancer cells growing in tissue culture dishes and a tumor-stimulating effect in the animal?

Two possible explanations immediately surfaced. Maybe DPPE was being broken down in the liver into a second compound that had different effects than the DPPE itself. That often happens with the drugs we take. Or maybe we were using too weak a dose of DPPE. We had arbitrarily chosen four milligrams per kilogram body weight in the rat because that was the effective dose to block the growth effect of estrogen in the rat uterus. We had settled on one milligram per kilogram body weight in the mouse based on the mistaken notion that, because the mice were at least four times smaller than the rats, we should decrease the dose accordingly.[33] What would happen if we repeated the experiments at higher doses? Would the tumors shrink rather than grow? The trouble was, I had no idea how much DPPE we could safely give to a mouse or a rat.

The second dilemma was both a business and an ethical issue: our patent. Based on what had just been observed in the animal experiments, the patent, which claimed the use of DPPE alone as an anticancer agent, appeared dead in the water. Who would develop, let alone market, a drug that could make cancer grow faster? Should I tell the University to forget the whole business and not spend any more money?

---

33 I was later to learn that, based on the formula of body weight divided by body surface area, for a drug dose in the mouse to be equivalent to a drug dose in the rat, approximately *twice* the dose had to be administered to the mouse as compared to the rat. We were way off in the opposite direction when we made our original calculation!

On the other hand, what if it were just a matter of finding an optimal dose, or some other way of administering DPPE that resulted in an opposite effect to the one we had just observed? Pulling the plug too quickly might be just as detrimental as pretending we had not seen what we had seen and continuing to waste the University's money prosecuting a useless patent. I made the decision right then and there to remain calm, to let the patent continue to percolate for the moment and to keep probing for an answer. As will become apparent, it was the right thing to do.

CHAPTER FIFTEEN:

Somersaulting Mice

I called Pat and Max into my office. "We need to order some mice and dose them with DPPE. How much can they tolerate? We don't know and we must find out." My two comrades agreed. Within a week we had our cages stocked with a new batch of "volunteers". Since we had already used the four milligrams per kilogram body weight dose without seeing any toxic effects, we decided to start by doubling the dose in batches of three mice. If there were no harmful effects in the first three, we would double the dose each time until we observed side effects. The highest dose that could be given without serious side effects (known as the "maximum tolerated dose" or "MTD") could then be used in future tumor experiments.

The first dose of eight milligrams per kilogram produced no visible effect after fifteen minutes. The dose was then doubled in the next three mice. No effect. On to thirty-two we went. The same. We looked at one another and shrugged. Three new mice received sixty-four milligrams per kilogram. Within a minute of being injected, all became a bit twitchy, their fur bristling for a few minutes. They then settled back to normal. "Let's go up a bit more slowly, to one hundred per kilo," I suggested.

Within five minutes of receiving that dose, three new mice were literally somersaulting in the air and bouncing off the walls of the cage. This incredible scene went on for about forty-five minutes and then stopped almost as abruptly as it had begun. With my weird sense of humor, I kept thinking that if Ed Sullivan were still alive, we could have booked them on his show as a lead-in for Topo Gigio. We all just looked at one another and laughed at the bizarre nature of what we had just witnessed.

Now recovered, the mice looked none the worse for wear and carried on normally as if nothing had ever happened. That was some trip, we all agreed. "Let's back down to fifty per kilo in another three," I suggested. The mice had absolutely no side effects with that dose.

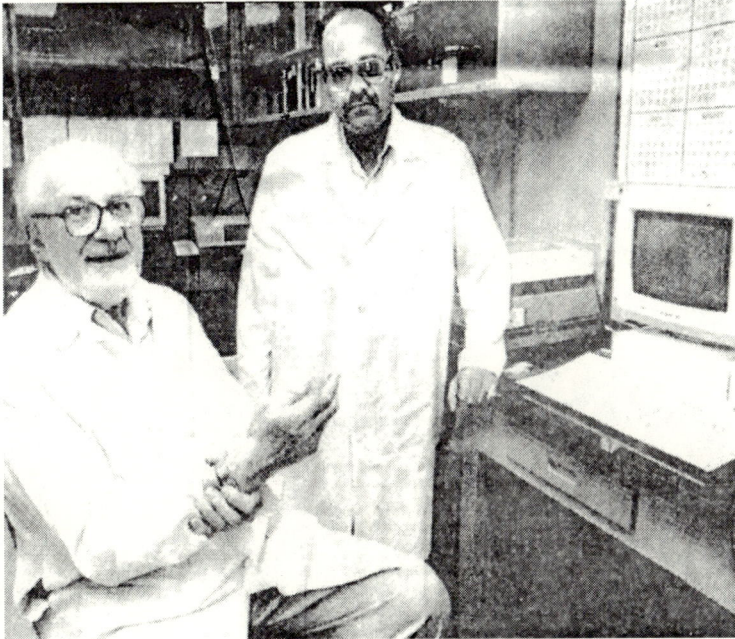

Carl Pinsky (sitting) and Ranjan Bose (Dept. of Pharmacology Archive)

We had found our MTD in the mouse: roughly fifty to sixty milligrams per kilogram. Up a notch and mayhem resulted.

"With DPPE, it is like suddenly going over a cliff," I explained to Carl Pinsky and his research associate, Ranjan Bose, the next day. As I described what we had observed at the sixty-four and one hundred milligrams per kilogram dose, the two neuropharmacologists smiled at one another and nodded knowingly. "It sounds typical for petit mal seizures,"[34] Ranjan suggested. "Wow, if that's petit mal, I'd hate to see grand mal," I replied. I did not know it at the time, but Ranjan's expertise would later prove vital in taming DPPE for human use.

---

34 Petit mal (or "absence") seizures in humans are associated with a short period of "blanking out" or staring into space, not at all similar to what we had observed in the somersaulting mice.

CHAPTER SIXTEEN:

The Incredible Random Event

Looking back on life, it is amazing how events often unfold. The years 1989-1991 proved to be pivotal to the DPPE and histamine story as several new players changed the landscape once and for all. I had never even heard of one of them, Rob Warrington, until I received a fateful call one day in mid-1989. It was from Ron Reid, a professor in the pharmacy faculty at the University's Fort Garry campus across town. His role in this story, although largely seren-dipitous, was key to everything that followed.

Ron was an excellent researcher who, like Ratna Bose, was interested in calmodulin. I had become acquainted with him some months earlier when I was invited by Dr. Chiu Ming Wong, a noted professor in the chemistry department, to give a seminar on my research. Ron was very outspoken. During my talk he interrupted frequently to express great skepticism about my his-tamine hypothesis. Chiu Ming, a gentleman's gentleman, seemed unhappy with his colleague's behavior that day, but I actually appreciated Ron's candor and we became friends. I could always count on him to give an honest opinion. He was a curmudgeon, but a straightforward curmudgeon.

The call from Ron went approximately as follows:

"Lorne. Ron here. Have you heard of a guy called Warrington in Saskatoon?"

"No."

"Well, he has some very impressive data showing that L-histidinol[35] markedly increases the ability of a whole bunch of different types of chemotherapy drugs to shrink cancer in mice. The combo actually seems to be curing them of leukemia. And get this.... histidinol also protects the bone marrow from the toxic effects of the chemo."

"You've got to be kidding, Ron," I exclaimed, thinking of the ulcer-protecting effects of DPPE that Gary Glavin had observed.

"No. I'm serious. I'm sending you a copy of one of his papers in the internal mail. You should have it by tomorrow. Call me after you've read it."

I was bowled over by this news because both Ron and I knew that *L-histidinol turns into L-histidine, which can be converted by histidine decarboxylase into histamine!* Could Warrington's findings be another link between "nascent" histamine and growth? Even *more importantly, could this be the clue on how to use DPPE in cancer therapy?*

I now had the luxury of asking these important questions, knowing that my laboratory would survive another year. Although (once again) my grant applications were turned down by the NCIC and MRC, I got lucky with the Manitoba Health Research Council, a provincial funding agency chaired by Dr. Frits Stevens of the University's biochemistry department. The MHRC had been established some years earlier as a result of Lyonel's efforts to help support scientific research in the province. On hearing of the

---

35   L-histidinol is the alcohol form and immediate precursor of L-histidine. Histidine is one of twenty amino acids that are the building blocks of proteins. Like all amino acids, histidine exists in left-handed (L-) and right-handed (R-) forms that are mirror images of one another.

award, I felt better knowing that at least some scientists thought my work was worth funding.

A large envelope from Ron arrived in the next morning's mail. In it was a copy of a 1986 paper in *Anticancer Research* written by one Robert C. Warrington of the University of Saskatchewan. It had a riveting title: "*A novel approach for improving the efficacy of experimental cancer chemotherapy using combinations of anti-cancer drugs and L-histidinol*". I immediately took it to my office, closed the door and sat down to read it. Like Kahlson's monograph, this manuscript was, for me, a "Eureka!" moment.

After I had finished, I immediately called Ron back. "How did you learn about this?"

"Pure chance. I was a visiting lecturer at Saskatchewan and Warrington was on my itinerary of people to meet. He told me about his work and gave me a reprint of one of his papers. I immediately thought of your crazy histamine theory. I think you two guys may be looking at the same thing, or maybe something close. Are you going to contact him?"

"Absolutely, but not yet," I responded. "He says in his paper that histidinol may work as a protein synthesis inhibitor.[36] I want to do some binding studies first."

I thanked Ron for this important lead, hung up the phone and then ruminated about life. Is our destiny governed by a series of random events? Or is there really Someone or Something up above who determines the Grand Design of what is, and is not, meant to be? "That, my friend, is what keeps us humble," I said to myself.

Having carefully read the Warrington paper, I calculated that, as compared to most drugs, a very high dose of L-histidinol was required to be effective in the mice with tumors. From the concentrations we found effective in our own previous experiments

---

36   It has long been known that amino acid alcohols interfere with the incorporation of the corresponding non-alcohol forms of amino acids into proteins. L-histidinol blocks protein synthesis by preventing the incorporation of L-histidine.

in the MCF-7 breast cancer cells, DPPE appeared to be a thousand times more powerful than histidinol. Our new binding assays might be an easy way to see whether that prediction held water.

Over the past few months we had switched from using brain membranes to liver microsomes, where the AEBS was originally discovered. To my relief, the binding studies using radiolabeled DPPE and histamine were identical in both preparations; the binding of large amounts of radiolabeled histamine in the liver was an especially important observation because, unlike the brain, conventional histamine receptors apparently do not reside there.

What we were observing was altogether new. Moreover, once again our computer program told us that the number of AEBS sites, identified by DPPE, and the number of histamine sites were of equal number. This again suggested that they might be closely associated. I was excited. In his less demonstrative way, Frank also seemed impressed.

We then went a step further. Although Frank was somewhat skeptical of the idea, I wanted to see whether histamine and DPPE also might bind to DNA in the nucleus, the main regulator of the cell. Our genes, containing the DNA blueprint of life, reside there in ribbon-like structures called chromosomes. It is ultimately from the DNA in the nucleus that signals emanate to tell cells what to do and when to do it, including when to divide. Dr. Jim Davie, a member of the biochemistry department, was an expert in removing the nucleus from the cell and purifying its components. He enthusiastically agreed to help Pat learn this complex procedure using our rat liver cells. It was time-consuming and laborious work, but eventually, to our delight, the results showed that DPPE and histamine bound in the nucleus and, particularly, in the DNA-containing part. Although it was still not direct proof, I believed that this finding was a giant leap forward in linking histamine and the AEBS to growth. Frank just shook his head in amazement as he reviewed the results. "The Lord works in mysterious ways," he philosophized.

I now called Patty, who was in Frank's lab, and asked her to come over to my office. When she arrived I gave her a copy of the Warrington paper and asked her to read it. "Order some L-histidinol from our supplier and let me know as soon as you receive it," I requested. She was to screen histidinol in the binding assays. I went out on a limb and predicted to her that the histidinol would interfere with histamine binding, but it would be substantially weaker than DPPE. "Let's see if I'm right," I told her with some hope that I knew what I was talking about.

Within a couple of weeks of my request, Pat came back with the answer on L-histidinol. My predictions were bang on. "How did you know this?" she asked. "Just a lucky guess," I answered with a smile. "Or maybe not," I said under my breath. It was now time to retest DPPE in mice with tumors, this time in combination with chemotherapy à la histidinol!

CHAPTER SEVENTEEN:

Dr. Warrington, I Presume?

Unfortunately, we found that our L5178Y leukemia cells had become overgrown with contaminating bacteria. A new batch from the other lab would take a few weeks to obtain. I was just too impatient to wait that long. Luckily, another colleague at the Institute, Dr. Arnold Greenberg, had tumor cells, called C-3, that were growing well in his laboratory. They were derived from a type of mouse cancer called sarcoma. Arnold told me that they were highly malignant and rapidly formed tumors when injected under the skin of genetically-identical mice. The scenario was essentially the same as with the L5178Y cells we had used previously. "That would be just great," I replied, thanking him.

This new task fell by default to the already-overburdened Patricia. After only a year, Max had just left to take up a teaching position at a local high school. I was happy for him but sad for us, as he had really begun to blossom and his work was excellent. As always, Patty was only too willing to do whatever I asked of her. She was a gem. I assured her I would hire a new technician to help us out as soon as I could.

Using a small syringe and needle, Pat inoculated several thousand sarcoma cells under the shaved skin on the backside of twelve mice. The next day she randomly separated them into two groups of six. Into the first group, she injected our newly-identified "maximum tolerated dose (MTD)" of DPPE, followed one hour later by an injection of doxorubicin, a powerful anticancer drug useful in treating several human cancers, including sarcoma. Into the second group, she injected placebo (saline) followed one hour later by the doxorubicin. Thereafter, the mice were examined every day for tumors; any that developed were measured.

By the end of the first week, Pat reported that every mouse injected with saline and doxorubicin developed small tumors, but she could detect nothing in the mice that had received DPPE and doxorubicin! I tried not to get overly excited by this news. Maybe another day or two and it would be a different story. A week later, nothing had changed in the group that had received DPPE and doxorubicin, while the tumors were growing larger in the other mice. Three weeks! Four weeks! Finally, after two months with no tumors, we had a little party for the six survivors and declared them "cured". I was beside myself with excitement. Patty saw me smiling from ear to ear. "You look very happy," she observed. "You can say that again," I replied. Was I happy or what?

Later that week I drove to the main University campus to update Marion Vaisey-Genser on our progress. Just as I sat down in her well-appointed, smoke-filled office, Janet Scholz stuck her head in the door to say hello and was invited in. "I have good news and bad news to report," I explained over a cup of tea. "First, the good news." I proceeded to tell them what we had just witnessed in the mice.

"That's just fabulous. And now the bad news, m'dear?" (Marion always called me "m'dear". I rather liked it.)

"The bad news is that we need to think about filing a completely new use patent for DPPE," I reported somewhat more solemnly. The original was definitely dead in the water. Marion was thrilled about the mice, but less thrilled about a new patent which would be an expensive proposition. She needed to think things over and asked me to leave it with her. As I went out, I gave both ladies a hug and told them to mark this day on their calendars. They definitely would, they assured me.

It was time to touch base with Rob Warrington, but not, as I had initially intended, by phone. I had just received a volume of abstracts for the upcoming annual meeting of the American Association for Cancer Research (AACR) which, that year, was being held at the Convention Center in New Orleans. Reading through them, I saw that Rob had submitted an abstract. It had been accepted for poster presentation, where the researcher is assigned to stand beside one of hundreds of poster boards in a large hall. The experimental results are tacked up on the board. Any interested person can come by to read and discuss the data with the presenter. I would attend Rob's poster in person and surprise him.

On the day and time that he was to present, I waited in the crowded room for him to appear. Five minutes…ten minutes…fifteen minutes went by. Most of the other presenters had already put up their data, but the board assigned to Dr. Warrington remained empty. "Oh, no," I thought, "don't tell me he's a no-show." That happens from time to time….a last minute cancellation for who-knows-what reason. It didn't help that I hadn't the slightest idea what he looked like. Just as I was about to give up and leave, a casually-dressed fellow entered the room. He had a very kind face under a well-trimmed beard and was carrying a hollow cardboard tube in which there was a poster. Could it be? Was it him?

Up to the assigned board he went. *Yes!!!* Without giving him a chance to finish putting up the poster, I went over, stuck out my hand and said, with great originality, "Dr. Warrington, I presume." As he turned around to shake hands, I continued to speak. "I'm Lorne Brandes from the University of Manitoba. I read your paper and I believe I know how L-histidinol really works."

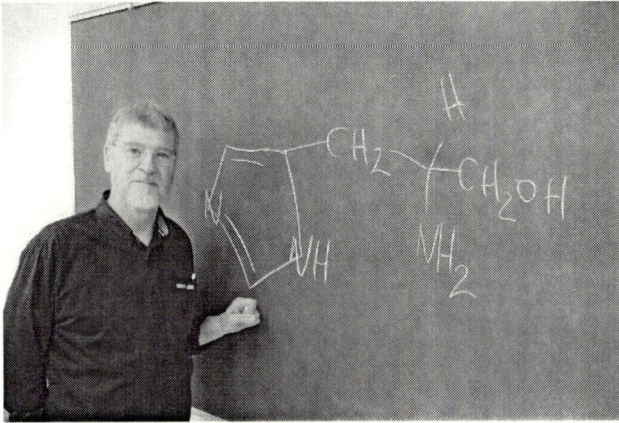

Rob Warrington standing next to a drawing of the L-histidinol molecule (Photo courtesy of Rob Warrington)

Hapless visitors to his poster fended for themselves as Rob and I huddled next to the wall, deep in conversation. He had not heard of our work but was captivated by the recent binding studies with L-histidinol and the preliminary tumor results with DPPE and doxorubicin. We agreed then and there to collaborate. I would test L-histidinol in our various cell assays and he would test DPPE to see whether he could reproduce its ability to mimic L-histidinol in mice with tumors. He would also determine whether DPPE could protect the bone marrow from the effects of chemotherapy. We exchanged phone numbers and promised to be in touch as soon as we got back to our respective labs. Needless to say, I was ecstatic over this development.

CHAPTER EIGHTEEN:

Vindication

That wasn't the only good news that year. As I flew home to Winnipeg, I thought about how 1989 had started with a long-overdue bang. Two months before my encounter with Rob, Frank and I were co-authors of a "breakthrough" histamine paper published in Frank's favorite journal, *Science*. It had all come together over the preceding year because of the interest and involvement of Jon Gerrard, a pediatrician and scientist at the Institute of Cell Biology, and two of his post-doctoral fellows, Satya Saxena, a recent arrival from India, and Archie McNicol, a personable Scot.

Jon's lab, across the hall from mine, was a going concern, researching platelets, the small sticky particles that circulate in the bloodstream to help prevent bleeding and bruising. As my work with Frank progressed, I would often pop into Jon's office to show him our data. One morning he called me over to his lab for a talk with Satya. Jon thought that the platelet might be a perfect system with which to test my AEBS/histamine hypothesis. The reason behind this was that, in the test tube, many substances are able to make platelets stick together to form clumps. This process, called aggregation, is how platelets stop bleeding at a sight of injury to a blood vessel. In effect, the tightly-clumped platelets act like little corks, or fingers in a dike, to staunch the flow of blood.

A chemical, called "PMA" for short, is very powerful to cause platelets to aggregate. PMA is also a "tumor promoter", meaning that it helps weak carcinogens become stronger to cause cancer. A few years previously, a Japanese scientist, Dr. Takehiko Watanabe[37] discovered that PMA turns on the production of Dr. Kahlson's old friend, histidine decarboxylase, the histamine-forming enzyme.[38] Therefore, Jon thought that Satya should investigate whether new histamine is produced by the platelets when they are caused to clump by PMA. If so, he would test DPPE and the other antihistamines to see whether they could prevent PMA from clumping the platelets, while Archie would carry out ancillary platelet studies to further test the hypothesis.

Two additional colleagues would lend their help to Satya. Allan Becker was a pediatric allergist and researcher who had recently obtained a piece of equipment to detect histamine in the blood. Coupled with a process that can separate out histamine from hundreds of other chemicals, Allan's detector would prove invaluable. Keith Simons, from the Faculty of Pharmacy, was an expert on measuring the levels of histamine and antihistamines in the blood. It sounded like an exciting approach. Frank and I were definitely out of their league when it came to platelets, but eager to help in any way we could.

---

37   Takehiko was to become a friend and colleague through my involvement with the European Histamine Research Society. At a 1990 meeting in Amsterdam, he told me that he had been one of the reviewers of the "Saxena" paper reporting on the role of intracellular histamine in platelet aggregation and had recommended it for publication in Science.

38   The fact that a chemical that promotes tumors to grow also makes platelets clump is not surprising. Blood clots are much more common in cancer patients than in the healthy population. I believe that the stimulation of histamine formation in both instances is unlikely to be a coincidence.

It took many months of often frustrating work by Satya, but he ultimately showed convincingly that PMA caused the platelets to produce a wave of new histamine, vital to their ability to aggregate. DPPE was stronger than the conventional H_1 and H_2 antihistamines to block this process. Most impressively, by using a detergent treatment to make their cell walls "leaky", excess histamine could be flooded into the platelets from the outside and overcome the effects of DPPE.

Then came the real clincher. Collagen, a natural substance that makes platelets clump in response to bleeding, also caused the platelets to make histamine. Once again, DPPE blocked the effect of collagen, while excess histamine overcame DPPE when the platelets were treated with detergent.

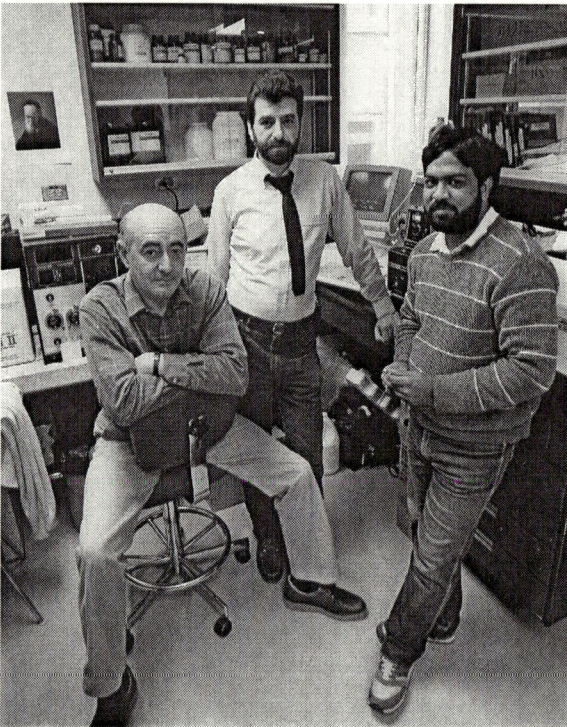

With Frank LaBella and Satya Saxena on the occasion of our Science paper
(CancerCare Manitoba Archive)

We concluded that histamine was acting as a "se
messenger"[39] inside the platelets by binding to an "unconvent
site" blocked most effectively by DPPE. This was a scientific "first",
and its publication in *Science* was cause for celebration among us
all. Take that, you nay-saying grant reviewers! I felt vindicated,
scientifically and personally. I could only hope that Dr. Kahlson
was loving it from "somewhere up above".

---

39 Many substances, including calcium, are known to be "second messen-
    gers" in cells. A second messenger is a chemical or substance that is
    formed in cells as a result of some preceding event, for example, estro-
    gen binding to its receptor. When the second messenger is formed, it
    helps the cell to respond to whatever has stimulated the receptor in the
    first place. This is a prime example of the elegant complexity of nature.

CHAPTER NINETEEN:

Speeding Up And Slowing Down

After returning from New Orleans, I immediately sent off some DPPE to Rob Warrington. I had new plans for histidinol as well. We had recently found a simple way of testing the effect of DPPE and other compounds on the growth of cells in the laboratory. When cells divide, they make a copy of their DNA blueprint and pass it on to their offspring. This process can be detected by adding a radiolabeled substance called thymidine, one of the four essential DNA building blocks, to the cell culture. As DNA is made, the labeled thymidine becomes incorporated into the structure of its "double helix". As a result, any new DNA becomes "hot" and its radioactivity can be measured.

In malignant cells, the uptake of radioactive thymidine by DNA is always very high because, unlike normal cells, they continuously divide without stopping; that is their nature and is what defines this disease. In contrast, normal cells do not usually divide in the test tube unless artificially stimulated to do so. If that occurs, their "cold" DNA then becomes "hot". As an example, normal immune cells (called lymphocytes), obtained from the spleens of mice, do not normally make new DNA unless they are stimulated to divide by exposure to a specific plant substance called a mitogen. When that happens, their DNA counts go way up for two or three days.

We had recently found that DPPE did something rather amazing (at least, to me) in this test. It prevented normal immune cells from dividing when they were exposed to the mitogen. As a result, no radioactivity went into their DNA. The cells had been put into a "resting state" by DPPE without injuring or killing them. In contrast, DPPE had the reverse effect on MCF-7 breast cancer cells: their already "hot" DNA became even hotter, suggesting that DPPE was *stimulating* them to divide even more than usual. Only when more DPPE was added did the radioactive DNA go down because, unlike the normal cells, higher amounts of DPPE killed the malignant cells rather than simply putting them to rest.

I believed these "test-tube" observations were accurate because they mimicked what we had observed in mice and rats, where DPPE made tumors grow bigger. However, even though higher DPPE doses killed cancer cells in the test tube, we had not observed that it could shrink tumors in the animals. "Perhaps it is not possible for DPPE to kill cells in the body except at toxic doses…remember those somersaulting mice…" I thought to myself. I then wondered whether the opposite effect of DPPE on DNA synthesis and cell division, depending on whether the cells were normal or malignant, might also explain Rob's findings with L-histidinol. That histamine-like compound made cancer cells more susceptible to chemotherapy but at the same time protected normal blood cells in the bone marrow.

As an oncologist, I had been taught that chemotherapy drugs kill dividing cancer cells by getting into the nucleus and damaging the DNA to such an extent that the cells actually commit suicide in a process called "apoptosis". As a general rule, rapidly-growing tumors tend to be more susceptible to chemotherapy than slower-growing tumors. Normal body cells that divide constantly to replenish themselves, such as the bone marrow, hair follicles and those lining the gastrointestinal tract (including the mouth) are also susceptible. That explains the most common toxic effects of chemotherapy, including low blood counts, hair loss, mouth sores and diarrhea. In tissues such as the brain, where cells do not normally divide, or divide infrequently, the effects of chemotherapy are usually much less pronounced.

A provocative theory quickly took form in my mind: to make cancer cells speed up and divide even more rapidly, but to slow down the division of normal cells, first administer a substance that binds to Dr. Kahlson's "unconventional" histamine receptor. Then administer chemotherapy. The result should be more killing of cancer cells and less toxic effects on normal cells. *That appeared to be exactly what we were observing with DPPE and histidinol: a new method to treat human cancer!*

I immediately gave Patricia and Balram Sukhu, a very welcome addition to our lab, their marching orders. They were to test histidinol in the "growth test" using the same cells we had employed with DPPE. In addition, using a fancy new detector we had recently purchased with a grant from the Winnipeg Foundation, Balram was to determine whether the cancer cells and the stimulated immune cells produced histamine as they grew. We knew from Satya's experiments that platelets formed new histamine when they were stimulated to clump; what about dividing cells?

After several weeks and repeated experiments we had our answers. L-histidinol showed the same effect as DPPE: it shut down DNA production in normal immune cells without harming them, while it stimulated already high DNA levels in the cancer cells until, at higher concentrations, it killed them. To achieve this result required about one thousand times more L-histidinol than DPPE. It fit with the doses Rob had to use in his mice, and with our studies showing L-histidinol to be one thousand times weaker than DPPE to interfere with the binding of radioactive histamine in the microsomes.

Balram's results were just as remarkable in their implication. As Dr. Kahlson originally observed, large amounts of new histamine were being formed and "kicked out" into the culture medium by both the cancer cells and stimulated normal immune cells! In my mind, this bolstered the possibility of a link between histamine production by dividing cells and the effects of DPPE and L-histidinol on growth. While this theory was very possibly correct, for further verification Rob would need to test DPPE.

I did not have long to wait. A few weeks later he called me. Although further experiments were required, the preliminary verdict in his mice was that, just like L-histidinol, DPPE increased the ability of two different chemotherapy drugs to kill a deadly tumor called melanoma. It also protected normal blood cells in the bone marrow from daunorubicin, a chemotherapy drug related to doxorubicin.

After the potential enormity of our combined results sank in, I asked Rob whether he had patented any aspect of his work. For example, did he have a use patent for L-histidinol? Regretfully, he never had a Janet Scholz to advise him. By the time a patent application was considered, he had already "spilled the beans" with his first publication. Interested drug companies had excitedly approached him at meetings where he presented his work, but their enthusiasm quickly evaporated when apprised that there was no patent protection.

I told Rob that I intended to take our findings into patients, a prospect that thrilled him as much as it did me. He was a PhD, totally dependent on medical colleagues for any clinical applications of his research. As an MD and practicing oncologist, I had the definite advantage. But before we could publish or move forward in patients, I needed to file a new DPPE use patent. Based on our joint discovery, I felt that he should be offered co-inventorship. His reply surprised me: DPPE was my discovery, just as L-histidinol was his. Rob was delighted to collaborate on these experiments but firmly declined to be included in a new patent. Rarely had I encountered such a selfless individual. In science, as in other of life's endeavors, new knowledge is often really not that new. Rather, incremental increases in our understanding are made on the shoulders of those who have come before us. Rob had very broad shoulders indeed.

I reported to Janet and Marion on the remarkable new findings, as well as my discussion with Rob Warrington, and requested that we now embark on that new use patent to protect DPPE. It would be based on the *Method of cancer treatment* theory that I had formulated. We now had a Toronto-based patent agent, Michael Stewart, with whom I could write a new application. If we were to have any chance of capitalizing on this discovery, we had to do it. However, as before, Marion hesitated when the subject of a new patent came up. "Just give me a bit more time, m'dear," she said. What choice did I have? "Please don't wait too long, Marion," I pleaded.

As I later learned, Marion did not procrastinate. She soon talked with Terry Falconer, the University comptroller. The cost would be high because of the need to file a completely new world-wide patent. "Can the University afford this?" Marion asked him. According to Janet, Mr. Falconer simply replied, "You said earlier that we have to start somewhere, Marion. It might as well be with this." Once again, the decision had been made without a lot of fuss. Bless those two University of Manitoba bureaucrats!

CHAPTER TWENTY:

Bernie and Eli

In the early summer of 1989, Arnold Greenberg, who had recently been appointed director of the Institute of Cell Biology, informed me that a representative of pharmaceutical giant, Eli Lilly, was touring various Canadian universities and would be stopping in Winnipeg. The company was looking for new innovations that might be commercially attractive and Arnold thought DPPE would be "a natural". Did I want to meet with this person? His question gave me pause to reflect.

In November, 1988, we had finally heard back from Julius Vida. Out of the blue, a fax suddenly arrived at Morris Silver's office. Morris immediately reached me in my lab and suggested that I come over to read it for myself. The letter was short and to the point. Julius regretted that DPPE was of no interest to the cancer research people at Bristol-Myers, not least of all because of its "lack of patent protection." *What???* He wished us continuing luck in our "efforts... to commercialize DPPE. With best regards....".

After all this time! Although I liked him, I was quite perturbed at the brush-off and decided to try to reach Julius at his

office. After two years MIA he was there. "Do you have a copy of
the letter you just faxed me?" I asked testily. "Yez, ov courze," he
replied. "Well put it in a file named 'Missed Opportunity,'" I told a
startled Dr. Vida.

I had now struck out twice. Would it be third time lucky?
"Okay," I finally replied to Arnold's question. A smile came over
his face. He knew what I had been through with drug companies
and granting agencies. He had an idea. He would like to present
the story to the representative himself. Coming from the head of
Cell Biology, it might carry more weight. I would be there with
him to field more detailed questions. I thought it was a good suggestion, made genuinely out of caring, and I agreed.

A few days later we sat down in a small medical school conference room with Dr. Bernard Abbott. After signing the obligatory
confidentiality agreement that had been prepared in advance,
Arnold told him about my research, the findings with DPPE and
its patent protection. Dr. Abbott's eyes widened appreciably. "Dr.
Brandes, if what Dr. Greenberg tells me is accurate, Eli Lilly would
definitely be interested in DPPE," he announced enthusiastically.
I told him he had heard right. Happy with Dr. Abbott's response,
Arnold took his leave and left me alone for further discussion.

"Call me Bernie," he suggested. "Okay, Bernie. Call me Lorne,"
I offered in kind. Bernie Abbott was an affable guy. He was about
my age, had a PhD, flew his own plane and had a research background before joining Eli Lilly at its head office in Indianapolis.
The official title on his business card was "Manager, Technology
Acquisition". Bernie told me that the university tour was his idea
and the company went along with it. Historically, drug development at Lilly had been strictly "in-house". But times were changing and pharmaceutical companies had come to realize that there
were many potential opportunities beyond their walls. This was
the same kind of thinking that led universities, such as Manitoba,
to protect intellectual property through the establishment of an
"Office of Technology Transfer", staffed by qualified people such
as Janet and Morris.

Bernie had several more people to interview that afternoon but his flight was not leaving until just before noon the next day. He was staying overnight at the Crowne Plaza and suggested we meet over breakfast for further discussion. "Sure," I replied. At 8:30 the following morning, I arrived to find Bernie waiting for me in the hotel restaurant. As we drank our coffee, he told me that he was very excited about what he had heard the day before. DPPE would be at the top of the list when he got back.

I had recently prepared a hefty summary of our work and offered to send it to him under the confidentiality agreement. "Would it be of value to you?" I asked rhetorically. "You bet it would." Bernie replied. He wanted this project to work and told me he would take personal responsibility for guiding DPPE through the company bureaucracy. Shaking hands with me as I got up to leave, he promised to be in touch very soon. Back at the lab, I put a copy of the summary, along with several reprints of our published papers, in a FedEx overnight envelope.

Bernie called me from his office the next day to say he had received the package and was distributing copies of the material to appropriate individuals within the company. He would get back to me as soon as he had feedback. He gave me his direct phone number. "Call me anytime if you have questions," he implored earnestly. Within a week my phone rang again. It was Bernie to tell me that there was "genuine interest" among his colleagues. He wanted to come back to Winnipeg to learn more about our whole group and the histamine project. Frank, Jon Gerrard, Gary Glavin, and Frixos Paraskevas, an immunologist with whom I had recently collaborated on the DNA studies in immune cells, were delighted with this news and eager to participate in the Bernie Abbott "road show".

When he returned to the city a short time later, we sequestered ourselves in a conference room and gave him a three-hour seminar. When it came time for Frank to talk, he announced that he would present his theory that the AEBS and histamine sites might be on P450 enzymes. Before he started, I suggested to

Bernie that what he was about to hear was very interesting but somewhat speculative. As soon as I said those words, I knew from the glint in Frank's eyes that I had overstepped the boundary and insulted him. Always the gentleman, Frank did not otherwise react and proceeded to give his talk, speculative or not.

After the seminar, I met with Bernie privately in my office to get his feedback. He was generally very impressed with everything he had heard. Above and beyond a licensing agreement for the "technology" (which I took to mean DPPE), he wanted to explore funding for the whole group with his company. All, that is, except for the "P450 stuff LaBella presented". Lilly would never fund that.[40] As we drove to the airport, Bernie once again reiterated that he was going to be our advocate within his company. He would get back to me shortly.

True to his word, he called within the week. It was time to arrange for me to visit Eli Lilly and meet directly with various senior people. I was excited by the pace of events. Bernie was definitely keeping the promise he had made to me over that fateful breakfast. "Third time lucky," I repeated over and over to myself. Of course I would be delighted to go, I told my advocate.

A few weeks later, on a cold, overcast, blustery, early October day, I stepped off the plane in Indianapolis. Bernie was there to meet me. It was mid-afternoon and my meetings were not scheduled to begin until the following morning. He suggested we drive to his house to relax, and talk over drinks and dinner. That was fine with me.

Bernie's gracious home was several miles out in the suburbs. Motoring down a rural road, we passed through the "small-town America" that dotted the Indiana countryside. I was especially taken by the number of churches we passed. There seemed to be not one, not two, but sometimes three at every intersection (the

---

40   To this day, Frank has never let me forget my gauche remark. Nor should he. On the P450 issue, I turned out to be dead wrong. Bernie Abbott lacked as much insight as I did. There will be more to tell about this later.

fourth spot seemed to be saved for gas stations or convenience stores). Everywhere there were road signs preaching salvation or warning of damnation. There was no doubt that we were in the "bible belt".

As we continued along, it started to snow. "Don't ever make fun of Winnipeg after this," I told Bernie. Even there we don't (usually) see snow in early October.

"We arranged this just for you so you wouldn't be homesick," he retorted. Dropping me off at the hotel after a pleasant evening, he instructed me to be in the lobby the next morning at nine. Before going to bed, I tried to dry the very wet soles of my shoes with the hair blower provided in my room. Of one thing I was sure: talk of the weather would make a good icebreaker with every person I met during my visit.

I had insomnia that night as I wondered what the next day would have in store for me. As my mind continued to race, I remembered with a smile the adventure Lyonel and I had during our visit to Burroughs Wellcome, and the calming influence he had on me during my talk. Too bad he had not accompanied me this time. Bernie would have to be his substitute. I restlessly paced the floor and went over and over what I would say at my presentation. Finally, exhausted, I laid down and drifted off to sleep.

The morning came all too quickly. Looking out the window, I saw to my amazement that the snow had continued all night. Several inches now covered the ground. This really *would* be a visit to remember. As promised, Bernie arrived promptly at nine. Sliding downtown in his car, we parked in front of several old, drab, buildings that housed various administrative offices and laboratories of Eli Lilly.

Entering a very large room at the top of a flight of stairs, we came upon scores of people milling about or sitting in small square cubicles fashioned out of six-foot-high fabric wall dividers. In contrast, along the left side of the room were expensively-furnished offices, their paneled walls adorned with various prints and oils. "Which one belongs to Bernie?" I wondered as we kept passing doors.

But Bernie continued right past all of them, crossing to the other side of the room and entering one of the homogenized cubicles that had his name embossed on a small plaque on the outside. It was now obvious that he was not as senior as I had thought! At least he was by an outside window. After slinging our outerware over a coat tree beside his desk, Bernie made a quick phone call. "That was Pat Roffey, one of our senior vice-presidents. I want to introduce you," he said, taking me back across the room to a large sumptuous corner office.

Although in the middle of a conversation with two other people, Dr. Roffey welcomed us with a smile and bade us come in. His message was short and to the point. "We at Eli Lilly are only interested in the cutting edge of research and I am told that you are very much on that cutting edge," he said. I thanked him for the compliment. He nodded. That was it. We left his office and went to a very large conference hall. End-to-end meeting tables stretched around its circumference. There was a small microphone in front of every chair.

The room quickly filled with a large number of people. And guess what? Most had pen and notebook in hand. Although it seemed to go well, my presentation, and the questions that followed, were largely a blur. I stressed my vision of DPPE as a potentiator of chemotherapy and protector of normal cells in patients with cancer. Afterward, I was introduced to various key players, including Homer Pearce and Jake Starling from the oncology division, and David Henry, who had a special interest in histamine and histamine metabolism.

The morning session over, Bernie and the others took me "upstairs" for lunch in the company dining room. It had its own chefs and service staff. The food was definitely first-rate. While we were eating this gastronomy, I spied two men seated at their own table, deep in conversation as they sipped generously-sized martinis. A waiter hovered nearby at the ready. The duo were well-dressed in expensive blue suits, striped shirts with French cuffs, silk ties and gold jewelry. They must have gone to the same tailor. One had a very florid face and, given his obesity, seemed to my clinical eye to be a likely stroke candidate. In total contrast, the other man was thin and quite pale. Compared to his table companion, he looked merely unwell. Nudging Bernie, I asked, "Who are those two guys?"

"Senior management," he whispered.

"Wow," I said, "not very good PR for an organization that is supposed to be promoting health." Bernie smiled but said nothing. A true company man was he.

After lunch, I visited the laboratories of other senior Lilly scientists. Potential collaborations were established as we discussed various aspects of the research published by me and my colleagues. Time flew by as I met person after person. Before I knew it, the end of the afternoon was fast approaching. At four, we were all supposed to meet at a local pub-type restaurant. I sure could use a cold beer. However, there was one final visit on my schedule. I was to meet with Dr. Stan Marshall, a senior Lilly scientist and VP. As Bernie explained it, Stan was a company icon, with a long and successful career in drug development behind him. After dropping me off at Dr. Marshall's office and making the introductions, Bernie left the two of us alone to talk.

Appearing to be in his late sixties, Stan Marshall was a physically-imposing figure. After putting me at ease with some small talk, he requested that I tell him more about my work. Only a sketchy outline had been provided to him. As I went on passionately about the studies on histamine and growth, and my hope that DPPE might make a difference in cancer therapy, he became very attentive. When I finished, something in his eyes told me I had scored points. After a moment or two of silence to digest my words he said, simply, "Dr. Brandes, I think we should help you find out whether or not you are right."

C H A P T E R   T W E N T Y - O N E :

Not Useful For Anything

Back home once again, Dr. Marshall's words kept running through my mind. I had been shown a very warm reception in Indianapolis and, over several rounds of beer and tacos at the end of my visit, was left with the distinct impression by Homer Pearce and others that there was great enthusiasm for the possibility that there might be a previously-undiscovered histamine pathway in cells that could be targeted by new drugs. And didn't Dr. Roffey say that our research was on the cutting edge? I optimistically reported to my colleagues that I believed we had an extremely good chance of getting research monies for all of us. Morale ran high, especially after Bernie called to tell me that he and a team from Lilly wanted to set up a visit to Winnipeg. I was to present a program summary. After that, they wanted to talk turkey.

"Those guys wouldn't do that unless they were serious," Frank remarked on hearing this news. He was still steamed about Bernie's statement that Lilly would not be interested in funding research on a potential link among P450 enzymes, the AEBS, and histamine binding. Yet, in his usual magnanimous way, he was genuinely pleased that a large drug company was on the brink of licensing DPPE and funding our team of investigators. "Any plan absolutely would have to include you," I told my partner. We both knew only too well that we desperately needed money to continue our collaboration.

Three weeks later, a team headed by Patrick Roffey arrived by corporate jet just before noon. Stan Marshall, Homer Pearce, Bernie Abbott and eight other company people sat around the long table in the Dean's conference room. Sitting along the back wall to provide me with moral support were Morris, Janet and Ed Kroeger, who had recently been appointed an associate dean. I had personally called to ask that he be present at my talk. He was thrilled about this development. Nothing would keep him away.

For an hour, under the watchful gaze of former deans of medicine whose portraits hung on the mahogany walls, I summarized the history of my research and the collaborations that had led to our many recent publications, including the paper in *Science*. Making eye contact with Dr. Marshall, I stressed the similarities that Rob Warrington and I had found between DPPE and L-histidinol and my belief that, based on these preclinical findings, DPPE had exciting potential in cancer therapy. I finished by asking for financial support for our entire group so that we could continue our work together. It was grueling. I was centre-stage, knowing that a business decision would be influenced by my performance and the things I said.

At the end of the presentation, there were the ubiquitous questions and much discussion. When we finally broke for coffee after ninety minutes, Morris and Janet gave me the "thumbs-up" sign. Ed, however, took me aside to tell me that during my introductory remarks I had been a little too self-deprecatory (that must have been a first!) when discussing my accomplishments; it was because of me that this meeting was taking place at all. I thanked him for his caring support and promised henceforth to be less humble. "Not too much less," he quickly countered.

Patrick Roffey then called the meeting back to order. After thanking me for illuminating everyone with my talk, he came directly to the point. "Eli Lilly's primary interest here is the science behind the 'intracellular histamine receptor'. That is what brought us all the way to Winnipeg today," he stated.

"It's a good thing Frank is three floors above, out of earshot," I thought to myself on hearing the word "receptor".

He continued, "Any funding will be directed specifically to your own studies."

"What about my colleagues?" I asked.

"We would have to think about that," he replied. That was not at all what I had expected to hear.

"What about a licensing agreement specifically for DPPE?" I asked.

"DPPE would be included as part of any deal." There seemed to be a certain non-committal blandness to his answer, so I pushed him a bit further.

"What about the specific application to cancer?"

"If it is warranted by our own studies. But first there would be a program to determine how best to come up with more active or selective agents."

Now the alarm bells were going off in my head. I looked across the room for support from my side. Only Morris and Janet remained, as Ed had another meeting and left at the coffee break. Both seemed to be on the edge of their seats.

"But my vision is to take DPPE into the treatment of humans with cancer as soon as possible," I pushed on.

And then came the statement that I will never forget as long as I live. "Dr Brandes," said Patrick Roffey, pulling himself up to his full level of seniority, "we at Eli Lilly have concluded that DPPE will not be useful for the treatment of anything."

"Including the treatment of cancer?" I asked incredulously.

"Including the treatment of cancer," he cooly replied, staring me straight in the eyes as he carefully repeated my words.

Quickly scanning the room, I first looked over at Stan Marshall. His jaw was clenched as he gazed straight ahead and not at me. Bernie appeared distinctly uncomfortable, his upper lip sweating. Homer looked down at the table. Morris's eyes were bulging, while Janet's face was flushed. Heaven only knows how terrible I must have looked at that moment!

I immediately understood Roffey's subtext. It was this:

"Dr Brandes, we are Eli Lilly. We know much more than you and are infinitely wiser as to any future potential of your discovery. You may think that DPPE is the greatest thing since sliced bread but we will discover new and better analogs. You only have use patents on DPPE, whereas we will obtain composition patents on our molecules. We will buy you off for a small amount of funding, which we know you badly need, and will control you through legally-binding agreements. You will publish only after we approve any manuscript you write. For all these things, you and the University of Manitoba should be eternally thankful. After all, it is not every day that a company of our stature spends all this time and money, risking the wrath of our shareholders to license your unproven technology."

The silence that followed was soon broken by Stan Marshall. "It's getting late and we have a long flight home," he announced as he looked at his watch. That was the cue. Everyone started packing their briefcases. Patrick Roffey thanked us for our hospitality and allowed that, following "internal discussions", we would be contacted by Bernie. Taxis were summoned. Less-than-robust goodbyes were said. After the last of our visitors was out the door, Janet looked at me and said, simply, "Well, at least we're still standing." I nodded soberly. As she turned to go into her office, I saw that the back of her sweater was moist and wrinkled; it was clear that she and Morris had sweated buckets for me.

As promised, Bernie soon wrote back with an official offer: two years of funding for me, amounting to about two hundred and thirty-five thousand dollars, and a ten thousand dollar consulting honorarium for each of my colleagues to "share their expertise" with the company. There would be no up-front payment for licensing DPPE and no commitment to its development. Breaking the bad news to Frank and the others was difficult, but necessary. There was anger and incredulity all around. All I could do was tell my colleagues how sorry I was and that I shared their feelings.

Janet Scholz told me that any "yes" or "no" would be my call. It did not take me long to come to a decision. I contacted Bernie to personally thank him for his effort on my behalf, but to tell him that we were not interested. He was flabbergasted. "I'm sorry, but it's an offer I just can't accept," I told him without lengthy elaboration.[41]

In the end, it was an easy choice. I really needed that funding, but I was not going to sell my soul or ruin my relationships with wonderful collaborators to obtain it. I also believed in the clinical potential of DPPE and was not going to allow an arrogant drug company to sidetrack my plan to test it in patients.

---

41   During the writing of this book, I sent Bernie Abbott, now retired, the "Eli Lilly chapters" for his review and comments: "...The events you recounted are similar, although not identical, to my recollections....Best of luck with your project. I have added 'tesmilifene' [DPPE] to my alerting service and hope to keep up with its development," he replied.

CHAPTER TWENTY-TWO:
Send In The Clones

It was now early 1990 and my grant money would run out in a few short months. Frank was also having to watch his budget. Even at the time our hopes were running high for a licensing agreement and funding from Eli Lilly, I had suggested to my colleagues that we hedge our bet by applying to the Medical Research Council. The MRC had a policy of considering new group applications for innovative projects. The timing appeared right as we had just been published in *Science* and written an invited review of our collective work on intracellular histamine for another prestigious journal, *Biochemical Pharmacology*. I had also just been invited to give a talk at an international symposium on histamine research that was being held outside Amsterdam that spring. Frank, Jon, Gary and Frixos were all in agreement to proceed with "Plan B".

We were first required to submit an abstract of our proposal which, if deemed worthy by a screening panel, would result in permission to formally submit a grant application. The first hurdle was passed. Many weeks were then spent writing our grant, entitled, *A multidisciplinary study of histamine as an intracellular second messenger.* Eight hundred thousand dollars in funding was requested. The MRC site visit was set for Friday, March 2, in the Cancer Foundation boardroom.

Despite my unhappy encounter there with the NCIC three years earlier, I was not superstitious. As it turned out, I should have been. With the exception of Jon's proposed studies in platelets, it would be an understatement to say that the rest of us received a tepid response from the four site visitors. In their critique of our proposed experiments, the words "superficial" and "uninformative" were used time and again. Once again, our biggest sin was not proposing to "clone the receptor" for histamine.

Gary received an especially rough ride from one of the reviewers, who vigorously took him to task for being unaware of one small piece of binding data that Frank and I had generated in our part of the application. In the written summary of the visit, the suggestion was made that this failure of communication "…indicates that such interactions apparently do not exist to any significant degree amongst these individuals and the rationale that this work should be carried out under the format of a Program Grant should be seriously questioned."

After reading this polemic, we all wondered whether someone came with their own agenda. The whole tenor of the review was hostile and seemed off-base. Unfortunately no appeal was possible. We were left with the perplexing question of how our work was good enough to be published in top journals, but not good enough to fund. There is an old saying that "Money talks." It certainly was not talking to us. So much for Plan B.

Just as things once again looked grim for the survival of my lab program, a benefactor named Margaret "Peggy" Sellers saved the day. Her late husband, George, a wealthy grain baron, had developed advanced throat cancer several years earlier. I, and a close friend, Dr. Wayne Beecroft, had taken care of him. Wayne was a fabulous surgeon but, unfortunately, there was little he could do. Mr. Sellers succumbed a short time after I gave him a futile course of chemotherapy. Nonetheless, Peg and her family were very grateful for the TLC he had received and decided to direct a portion of the family fortune towards philanthropic causes at the medical school.

After first establishing the G. H. Sellers Chair in Medicine, Peg wanted to endow a Sellers Foundation that would fund cancer research and help support worthy programs at the Institute of Cell Biology. She was greatly enamored of Lyonel, whom she once described to me as a "real hunk". Aside from Lyonel's wife, Esther, Peg was probably not the first woman to feel that way about the handsome, athletic and charming Lyonel Israels. He helped her establish her wish to the tune of over one million dollars. Along with four of her trusted advisors, Peg asked Lyonel, Wayne and me to sit on the Sellers board to oversee the awarding of yearly grants. We met every six months over lunch in my favorite Cancer Foundation boardroom.

Shortly after the fatal MRC site visit, I explained my dire funding predicament to my fellow board members and asked whether there would be a conflict of interest if I applied to the Sellers Foundation for help. I would use the money specifically for research on DPPE, with the aim of taking it into human clinical trials. Peg immediately asked Lyonel for his opinion. He backed me to the hilt, saying that if ever there was a worthy project, it was this. My fellow board members agreed. Chairman, Lorne Campbell, Peg's crusty downtown lawyer, called for a vote. I recused myself. The "ayes" had it. I was invited to apply. A notification arrived a month later telling me that I was successful. Safe for another year.

CHAPTER TWENTY-THREE:

Someone In The Department

Sometimes good news begets good news. Rob Warrington called a few days later to report that DPPE protected the bone marrow from the toxic effects of a second chemotherapy drug, 5-fluorouracil. I had equally good news for him. We had again achieved "cures" as a result of combining DPPE with doxorubicin in mice with sarcoma tumors. We also observed what is called a "dose-response", meaning that the number of cures increased as we upped the dose of DPPE. The best result was seen at the fifty milligrams per kilogram dose, near the top of the "safe range" for the drug. Rob had likewise observed a dose-response for DPPE to cure mice with melanoma.

The fact that two different laboratories had found the same thing was a very powerful argument in favor of a true effect. There was now enough good evidence to write up our results for publication. However, before we could proceed, I needed to be sure that we had our new use patent filed. This would take some time. After his experience with L-histidinol, Rob understood only too well and told me to take as long as was needed.

I soon had the opportunity to meet with our patent agent, Michael Stewart. Janet Scholz had invited him to Winnipeg to meet various investigators who might have patentable innovations. She put me at the top of the list. During our discussion about my proposed "method of treatment" patent, I explained that so far we had only treated mice, but I was planning human studies. Michael believed we would have a much stronger chance of success with the patent office if we had human data, no matter how preliminary. It was now April, 1990. I decided it was time to call the Bureau of Prescription Drugs at the Health Protection Branch in Ottawa.[42]

There is a common stereotype we all too often conjure up when thinking of government bureaucrats: all cut from the same mold; no interest or imagination; do everything strictly by the book; go home exactly at quitting time. That was the image in my mind as I called the number that had been provided by the operator. Several rings later I was connected to the main switchboard. With whom did I wish to speak? "I don't have a specific name," I replied. To which area did I wish to be connected? "Prescription Drugs," I answered.

"One moment, please."

"Bonjour," said a pleasant voice en français. I gave the woman my name and asked to speak to "someone in the department" about developing a new oncology drug. Immediately switching to English, she asked me to please wait and she would try to get someone to help me. After being placed on hold for a good five minutes, I was about to give up. Just in time, a new voice came on the line. "This is Agnes Klein. Can I help you?"

As it turned out, Dr. Agnes Klein was not just "someone in the department", but head of the combined Gastroenterology/Hematology/Oncology Division. She listened patiently as I told

---

42 The Canadian drug regulatory agency is equivalent to the FDA. In those days it was called the Bureau of Human Prescription Drugs, The Health Protection Branch, Health and Welfare Canada. Today it is known as the Therapeutic Products Division, Health Canada.

her about the promising results with DPPE in mice and my hope that we could get permission to test it, in combination with chemotherapy, in humans. I offered to send her the extensive summary that I had previously couriered to Bernie Abbott. Dr. Klein's answer was at once as hopeful as it was unexpected. It might well be possible to do this. *What? Did I hear right??* Please send her the information. She would give it her full attention. Please be patient. She would call back in two or three weeks at the latest. *Wow.* The only thing stereotypical here had been my thinking.

True to her word, Agnes Klein called me three weeks later. "What I have read is very interesting and potentially exciting. I want to help you," she said. "However, first there are some tests that you must carry out." She gave me a short list of toxicology studies. The highest dose of DPPE that had no side effects was to be injected into groups of mice, some daily for a week and others weekly for a month. We were then to kill the mice and perform autopsies by removing the organs and examining them under the microscope for possible toxic effects of DPPE on the tissues. There must be control groups treated with saline instead of DPPE. Since I was proposing to give the drug by vein in humans, we would also have to find the highest safe intravenous dose in rats. I was to get back to her once I had the results. Invigorated by a sense of optimism that we were in striking distance of human patients, Patty, Balram and I spent the next two months carrying out the required rodent studies.

To provide an expert report on the various tissues, I enlisted the help of my favorite retired pathologist, Dr. Georgina ("Georgie") Hogg. Georgie was a crackerjack with a microscope. A diminutive woman, weighing no more than ninety pounds, she was a giant, both among her colleagues in the pathology department and among clinicians who counted on her advice to make a diagnosis in their patients. If ever there was a difficult biopsy to be interpreted, Georgie was everyone's first choice. When she finally retired in her seventies, the loss to the medical community was palpable. Even after she left, I remained in close touch and called or visited her as often as I could. She remained very interested in my research, so that after the requisite "hospital gossip" we would talk about the latest lab developments over a pot of tea in her small living room.

Georgie had recently broken her hip and was largely confined to her apartment in the Osborne Village area. I called to say I needed a favor. Could I come over? We made a date for the coming Saturday. Over tea, I told her of my contact with Dr. Klein and broached the subject of the mouse autopsies. To my delight, but not necessarily surprise, Georgie said she would take on the project if I could get her a microscope.

I contacted Dr. Colin Merry, head of the hospital hematology lab and longtime friend to Georgie and me. Within a week, Colin had located a good microscope, personally brought it to her apartment and set it up on the dining room table. The pathology lab was not funded for medical services to rodents but, out of deference to Georgie, agreed to cut up the organs and stain the necessary tissue slides for her to examine. I doubted that toxicology studies on any new drug had ever been carried out in quite this manner and setting, but who cared? We were in business.

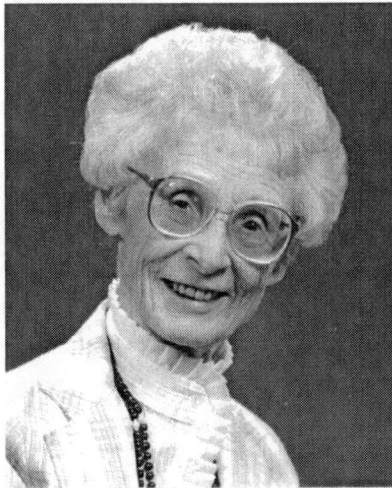

Dr. Georgina (Georgie) Hogg (Dept. of Pathology Archive)

Georgie suffered from a chronic eye inflammation and looking down a microscope was hard on her peepers. She had to stop frequently due to the burning and put a Kleenex to her eyes. Although this slowed her down, I could not help but admire her remarkable resiliency. During her long career she had overcome many health obstacles, including tuberculosis and breast cancer, rarely missing a day of work when her health permitted. This was but one more example of her grit and determination, proof that women are definitely the stronger sex.

She finished her work within two weeks and called me to come to her apartment to discuss the findings. Georgie had found little effect of DPPE on the tissues except for one potentially-concerning finding. The lung tissue from some of the mice showed quite a lot of inflammation around small blood vessels. Wisely, she had gone back over the same lung tissue in the control mice who received only saline. Some of them also had this blood vessel finding, but the inflammation was noticeably less than in the DPPE-treated mice. It appeared to Georgie that this strain of mice was naturally susceptible to low-grade blood vessel inflammation in the lungs and that DPPE may have made it worse.

I immediately remembered Gary Glavin's ulcer experiments that had suggested DPPE was affecting the prostaglandins; some are protective to cells, while others cause injury and inflammation. Perhaps DPPE was increasing both "good and bad" prostaglandins. I called Agnes. She recommended that we repeat the DPPE and saline injections in a different strain of mice. If no problem was encountered, she would be satisfied.

A few weeks later, I sat nervously on Georgie's sofa as she scanned the new slides of lung tissue. "I don't see anything abnormal in either group," she reported. We both let out a sigh of relief. It was now likely that DPPE did not have any intrinsic effect on normal lung tissue or blood vessels, a toxic profile that could result in its rejection by regulatory agencies that have to approve drugs as safe, in addition to effective, for human use. However, while DPPE itself did not cause inflammation, it appeared to make existing inflammation worse. I realized that this could be a potentially important issue in selecting patients for treatment. For example, DPPE might make rheumatoid arthritis worse.

The great thing about scientific research is that observations raise questions that require more testing to get answers that in turn raise more questions....and the cycle continues. As a result of the lung findings, I had an idea for an experiment to look more specifically at the effect of DPPE on inflammation. I would need Georgie's help just a little bit longer. That was fine with her. She was enjoying this facet of her "retirement".

We would once again use "PMA", the chemical that activates histamine formation, and makes platelets clump and tumors grow. PMA is a constituent of croton oil. It has been known for decades that when croton oil is painted on an area of shaved skin in rats, it acts as an irritant and produces inflammation and cell division. If painted on the skin chronically, PMA itself can cause malignant tumors. Inflammation is an important factor in the evolution of cancer. As proof, the cancer-promoting effects of PMA in the skin can be blocked by cortisone and anti-inflammatory drugs.

What would DPPE do in this situation? In platelets, Jon and Satya had found that it blocked the clumping caused by PMA. Based on this finding, one scenario was that DPPE might block the skin inflammation. On he other hand, based on the first set of lung slides, DPPE might make the PMA-induced inflammation worse. We would soon find out.

Luckily, Georgie was an expert in skin pathology. Over the years she had often been exasperated when trying to make a diagnosis on poorly-prepared skin biopsy slides. She developed a simple protocol to remedy this problem. After removal, the specimen of skin must immediately be smoothed out, tacked down at the corners with pins on a small piece of heavy paper and put into formaldehyde preservative. This would keep the specimen flat and allow the pathology lab to make optimal tissue slides for her to examine under the microscope. I would need the services of a surgeon to give Georgie exactly what she wanted. Wayne Beecroft would be perfect. He always loved to help out his old pal.

Balram prepared the rats by shaving the skin and painting it with PMA dissolved in acetone. One group of PMA-painted rats then received three daily injections of DPPE into the belly, while a second group received three daily injections of saline. A control group had only acetone applied to the skin, followed by three days of DPPE. Even before the biopsies, it was evident to Balram and me that the skin of the PMA-painted rats that received DPPE showed the most redness and swelling, whereas there was no obvious effect of the drug in the control rats that had been painted only with the acetone.

As planned, Wayne came by on the fourth day to operate on his "patients". He carefully cut out the treated area of shaved skin, smoothed it and then tacked the specimen to the paper according to Georgie's recipe. He had always wanted to do research himself but his clinical practice was just far too busy. Enjoying the opportunity to help out in our rat experiments, he smiled and joked as he performed the biopsies, just as he always did with his patients. They universally trusted and adored him. He was so facile when operating on the rats that I suggested he was wasting his talents on people. All these years later, I can still hear him laugh at that comment. Wayne was definitely a people person.

A few days later, Georgie confirmed our clinical suspicions. Under the microscope, the degree of inflammation and cell division caused by PMA in the skin of DPPE-treated rats was quite extreme as compared to skin from control rats that were painted with PMA and injected with saline. DPPE did not cause any skin inflammation in the rats who were painted only with the acetone. The implication was that, by increasing inflammation and cell division, DPPE might make PMA an even stronger tumor promoter. To my mind, this confirmed, in a different way, the stimulation of tumor growth in mice by DPPE. More than ever I believed it should help chemotherapy drugs kill cancer cells. The old saying, "Fight fire with fire", definitely applied here.

Next, I asked Carl Pinsky and Ranjan Bose to formally assess the neurological toxicity that I had described to them in mice that received high doses of DPPE. The information would be important for Dr. Klein. A few days after providing Ranjan with some mice and DPPE, he confidently told me that the seizure pattern was typical of the petit mal type. He could prevent the seizures by administering a dose of diazepam (Valium) a few minutes before giving the DPPE. Moreover, giving the diazepam to seizuring mice after they had received a high dose of DPPE was still effective to rapidly end the attack. This was good news because, if required, we could use this type of pre-treatment in patients receiving DPPE.

Taking Ranjan's finding one step further, I wanted to see whether seizures could be prevented or modified without the need for diazepam by giving the DPPE over a longer time, rather than rapidly into the belly. Why? When given slowly, the drug might not reach a high enough level in the brain to cause seizures. That is exactly what we found. One hundred milligrams per kilogram of DPPE, given over a few seconds, caused the mice to seizure within minutes. However, when the same amount of DPPE was divided into four equal doses of twenty-five milligrams per kilogram, and injected every fifteen minutes over one hour, there were no side effects whatever. This finding was of great importance. I now had reason to believe that intravenous treatment over sixty to ninety minutes might be the safest way to administer our drug to patients.

I prepared an official report of our toxicology findings, complete with documents signed by Georgie Hogg and copies of our lab sheets, and sent them to Dr. Klein. She called back within two weeks to tell me she was satisfied. Only five months had elapsed since I had first approached her. However, we still had three hurdles to pass before a "No objection" letter could be issued.[43]

---

43 By Federal regulation, the Health Protection Branch has sixty days to officially object to a formal application. If there is no objection to proceed, the applicant is advised of this in a letter.

First, who would supply the DPPE? There was very little choice here. With no drug company to sponsor me, I would have to make it myself. I explained to Agnes that the process was actually quite simple using purchased chemicals. With Asher Begleiter's help, I could make some simple procedural modifications that would increase the output of DPPE. A modern externally-vented fume hood in my laboratory would be scrubbed clean and dedicated to production of the drug. I would follow "good manufacturing practice" to the best of my ability. We had an excellent analytic facility at the main University campus that would easily be able to check the batches of DPPE for purity. That all sounded acceptable to Dr. Klein, but I would still have to satisfy the experts on drug standards at the Health Protection Branch when I formally presented my data to officials in Ottawa (Gulp!).

Second, I required an official treatment protocol that must garner approval both by the Human Ethics Committee at the University and by her department. Dr. John Maclean, the ethics chairman, and I would work closely on getting the institutional okay, while she and her colleague, Dr. Ivo Hynie (pronounced "Heen-y-a"), would do the same at their end. Ivo, the agency's clinical trials assessment officer, had a lot of experience in such matters and would advise me on the DPPE dosages to use in my studies.

Third, I would have to work with the hospital pharmacy to devise a plan for labeling and dispensing DPPE. Since it was a powder that required dissolving, a special filtration process would have to be employed to remove any bacteria. Initial samples would have to be tested by the hospital microbiology lab to make sure the preparation was sterile.

After hanging up, I felt elated. I was on my way. Agnes Klein was an absolute hero. Just imagine. A "bureaucrat" was helping to make this happen in record time. There would be a few more months of hard work putting everything in place, but none of the requests were problematical. I would do whatever it took. I reported my progress to Lyonel. He was delighted. He had already spoken with his new board chairman, Arnold Portigal, a success-ful businessman who had previously served in the same capacity with another hospital in the city. Arnold was very excited that a project of this magnitude had its roots in Winnipeg and gave it his full support.

Frank was next on the list of people to tell. He expressed his admiration for my chutzpah in moving forward with the clini-cal development of DPPE. He had been incredulous on hearing reports of Patrick Roffey's statement at that fateful visit by the team from Eli Lilly. I assured him that no matter how long it took, I would find out which of us was right. I believed it would be me. While much of my time and energy would be diverted to making DPPE and writing protocols, I was anxious that we carry on with our studies.

Frank assured me that he would continue to oversee the research. He then took advantage of the moment to again suggest that we test his hypothesis that DPPE and histamine were actu-ally binding to one or more members of an important family of metabolizing enzymes that are heavily concentrated in liver microsomes, the very tissue component we were using for our binding studies.

"Are you aware that P450 enzymes are found in almost all cells, including blood platelets and cancer cells?" he asked. I had thought they were concentrated mainly in the liver and, like a lot of doctors, was focused solely on their role in detoxifying the drugs I prescribed to patients. Frank then pointed out that P450[44] are also integral to making hormones and prostaglandins involved in cell division and growth. A scientist by the name of

---

44 The "P" is derived from "protein". The "450" refers to the approximate wavelength of light that is "shifted" when light-sensitive instruments are used to measure the enzymes. The protein itself resembles part of the iron-containing hemoglobin molecule that makes our blood red. "P450" is synonymous with the enzymes that both detoxify foreign substances such as drugs, and make important hormones and prostaglandins.

Daniel Nebert had written a scholarly paper on this whole subject. Frank handed me a copy and suggested I read it.

That night I did. Dr. Nebert pointed out that P450 enzymes had been around since creation, while drugs were largely a twentieth-century discovery. Nature obviously had a far greater plan for this enzyme system!

What Frank was trying to tell me a few months earlier now made total sense. Maybe histamine was binding to the P450 enzymes and somehow affecting their production of hormones and prostaglandins. If the AEBS that binds DPPE was associated with these same enzymes, in close proximity to where histamine was attached, that might explain the potent effect of DPPE to increase the levels of both protective and pro-inflammatory prostaglandins. If Frank was right, we just might have identified the nature of Kahlson's unconventional histamine "receptor" without cloning it!

CHAPTER TWENTY-FOUR:

Very Bad News

The weeks flew by. In between seeing patients in the hospital and in my outpatient clinics, I started yet another grant application, wrote a treatment protocol for submission to the ethics committee, and made three batches of DPPE per week. Somehow, time was juggled to prepare a presentation for my "debut" on the international stage of histamine research. Professor Hendrick "Henk" Timmerman, an internationally-recognized pharmacologist and head of the department at Vrije (Free) University in Amsterdam, had read my papers. He was organizing a summer meeting of leading histamine researchers at a former monastery in Noordwijkerhout, fifty kilometers outside the city, and invited me to present my findings. I was actually more nervous about that lecture than anything else, but was thrilled to have been asked to participate and was also looking forward to taking Jill with me. We planned to spend three days in Amsterdam before going to the meeting in Noordwijkerhout. After that, we had booked a week's bus tour through the Alps. Both of us could certainly use a vacation and, exciting or not, I definitely needed a break from my work.

In the early morning hours of July 2, 1990, our Air Canada 747 lumbered its way through the night sky at thirty-five thousand feet, eastbound to Heathrow, where we would pick up a morning KLM connection to Amsterdam. We had taken off from Toronto about four hours earlier and were now approaching mid-Atlantic. The drinks and meals had long ago been served and the remnants cleared away. The cabin lights were turned down as many passengers fitfully tried to get some shuteye. Jill was resting in the seat next to me, her head sideways on a small pillow and legs covered by one of those thin wool airline blankets. My overhead light was on as I went over my talk, yet again. All was well.....

The quiet hum in the cabin was suddenly broken by a jarring announcement from the cockpit. "Ladies and gentleman, this is your captain. I'm afraid I have some very bad news." All eyes popped opened simultaneously. During the next few milliseconds, I quickly recapped his words. "Afraid". Not just "news", not just "bad news", but "v-e-r-y bad news"! Eyes bulged. Throats tightened. Jill grabbed my arm.

The captain continued. "As you probably could tell, we have made a one-eighty degree turn." *We did? You sure could have fooled me.* "The good news is that the left inboard engine fire has now been completely extinguished." *Did he say a fire?* "The bad news is that, even though we were within five minutes of our point-of-no-return, aviation law requires us to turn back to the nearest terra firma, which is Canada. Another fifty nautical miles and we could have continued on to London. I hope to land in Gander where we will pick up a new aircraft. We should be there in a little over ninety minutes. I'll keep you posted as we get closer."

We spent the next four hours in semi-darkness without any further word from the cockpit. Boy, was this guy a PR disaster. "We're done for and they're not telling us," whispered Jill, always the optimist. Finally, after what seemed like an eternity, a crew member announced over the cabin speaker that we were landing at Montréal's Mirabel airport. What happened to Gander? Who knew? Everyone was now too relieved to care about the eight and one-half hour flight from Toronto to Montréal!

As we touched down, fire trucks lined the runway. Luckily, we did not need them. A few minutes after the jumbo came to a stop, we were all hustled out the door. Walking across the tarmac, we saw that a team of technicians had already removed the fire-charred cowling and was closely examining the blackened engine and pylon under floodlights in the dark of night. From the looks of it, there was no doubt in my mind that we had come close, surviving a potentially disastrous engine fire over water. "That could have been one bad random event," I murmured. Then again, maybe there really was a master plan that included DPPE.

We finally arrived a day late at our charming old hotel on Amsterdam's Prinzengracht canal. Tired, but happy to be there, we walked and walked. Just down the way was Anne Frank House. Climbing those narrow stairs to the family's tiny hiding place on the second floor above Otto Frank's business, we could feel the hair rise on our necks and arms. It was an all too sobering and very personal reminder of the Holocaust, the ultimate obscenity of the twentieth century. Here I was, a doctor, dedicating my life to saving others, yet realizing that such efforts are dwarfed by man's inhumanity to man. Strangely, I felt renewed by the experience of being in the same room as the world's most famous and tragic young girl. If my drug could end up saving just one life, it would diminish the madness of the genocide represented by this place.

CHAPTER TWENTY-FIVE:
Centre Stage

Two days later we took a bus to the monastery. Henk Timmerman graciously introduced himself to Jill and me and welcomed us to the meeting. Over beer and pretzels we met, for the first time, many of the scientists who were to become dear friends, including Pier Francesco Mannaioni, from Florence, who headed up the European Histamine Research Society (EHRS); Wilfried Lorenz from Marburg; Walter Schunack, from Berlin; Takehiko Watanabe, from Sendai; and Jack Peter Green, accompanied by his showbiz wife, Arlene (who, some years earlier, appeared with Robert Preston in *Music Man* on Broadway), from New York.

Jill, herself a New Yorker and talented singer, immediately charmed the Greens, especially Jack Peter, who spent the rest of the evening telling her his life's story. As this new friendship was unfolding, Pier, always the suave Italian, congratulated me on my beautiful wife. He immediately invited me to attend the yearly EHRS meetings; the next would be organized by Wilfried Lorenz in Marburg. I gladly accepted. It would be the first of many EHRS meetings Jill and I would attend.

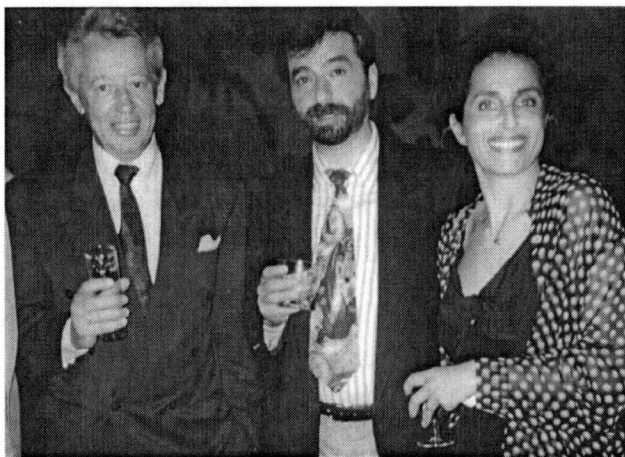

Henk Timmerman, me and Jill at Noordwijkerhout (Personal photo collection)

Takehiko, one of the major players in histamine research, told me that he had refereed our platelet paper and recommended it for publication in *Science*. He had a longstanding interest in Kahlson's work on growth and had been the first to publish the link between the tumor promoter, PMA, and histamine formation in the skin. I told him of our recent experiment with DPPE and PMA, based on his paper, and then proudly gave him a copy of the review article on our work that had just been published in *Biochemical Pharmacology*.

Soon, Wilfried Lorenz, a gregarious Bavarian, walked over, introduced himself and shook my hand. He was a real character... a warm person one could not help but like. However, he also carried a dark melancholy about his past. He revealed to me that his late father had been a member of the Nazi party and was an SS officer in the war. That horrible stain caused Wilfried to seek out and associate with Jewish scientists all over the world, especially in Israel, a country that he loved and often visited. I believed he was reaching out to me in the same manner. It was his way of continually trying to atone for the sins of his father. I greatly respected him for that.

After the war, as a young student, Wilfried had worked in Kahlson's lab. He regaled me and the others with his many stories about those years. Wilfried wanted me to be sure to meet Börje Uvnäs, from Stockholm, who would receive an honor for his contributions to histamine research at the next EHRS meeting. Börje had also worked in Kahlson's laboratory and had befriended Dick Schayer, the American researcher who had developed the histidine decarboxylase assay, vital to Kahlson's work. Listening to all of this, I stood transfixed with a smile on my face. Here I was, meeting in the flesh some of the very people who had been part of the "histamine story". *Was this really happening? Pinch me.*

The next morning I gave my talk. Takehiko, who chaired the session, introduced me. Although I felt nervous, my presentation seemed to go well. There was much interest in my topic about histamine and growth, especially my data showing histamine binding to the DNA-containing chromatin of the nucleus. This had never been demonstrated previously. I announced that our group was now tentatively calling our histamine "receptor" H_{IC}, to denote its intracellular location. After answering some questions at the end of the slides, it was all over. I had more than survived the moment.

At lunch, many people came over to congratulate me on my work. One of that day's speakers, Dr. Allen Barnett, an American from Bloomfield, New Jersey, briefly sat at our table. He told me he was involved in the development of a new H_1 antihistamine, loratadine, for Schering-Plough. Following further pleasant discourse we said goodbye to one another. Little did either of us know that, a few years hence, my research findings would cause him and his company much angst about loratadine.

Later that evening, I tried to engage Jean-Charles Schwartz, discoverer of the H_3 brain receptor, but noted a certain Gallic standoffishness. Thinking that perhaps he was annoyed with my earlier reference to the AEBS as a possible H_3 receptor in the *BBRC* paper, I told him I was sorry for the unintentional faux pas....chalk it up to my being new to the field. This mea culpa had no effect. He just looked through me.

I later learned from Henk that J.-C. did not think I had discovered a histamine receptor of any kind, let alone a mistaken H_3. He was certainly entitled to his opinion. After all, based on my grant reviews, he had a lot of company. Undaunted by his rejection, I remained convinced that we were on to something, especially with the possibility that our histamine "receptor" was actually on P450 enzymes. Now that I knew they were major players in growth, the word "unconventional", as it applied to our newly-named H_{IC}, loomed larger than ever. I liked that. Schwartz and all the others could believe me now or believe me later.

The meeting over, Jill and I said goodbye to our new-found friends and embarked on our bus tour. The Alps were a magnificent antithesis to the flat prairie that makes up much of Manitoba. Arriving in Lucerne, we called home to see how our kids were doing. Carolyn sounded upset. She told me that my seventy year-old mother had just been diagnosed with breast cancer, but did not want us to find out while we were away for fear it would spoil our trip. I decided to wait until the tour ended before contacting her.

As soon as we reached our London hotel, I called mom to be told matter-of-factly that she had found a lump, was recovering from surgery, and would be undergoing radiation to her breast followed by tamoxifen therapy. "Don't you worry," she said, "I'll be fine." I could only hope she was right. Suddenly, my research took on a greater urgency.

CHAPTER TWENTY-SIX:

The Ecstasy And The Agony

By September, I had finished writing two grants, one, a further exploration of the role of histamine in growth, and the other, to further assess DPPE as a potentiator of chemotherapy. I attached all of our latest published papers to buttress my planned research and sent off both applications to the NCIC. By this time, I was hardened to the reality of failure and had no expectations. I kept several local funding groups in mind if I needed them come the annual rite of springtime rejection.

On the up side, Michael Stewart had filed the new "Method of Treatment" patent. I notified Rob Warrington and Frank that we could now proceed to write up our study. I suggested we send it to the prestigious *Journal of the National Cancer Institute*. The editor might be favorably disposed to consider it since the journal had recently published a paper on histidinol that validated much of Rob's data. I told Wayne and Georgie that I would try to get to our "PMA" paper as soon as I had some time. "You mean I'll finally get my name in lights on a real research paper?" Wayne asked, smiling that big smile of his. "Absolutely!" I assured my pal.

I now put the finishing touches on my Ottawa presentation for Dr. Klein and her group. I had received good news from Kirk Marat at the University that the several batches of DPPE I had provided him were 99.9% "clean". He even provided me with impressive overhead transparencies showing the results of his method of analysis, called "nuclear magnetic resonance". This technology allowed him to look inside the chemical structure of DPPE, akin to an MRI scanner looking inside the structure of the human body.

There was one hurdle to overcome, however. The scientists involved with drug standards at the Health Protection Branch notified me that, since one of the two chemicals used to make DPPE was highly toxic, I would have to show that it was not the major component of the 0.1% impurity. That would require a different type of analysis.

As luck would have it, Jiangang Tong (he preferred to be called Tong), who had recently replaced Balram[45], knew a professor in the chemistry lab who had a special analytical device that could measure very tiny levels of impurities. Working nights in the professor's lab, Tong was able to demonstrate convincingly that the toxic chemical was not present in DPPE. The last hurdle having been passed, it was time to have my fateful tête à tête with Agnes Klein et al.

A week later I sat outside her corner office at the Bureau of Human Prescription Drugs, my folder of overhead transparencies resting on my lap. Dr. Klein was delayed in another meeting but would be with me shortly, her very pleasant secretary told me. She was the one with whom I had talked on the phone the day I had first called to speak to "someone in the department". Looking through the open door of Agnes' office, I saw a desk jumbled with

---

45 Although trained as an MD in China, Tong was unable to qualify in his chosen profession in Canada. Like so many other foreign medical graduates, he had to pursue an alternative career, in this case, as a laboratory technician. I felt badly for him as he appeared to have good medical skills.

dozens of thick worn folders. I assumed that one of them contained my file.

Within a few moments she came down the hall. I don't know what I was expecting to see. Perhaps a goddess with a sword? Quite the opposite, Agnes turned out to be the nurturing grandmotherly type, short with glasses, often stroking her hair with her hand to keep it from flopping over her eyes. I should have known. She immediately put me at ease with her smile and sense of humor. She was no longer a faceless bureaucrat. As we talked, Ivo Hynie joined us in the procession to the conference room where I was to review the whole DPPE project from A to Z.

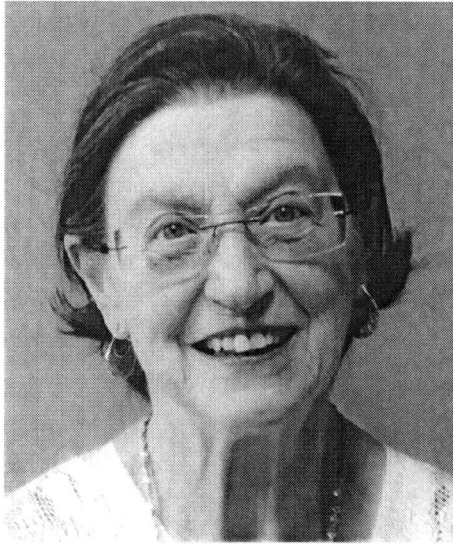

Dr. Agnes Klein (Photo courtesy of Agnes Klein)

The small room was packed with regulatory people.....requisite pens and notebooks in hand. I was soon at ease as the presentation proceeded. My sixth sense told me that, this time, the folks in the room were on my side. When it came time to present the purity analysis, I saw smiles and nods of approval from the drug standards people. At that moment, I knew I had won. This project was going to be approved. Flying back to Winnipeg later that afternoon, I was on such a high that I could have got there without the plane.

Over the next month, I worked closely with Agnes and Ivo by phone, and locally with Dr. John Maclean, to refine the patient protocol. To cast as wide a net as possible, we decided that the patients could have advanced cancer of any type. As with all drugs undergoing development for cancer treatment, the initial studies could only be done in people who had already been through other treatments, including chemotherapy, and had no remaining options. They would be required to sign a consent form telling them that this was an experimental treatment and that no guarantees could be given about either safety or efficacy.

The final paper work was agonizingly slow. Assuming no objections were raised, permission to begin our great adventure would likely come sometime in December, sixty days from the official application, and a mere eight months since my first contact with Agnes. One night in October, I worked late into the evening, making ever more DPPE for the trial. As some of the synthetic steps took half an hour or longer, I decided to leave the lab for a short time to visit a patient I had just admitted to one of the hospital wards.

Walking down the hall, I suddenly bumped into Wayne Beecroft, his wife, Heather, and son, Christopher, in tow. Wayne was carrying a small suitcase. Something was not right with this picture. "Are you visiting someone?" I asked, trying to be nonchalant. "Yeah. Me. I'm in that room across the hall." This time he was not playing the jokester. I just looked at him. "Come on, you can't leave me hanging like that."

We went into his assigned room. He sat on the bed and gave me the goods. He had been having some vague abdominal pain for a month or two. The minute he uttered those words, I remembered that a few weeks earlier we and our wives had gone out for a fancy dinner. Afterward, he had complained of some "heartburn" radiating to his back. The symptom persisted, so yesterday he had an ultrasound. He thought he might have gallstones. The gallbladder was fine but something was seen on his pancreas. It was probably just a cyst, but he was scheduled for an exploratory operation at eight o'clock in the morning. He was optimistic that everything would be fine. "I'll check on you as soon as you're out of the OR," I assured him. A cyst? I left the room feeling sick with concern.

The next day I checked with the ward just before lunch. He was already back from the operating room. The procedure had been relatively brief, not a good sign. Through his shock and grief, Wayne told me that he had inoperable cancer of the pancreas that had spread to his liver. He was determined to have "whatever it takes" to treat the tumor.

Pancreatic cancer is usually fatal in six months. It responds poorly to chemotherapy. Even today, only one or two mildly-effective drugs are available. In 1990 there was virtually nothing that had a track record. "Get that trial going," my pal told me. "I certainly will," I replied, pondering the irony that he might be a candidate for DPPE. I desperately wanted him to be around for that paper we would be writing.....and far beyond that. But I was a realist who believed there was no justice in this world. My dear, dear friend. It was one of the worst random events life could bestow.

CHAPTER TWENTY-SEVEN:

We Have No Objection

I received the "No objection" letter from Agnes Klein on December 5, 1990, a week before the sixty-day limit. Thanks to John Maclean, ethics approval was also in place. This was going to be what is called a combined phase 1, phase 2 study. Agnes preferred a more simple designation: a pilot study. Regardless, it still tested the classical endpoints of drug safety, including how much DPPE could be tolerated and what side effects it caused (Phase 1); and efficacy, in this case whether it helped doxorubicin shrink tumors (Phase 2).[46]

However, our study was significantly more complicated than usual for two reasons. First, it appeared from the mice and rats that DPPE could stimulate the growth of tumors. To determine its optimal dose and side effect profile, the initial patients had to first receive DPPE alone. This would be followed a week later

---

46 Phase 1 and 2 studies do not normally have a comparison group. If a drug completes phase 1 and phase 2 successfully, it then goes into phase 3, a more stringent test that involves a large number of patients who are randomly allocated to receive the new drug treatment or another established treatment to see which is better.

by DPPE plus doxorubicin. In that first seven days, we had to be on the lookout for any quickening of the pace of cancer growth. The patients would have to understand this risk. However, hitting the tumor with DPPE plus doxorubicin one week later might hopefully undo any potential damage and even result in a better outcome.

Second, we were also looking to see whether DPPE offered any protection against the expected side effects of doxorubicin, including nausea and vomiting, and low blood counts. For example, we did not plan to give any drugs to treat nausea unless it became apparent that DPPE was not preventing these symptoms. In another wrinkle, Gary Glavin's experiments had implicated a stimulation of prostaglandins by DPPE that resulted in protection against ulcers in the gut. As a result, we asked patients to avoid taking aspirin, or related "NSAIDS" such as ibuprofen (Advil), for fear they would block prostaglandins and work against any protection offered by our drug. On the other side of the coin, we would not treat anyone with underlying inflammation since DPPE might make it worse.

Before proceeding, Ivo primed me on the difference between mice and humans when it comes to calculating doses. Basically, if the maximum tolerated dose of DPPE in a mouse is sixty milligrams per kilogram body weight, the equivalent human dose is six milligrams per kilogram body weight, seemingly ten-fold lower. However, when species differences in body weight divided by body size are factored in, the doses in humans and mice are actually the same.[47]

---

47 When the dose is standardized to reflect the difference in the ratio of body weight to body surface area between a mouse and a human, the amount of drug administered is actually the same. The ratio of the two parameters in the mouse is 4 to 1, whereas in the human it is 40 to 1. In other words, a human weighs ten times more for his or her size than a light furry mouse. Therefore, in the mouse, 60 mg/kg x 4/1 = 240 milligrams DPPE per square meter of body surface. Similarly, in the human, 6 mg/kg x 40/1 = 240 milligrams DPPE per square meter of body surface.

He suggested that to be safe, we start low, at one milligram per kilogram of DPPE. It would be given intravenously over one hour, with close monitoring. We would treat two patients at that dose. If all went well after a week of observation and blood tests, the patients would be treated with the same dose of DPPE over one hour, followed by doxorubicin.

Then, if after a standard observation time of three weeks, there were no problems with the combination, we would double the dose of DPPE in the next two patients, followed by the drugs in combination a week later, and so on, until we observed significant side effects of DPPE, indicating the maximum that patients could tolerate. Once we had our answer as to the safe dose range of DPPE, we would skip the DPPE-alone step and treat all subsequent patients with the combination of DPPE and doxorubicin every three weeks.

However, there was one further variable that I wanted to assess. A recently-published paper from another laboratory had tested Rob Warrington's protocol for histidinol in mice. It was found that giving histidinol for an additional twenty-four hours after the chemotherapy proved more effective than the shorter schedule that Rob had used. This raised the question of whether extending the DPPE treatment for twenty-four hours, or longer, after the doxorubicin also might work better. We decided to feel our way along before making a decision on testing DPPE in this way. Ivo and Agnes were certainly willing to be flexible as long as there wasn't a safety issue. Time would tell.

The fateful day to begin human treatment arrived at last. Our first patient was an emaciated young man named Robert Fisher. He had advanced colon cancer. Robert was under no illusions about his chance to respond at this late stage, but was eager to be our first "guinea pig". I cannot adequately describe how I felt when the pharmacist handed me the bag containing my drug. Stuck to it was a label. Below the patient's name, ward and hospital number was typed, "DPPE, 48 mg. in 250 mL normal saline. For intravenous administration over 60 minutes. Dec. 8, 1990. Dr.

L. Brandes". We were about to make the quantum leap from the laboratory mouse to the human. W-O-W!!!

Susan (Susie) Bracken, my longtime clinic nurse who now administered chemotherapy, accompanied me up to the ward. She was an extraordinary person, with great patient and nursing skills. Picking her to assist me in the study was a no-brainer. Walking down the ward, the bag of DPPE and intravenous paraphernalia in hand, we both had a great sense of mission. "Here it is!" I exclaimed to Robert and his wife as we entered the room. Inspecting the labeled bag, they both nodded in anticipation. As the people at NASA would say, we were a go for launch.

Susie inserted the i.v. needle with ease, connected it to a thin polyethylene i.v. line and pushed the pointed connector at the other end into the bag, now hanging from a pole at the bedside. An EKG monitor was hooked up. "Any time you want to start," I told her. It was about five minutes before one o'clock. With a great sense of occasion, Susie decided that we should wait for the minute hand to hit twelve. I humored her. It may have been the longest five minutes of my life. Finally, the infusion was underway. Continually adjusting the i.v. rate to run over exactly one hour, Susie monitored his temperature, pulse, respirations and blood pressure every fifteen minutes and charted the findings. I kept my eye on the green-colored blips of heart activity that continually crossed the small monitor screen from one side to the other.

In the end, it was anticlimactic. There wasn't a hint of a side effect or an abnormal finding. I was not that surprised, given that we started at a low dose. Nonetheless, relief was evident all around. Elated, I left Susie with the patient and went to the phone to call Ottawa. "Agnes, we just finished giving DPPE to our first patient and all is well. Tell Ivo," I reported. Dr. Klein was pleased.

CHAPTER TWENTY-EIGHT:
Of Mice And Men

After observing the same "non-event" with patient number two, it was time to double the dose to two milligrams per kilogram. Once again, no side effects were observed in either patient. We moved on to four milligrams per kilogram. At the end of receiving this dose, one patient felt slightly light-headed and another felt mildly nauseated. However, both settled down quickly and in neither case was there a definite "event" that would suggest a maximum dose had been reached. Nonetheless, while the protocol would allow me to double the DPPE dose again, remembering those infamous mice going "over the cliff", I hesitated and called Ivo to ask his advice about implementing a lesser increase, to six milligrams per kilogram, in the next two patients. "That would be fine," he counseled. Better safe than sorry, we agreed.

All was going well with patient number five, a seventy-seven year old male. We had just completed the first forty-five minutes of his planned one hour DPPE treatment. As always, Susie was closely monitoring him while I watched from the sideline. Suddenly we saw some muscles twitch in his arms. Nothing major, just a bit of mild twitching. "His temperature has dropped a degree," Susie reported. His pulse, respirations and blood pressure were fine. "Let's keep going," I told her, closely watching for anything more serious.

Another five minutes went by. "Feeling okay?" I asked my patient.

"Yup. But why are you talking so loud?" he inquired.

"I don't think I am," I replied.

"Well you sure sound loud to me." Now both his legs were twitching as well.

"Stop the i.v. for a moment," I instructed. Susie nodded and immediately closed the valve, shutting down the flow in the i.v. tubing. I knew that we were on the cusp. In addition to signs of involuntary muscle movement, the patient had "hyperacusis", a medical term meaning "loud hearing". That meant that the auditory nerve that controlled his hearing was being over-stimulated, a sign of early neurological toxicity. Just at that moment he complained of nausea and then vomited.

That was the end of that infusion….stopped at fifty minutes. One hour later, our patient was feeling fine, symptoms almost all gone. Within another hour he was completely back to normal. I reported the finding to Ivo. It sounded as though we had reached toxicity at six milligrams per kilogram. However, as a much younger man was scheduled to receive his first dose of DPPE the next week, we decided to see whether he would do better.

"Tell us immediately if you are having any problems," I instructed as we started the treatment. Thirty minutes went by without a problem. At forty minutes, he reported feeling a bit light-headed but otherwise okay. Forty-five minutes….was that a muscle twitch in his arm? Yes. There it goes. "Temperature down one and one-half degrees. All other signs are normal," Susie reported.

"Keep going, I replied."

"I hear a radio playing," my patient reported at the fifty-minute mark. Susie and I looked at one another. We didn't hear anything.

Suddenly his right hand started to wave, snakelike, in the air, like a belly dancer. This was an involuntary movement called "choreoathetosis". Derived from Greek, it means, "a constant dance". Suddenly he sat bolt upright and vomited. An hour later everything was fine. We had definitely reached a toxic dose of DPPE in two of two subjects. Thank goodness there were no somersaults!

"It's a good thing we didn't go directly to eight milligrams per kilogram," I told Ivo. My colleague agreed. "Both are due for DPPE plus doxorubicin next week. Would you mind if we deviated slightly from protocol and gave them the same dose of DPPE, but over two hours instead of one?" Normally, we would have backed off to the previous, non-toxic, dose of four milligrams per kilogram. Ivo understood what I was getting at. Slowing the time over which a toxic dose of DPPE was given to mice prevented seizures. "Okay, as long as the patients agree," he said.

Both did, and received the same DPPE dose over two hours. Neither turned a hair. What struck me the most was how predictive our mice had been in every respect. If ever there was a good example of the value of testing candidate drugs in laboratory mice and rats, this was it. Side effects in humans occurred at the same relative dose as in mice, the brain appeared to be affected first in both species, the effects wore off quite quickly and giving the drug over a longer time prevented the side effects. "Let's hope they are just as predictive of an improved result using DPPE with chemotherapy in patients with cancer," I immediately thought.[48]

---

48 For some years, animal rights activists have campaigned vociferously to abolish laboratory research involving rodents and other animals, arguing that cell-culture (in vitro) experiments can give us all the information we need. While in vitro studies play an important role, only animals can be truly predictive of what effects drugs may have in humans.

CHAPTER TWENTY-NINE:

Six Months

As December quickly came to an end, I felt very pleased and "mellow" about our rapid progress. In only three weeks, we had accomplished our first goal of finding the appropriate dose range for DPPE. The first few patients had also received their followup treatment with the combination of DPPE and doxorubicin. The lab and clinic then closed between Christmas Eve and New Year's Day. I was happy to have time off for R and R and to light the Hanukkah candles with my family. At the same time I looked forward with great anticipation to what lay ahead. What would the coming year hold for my project?

Every Christmas season, Ernie Ramsey, head of the urology department, and his wife, Diane, a family physician, invited us to a night of wine, cheese and singing. Other yearly attenders included Lyonel and Esther Israels and the "Irish mafia", physicians, mainly, and their wives, who had immigrated to Manitoba from Northern Ireland. Come mid-evening, Ernie would sit at his prized grand piano and accompany the group in carols, followed by broadway music. Among several talented performers present,

Jill would invariably sing "solo" to Ernie's accompaniment, much to everyone's delight and approval. I usually followed her with my rendition of Gene Autry's *Back in the Saddle Again*. By the time I finished trying to sing it, Ernie would be laughing so hard that he often missed the keys.

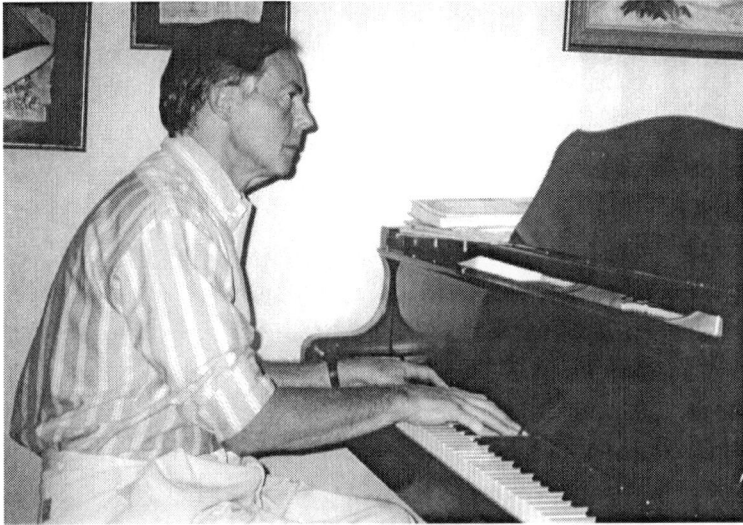

Dr. Ernie Ramsey (Personal photo collection)

Ernie, who had trained in Belfast, arrived in Winnipeg a year after I did, in 1972, and spent time along side me at the bench, doing research at the Institute before taking up his clinical duties. We worked well together and managed to publish two papers reporting our results. I realized from the very beginning that he was a special guy: cultured, musical, athletic and quite brilliant. We became very close. Over the years, we had a lot of laughs as we constantly reminisced about our adventures together.

Ernie's favorite "Lorne story" involved an eight o'clock invitation around the pool at his place one warm summer evening. Somehow, I misunderstood and did not realize that dinner was being served so, before going over, I barbequed steaks while Jill made a Caesar salad. We arrived at the Ramseys in time for....

barbequed steaks and Caesar salad. I said nothing as I slowly picked away at my second identical meal of the evening. However, Jill, unamused by my mistake, let those present know that, in the future, all dinner invitations should be vetted through her.

My favorite "Ernie story" was how I had got him involved in one of my lab experiments. After finding that DPPE prevented normal stimulated immune cells from dividing, I had a brain-storm that this might be "the" solution to organ rejection. When a person receives a transplant from anyone but an identical twin, the immune system "turns on" and attacks the foreign trans-planted tissue unless strong anti-rejection drugs are administered. Maybe DPPE would be a simpler and less toxic solution. To test the idea, I decided we should take skin from black mice and graft them on to genetically-unrelated white mice, with half getting a daily DPPE injection and half getting saline as a placebo.

As Ernie was the head of the kidney transplant program at the hospital, I collared him for the job of grafting the mice and assisted him as he carefully cut out and then sutured the skin from each to the other. Working away, we joked on the square that if this panned out, we would be shoo-ins to share the Nobel Prize. "Keep a bag packed for Stockholm just in case," I advised him. After about two weeks of injecting the mice, the grafts were all rejected and fell off. I called Ernie at home late one night.

"Do you have that bag packed for Stockholm?" I asked, feign-ing great excitement.

"Sure," he replied. Then a pause. "Are you *serious*?" he inquired.

"No. Unpack it," I answered, confessing that our experiment had bombed.

After he finished laughing, Ernie joked, "Maybe we should repeat the experiment using a black marking pen."

"That's already been tried unsuccessfully," I reminded my colleague.[49] He guffawed about this episode for years. We really loved one another.

This particular Christmas, 1990, Wayne and Heather Beecroft were invited to the Ramseys. Ernie was also close with Wayne and, like everyone else, was devastated by the news of his pancreatic cancer diagnosis. Wayne looked thin but was in good spirits. He had recovered from his surgery and was undergoing chemotherapy. Seeing him come into the room, I walked over, hugged my pal and kissed him on the cheek. We spent the evening trying to act as though everything was normal. Standing side by side with Wayne, sharing a sheet of carol music while Ernie played and everyone sang, I could not help but have a great feeling of sadness. If statistics held true, this would be his last Christmas.

The holiday season held additional significance, as Jill and I had married on December 25, 1966. In this, as every year, our family joined former neighbors, and still close friends, Susan and Tony Russell and their children, Carolyn and Peter, for a lavish Christmas cum anniversary dinner, complete with turkey, stuffing and my favorite Figgie pudding for dessert. Following British tradition, we and the kids wore paper crowns and, before eating, pulled "crackers" that, on making a bang, released a little toy or ornament along with a small paper on which was printed a

---

49 One of the biggest scientific scandals of the 1970's involved William Summerlin, a graduate student of famed Sloan-Kettering immunologist, Dr. Robert Good. After first maintaining skin tissue in culture for several weeks, Summerlin had carried out a similar graft experiment from black to white mice that apparently worked on the first try without the need for anti-rejection drugs. The finding was immediately played up by Good and word of the "breakthrough" spread like wildfire. Unfortunately, the hapless Summerlin could not reproduce the result in follow-up experiments. Rather than risk the ire of his boss, he used a black felt marker, painting the skin of the white mice to mimic a successful graft and reported further success. Good then continued to tell the world of the breakthrough. The fraud was eventually discovered by other lab workers who blew the whistle. The episode ended the young doctor's research career and severely tarnished Good's illustrious reputation.

fortune. Mine read as follows: "Your work will bring you much happiness." If only it were that simple, I thought.

With 1991 officially begun, it was back to work and full steam ahead with our clinical trial. A welcome addition to my little "team" was Kerry McDonald, an oncology nurse practitioner with an exceptional ability to monitor the patients for side effects in the days and weeks after each treatment. After further discussions with Ivo in Ottawa, I decided to test the remaining patients over a range of DPPE doses from low (two-tenths to one milligram per kilogram) to middle-of-the-road (two to three milligrams per kilogram), where the drug itself caused no side effects. I was also authorized to give the DPPE for an additional twenty-four to seventy-two hours after the doxorubicin chemotherapy. The idea was to see whether, as compared to one dose or duration of DPPE, another might prove best to decrease the side effects of doxoru-bicin, or to help it shrink tumors. The more I thought about it, the more I agreed with Agnes' designation of this first trial as a "pilot study". At this early point, we were really just feeling our way along, probing. It was unstructured and unconventional, perhaps, but fine with me. After all, "unconventional" was a word with which I was all too familiar.

When treating these patients, I also continued to keep an eye out for any accelerated growth of tumors. One of the early sub-jects had a spread of tumor to the skin of his chest, right over the breast bone. He was in the first group that was treated with DPPE alone before receiving it in combination with doxorubicin one week later. Within five days of receiving DPPE, there was a very obvious increase in size of the chest tumor which, up to that time, had remained rather quiescent and small. Coincidence? Maybe, but I was suspicious.

Even when giving DPPE together with doxorubicin, stimula-tion of growth theoretically might occur if a particular tumor was resistant to the killing effects of the chemotherapy drug; in such a scenario, DPPE might exert an unchecked stimulating effect. I told this to all the patients but, without exception, they were brave enough to want to go ahead with the treatment. Only time would tell whether this would turn out to be a significant problem. It is one thing to treat groups of mice with tumors in the confines of the laboratory, but quite another to treat individual human beings in the real world.

At virtually this same time, a "random event" in the clinic added a whole new texture to the issue of tumor stimulation. It also greatly complicated my life. Here are the details. Despite frequent reassurances by me that her breast cancer remained in remission following surgery and chemotherapy three years previously, a fifty-year-old woman was having great difficult in coping. Her family doctor thought that she was depressed and prescribed amitriptyline. This drug belongs to an older family of antidepressants called "tricyclics". Chemically, it has much in common with DPPE and H$_1$ antihistamines.

Within two months of starting the amitriptyline, her cancer recurred and metastasized. On examining her, I was quite amazed at the rapid growth of her tumor in such a short time. Thinking about her situation, I was suddenly struck by a frightening thought. If DPPE could stimulate the growth of cancer, what about chemically-similar amitriptyline? Then again, what about many other chemically-similar drugs that we use in the clinic? However, cancer and depression are both common diseases. Cancer can recur and spread for any number of unknown reasons. Any association of rapid growth and starting on an antidepressant could be apparent rather than real. "Don't jump to hasty conclusions," I told myself, quietly parking the observation in the back of my mind.

It didn't stay there for long. Over the next two months I believed I saw this same scenario in two other patients. One, with no identifiable risk factors, such as a family history of breast cancer, had developed an aggressive form of the disease within six months of going on a tricyclic antidepressant similar to amitriptyline. The other patient was similar to my first; soon after being placed on a newer class of antidepressant (fluoxetine; Prozac) for depressive symptoms, her disease suddenly recurred and spread.

I was aware of a decades-old controversy surrounding a possible link between depression itself and the development of cancer. Some studies were "positive", while others were "negative". But what if any link was, instead, between taking an antidepressant drug and stimulating the growth of an underlying cancer that may, or may not, have been previously diagnosed? My research with DPPE told me that this could be possible. There was a way to find out that I knew all too well. I spoke to Frank about my concerns and what I intended to do about them in the lab. As a result of his longtime interest in the effect of chemicals, pesticides and pharmaceuticals on the health of the population, he was in complete agreement.

"I want you to do binding studies on amitriptyline and fluoxetine," I told Patty. Obtaining the amitriptyline was easy, as it was long off-patent and available as a pure powder from the chemical supply house. Fluoxetine was a bit trickier. At that time, it was on patent and available only in commercial form. We therefore had the choice of testing a capsule or liquid emulsion formulation. With commercial preparations, additional substances, such as preservatives, are often added by the manufacturer. Their presence could make testing difficult. The liquid preparation obviously contained coloring dyes, flavorings, and who knew what else. It was out.

Luckily, we found out that, in addition to the active drug which, like DPPE, was in a water-soluble form called a "salt", the only other component of the capsule was an insoluble cellulose filler. By gently opening the capsules, spilling their contents into a small test tube containing a few ml of saline, and spinning the solution in a centrifuge, we should then be able to pour off the saline in which the drug had dissolved, leaving the cellulose filler behind at the bottom of the test tube.

"Who makes Prozac, anyway?" I asked our hospital pharmacist.

"Eli Lilly," she responded.

"Oh, brother," I murmured to myself, thinking of all that had transpired between me and that company. However, this was about science and human health, not politics or big business. If there was a potential tie-in between some, or all, antidepressants and cancer growth, I was determined to get to the bottom of it. I was certainly not out to pick on Eli Lilly or any other drug company. After all, the "problem", if there was one, appeared more likely to be generic than specific. In other words, more than one drug, or class of drugs, brought to market by many different companies, might be suspect.

I also realized intuitively that if a cause and effect were found, this would become a humungous bag of worms. I strongly believed that antidepressants are both valuable, and often necessary, in the treatment of the debilitating symptoms of depression. Moreover, depression in patients with cancer is often a natural consequence of the stress involved in dealing with a very scary diagnosis. This is an important "quality of life" issue that cannot be overlooked or undertreated, but if antidepressant drugs were linked to cancer growth, how would we deal with the issue in depressed patients with cancer?

There was a further issue that concerned me just as much. In the early 1990s, physicians were increasingly prescribing antidepressant drugs, such as Prozac, to literally thousands of people who were not clinically depressed, with the stated benefit of "smoothing them out". For example, aggressive behavior at home or work might be made to vanish with a daily dose of Prozac. Would this approach really help some of these people? Possibly. But what about unintended consequences? There is no such thing as a totally safe drug.

It was now early February, 1991. As Patty toiled away in the lab, Susie and I continued to add new patients to our clinical study. Definite trends were beginning to emerge. The lower doses of DPPE, especially when given for up to seventy-two hours, seemed to substantially protect patients from the nausea and vomiting, as well as low blood counts, associated with doxorubicin. In contrast, as compared to the lesser doses, the higher doses of DPPE actually increased doxorubicin-induced nausea and vomiting, and the blood counts were lower.

Despite that negative, the higher DPPE doses, especially when given for up to seventy-two hours, seemed to be helping doxorubicin shrink tumors more effectively than the lower doses. Some patients with breast cancer who were treated with the higher doses of DPPE and doxorubicin, had a complete remission of their disease. Ultimately, if I had to choose between lowering side effects or increasing the chance of remissions, it would be the latter. After all, we had other effective drugs to prevent chemotherapy side effects. Moreover, they could be used to counteract the side effects of higher DPPE doses. However, before reaching a final conclusion on how we should proceed, I needed more patients and more time to follow them up.

March arrived with both very good and very bad news. On the bad side, Wayne was failing quickly. He had stopped chemotherapy as, all too predictably, it was not helping him. I had gone over to his home that weekend to find him sitting in the living room in his leather easy chair, crying with pain. A few weeks earlier, Heather had called to ask me to help her buy Wayne a "really good" stereo system. She hoped the music would be therapeutic and soothing. I gladly obliged her. When we brought the components and speakers into the house and wired them up in the living room, he was very grateful and immediately played around with his new system. However, that morning, there was no music playing.

Wayne and Heather seemed lost, helpless to know what to do. I quickly arranged for him to get oral morphine and made a call to connect him with one of our medical colleagues in the pain clinic. Wayne was trying to console himself reading passages from the bible. The three of us sat there for the longest time, holding hands and talking. Soon the crying passed. It was just so tough. I promised to check back often and told him to call me any time day or night if there was a problem with which I could help. As I drove out of his long driveway, the tears welled up in my eyes. "There is no justice in this life," I concluded.

Monday morning had a decidedly different tone. As I walked down the hall towards the Cancer Foundation, Henry Friesen was coming towards me and we stopped to talk. I could tell he was happy about something. "Hi, Lorne," he greeted me with a wide smile. "I've just come back from the NCIC. I can't tell you anything official….except that you will be receiving some very good news." He then walked away, still smiling. Normally not a demonstrative person, his demeanor told me everything I needed to know. Henry was NCIC president at the time and knew the decisions of the grants panels that met biannually to assess the applications. Now I assumed the decision would be positive for funding at least one of them. It was extremely kind of Henry to give me a "heads-up" without breaching confidentiality. That was just like him. He was as politically savvy as Lyonel.

A few days later, the "very good news" arrived in the mail in the form of two thick envelopes from the NCIC. The enclosed letters and forms indicated that both grants were highly rated and funded in full for two years. I was back on track! I would have money! I could hire new people in the lab! Last year, histamine and DPPE were losers with the grants panels. This year those same panels said they were winners. Go figure.

That same week, I received further very good news of a different kind. An envelope arrived from the Editor of the *Journal of the National Cancer Institute*. Our paper, written with Rob Warrington, was acceptable for publication pending some very minor revision. I made the suggested changes and sent the paper back. Counting out the months on my fingers, I assumed that, all being well with the modified version, it could "hit the stand" sometime between July and September, still a few months off. Everything seemed to take so long. Nonetheless, I and my co-authors were delighted. The paper would be widely read, as *JNCI* was very popular with doctors and researchers in the cancer field.

In early April, Patty came to my office with the results of the antidepressant drug binding studies. First she showed me the data for amitriptyline. Although somewhat weaker than DPPE, it nonetheless bound to the AEBS and also competed for radio-labeled histamine binding in the liver microsomes and nuclear preparations. "Wait until you see the results for fluoxetine," she said, handing me the graph and printout. My eyes widened as I observed both of its very powerful binding curves, slightly stronger than DPPE on all counts. After she left, I sat in my office, thinking about the potential importance of what I had just seen. "Wow. This is getting scary," I told myself.

The next step would be tumor studies in mice and rats. But before I could proceed, I needed to hire two additional people to help with the experiments. I had already decided that one of them would be Randi Arron, a first-year medical student who had shown interest in working in my lab for the summer. I had known her family for years; her mom and dad, Gerry and Phyllis, were the first to befriend us when we moved to Winnipeg. Gerry was my lawyer. Randi was bright and I believed she could do a good job if properly supervised. She could start in mid-May, once her exams were over. That would be fine. I suspected that she would be in for a surprise when I told her the nature of her project.

The third week of April brought with it the inevitably sad news that Wayne had been admitted to hospital with increasing jaundice. His only brother, John, a physician, flew in from Toronto. Together with Heather and Christopher, he stayed constantly at the bedside. The three of them, and all of us, comforted Wayne as best we could. Within a few short days he was gone, almost exactly six months after the diagnosis was made. He was only forty-four years old, cut off in the prime of his life. Those terrible statistics were all too accurate.

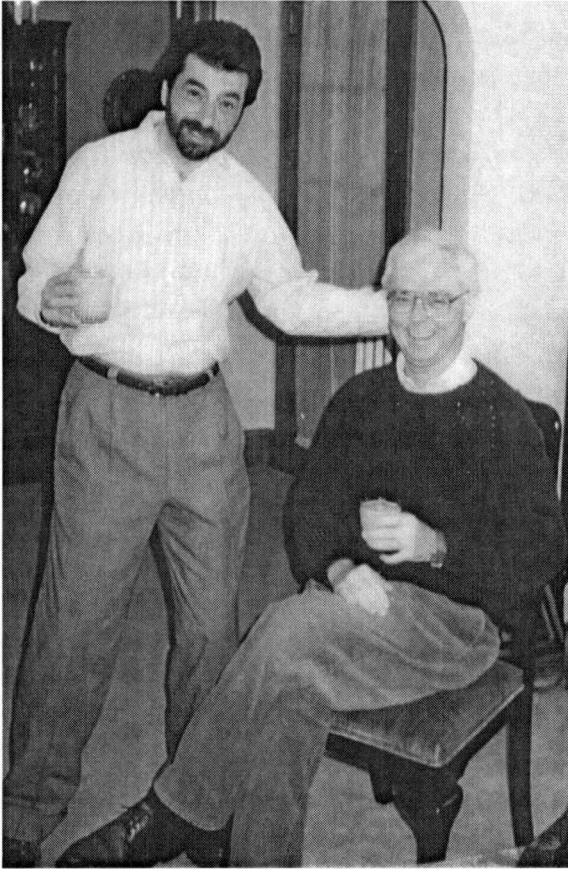

With Wayne Beecroft (Personal photo collection)

The church funeral was very large. Everyone was there: Lyonel, Ernie, Peg Sellers, the medical and lay community at large, and innumerable grateful patients to whom Wayne had given so much care and compassion. Asked by Heather to take part in the eulogies, I chose a verse from Psalm 103 that reads, in part, "The days of man are as grass; he flourishes as a flower in the field. The wind passes over it and it is gone, and no one can recognize where it grew." That passage notwithstanding, Wayne would never be forgotten by me or anyone else with whom he had come into contact. More than ever, I owed him that research paper.

A month later, it was written. With Georgie's blessing, I decided to go back to the well one more time and submit the paper to *BBRC*. Noting with regret that my old "friend", Dr. McElroy, was no longer listed as an editor, I took a chance and picked Dr. Daniel Lane at Johns Hopkins. Fortunately, he proved as receptive as Dr. McElroy. The paper was accepted in June and published in September. At the end was this acknowledgment: "We dedicate this paper to the memory of our co-author and esteemed colleague, Wayne Arthur Beecroft (October 12, 1946-April 24, 1991) - LJB and GRH." I had kept my promise. His name was in lights.[50]

---

50 Brandes LJ, Beecroft WA, Hogg GR. In vivo stimulation of tumor growth and phorbol ester-induced inflammation by N,N-diethyl-2-[4-(phenylmethyl)phenoxy]ethanamine.HCl, a potent ligand for intracellular histamine receptors. Biochem. Biophys. Research Commun. 1991; 179:1297-1304.

CHAPTER THIRTY:

Don't Shoot The Messenger

We mourn and then life goes on. It has to be that way. Jill and I were off in mid-May to our first European Histamine Research Society meeting in Marburg, Germany, hosted by Wilfried Lorenz. This was the annual conference to which I had been invited a year earlier by Pier Mannaioni when we first met at Henk Timmerman's histamine symposium in Noordwijkerhout. Thankfully, this time our trans-Atlantic flight was completely uneventful.

As promised, Wilfried introduced me to Börje Uvnäs, then in his late seventies. Decades earlier, as a graduate student, he had worked in Professor Kahlson's laboratory where he had befriended Richard "Dick" Schayer, the American scientist who had perfected the histidine decarboxylase assay that enabled Kahlson to detect the formation of histamine in growing cells. Although his life's work focused on the enigmatic histamine-containing mast cells, Börje was pleased that I had taken up where his old boss had left off. I told him about DPPE and promised to send him some reprints. It was the beginning of a beautiful friendship.

At the meeting, I presented my latest findings and got to know many new researchers. One of them, Manuel Garcia-Caballero from Malaga, Spain, had also been looking at the role of histamine in growth. He invited me to present a lecture at the following year's meeting that he was organizing in nearby Torremolinos, a favorite tourist destination noted for its stretches of beach and sea food restaurants along the shores of the Mediterranean. I was delighted to accept. Jill was even more delighted. We had spent a wonderful week there on a delayed honeymoon in 1968 and always talked about going back. Now we would.

The highlight of Wilfried's conference was the final banquet, held in the ancient Marburg Castle, on a hilltop overlooking the city. Every year at the end of that gala dinner, the members would sing the "official song" of the Society, to the tune of *Polly Wolly Doodle* (!). Tradition dictated that a new verse be added to commemorate each meeting. By now there were many. It was charming in a corny sort of way. Late that night we bade goodbye to all our new friends and promised to see them in Spain the following year.

Freshly home, I came into the lab the following Monday to find Randi Arron waiting for me, her exams now over. I sat down with her in my office and reviewed what we had found with DPPE and histidinol. I then told her about the recent binding studies with the two antidepressant drugs and my concern about the implications. "How would you feel about injecting some mice?" I asked her.

"No problem, as long as you teach me how," she replied. I liked her spunk.

Then and there, we designed our first "quick-and-dirty" experiment. Randi would inject sarcoma cells, obtained from Arnold Greenberg's lab, into the shaved backs of twenty numbered mice[51] and then divide them into two groups of ten. She was to label the cages of the treatment groups as either "A" or "B". One group would be injected daily with amitriptyline, the other with saline

---

51   The mice were numbered on their tails using a marker pen to make a series of dots or dashes, similar to a Roman numeral system.

as a placebo, but I was not to know which. In mouse terms, the daily dose of each drug would be the same as a human would take. Over a ten day period, all the mice should develop tumors. I was looking to see whether, after the injection of cells, visible tumors appeared earlier in one group than the other. The scientific term for this interval of time is "latency".

Each day after Randi had finished her injections, I examined the numbered mice in each group for tumors and recorded my findings on a sheet of paper. Within the first five days, I observed a clear difference between "A" and "B". One group had already developed four tumors, while the other had none. I kept this information to myself to prevent any bias that such knowledge might confer on Randi. By ten days, as expected, virtually all the mice had developed tumors. The experiment now ended, we met in my office.

"Okay," I said. "There was a definite early difference in latency. I will go out on a limb and predict that 'A' received amitriptyline and 'B' received saline."

Randi's eyes widened. "Get out. I don't believe it!" she gasped, clearly impressed.

"So am I right?" I asked. I was, she said.

We repeated the experiment, this time with fluoxetine and saline. As before, by the fifth day there was a clear difference between "A" and "B": I scored it five to nothing. At the end of the ten days, Randi and I again met in my office.

"I will once more go out on a limb and predict that 'A' received fluoxetine and 'B' received saline," I said, showing Randi the yellow piece of lined paper on which I had charted my daily observations.

"Unbelievable," she said. I was two for two.

The next step would be unpopular with my assistants. I called Patty, Tong and newly-hired technician, Cheryl Zaborniak, into my office and told them of the preliminary findings. "We have to find out whether human-equivalent doses of the antidepressants stimulate the growth of breast cancer in rats treated with DMBA," I told them. Patty's eyes seemed to glaze over as she remembered her last encounter with rats in the same carcinogen test with DPPE. Tong made the scenario more agreeable by offering to assist in administering the DMBA. Bless his heart.

As with the latency experiments, this one had to be "blinded" to prevent any human bias. Tong would perform all the Monday to Friday injections, and only he was to know what treatment the rats received (amitriptyline, fluoxetine, or saline). The cages were to be coded to keep Pat and Cheryl in the dark when they examined each rat for tumors once a week. While that was going on, Randi would learn how to measure radiolabeled thymidine uptake into DNA so that she could determine whether the two antidepressant drugs, like DPPE, increased cell division in breast cancer cells.

After the group left my office, I went to Arnold Greenberg and showed him what we had found with his sarcoma cells. His reaction was one of simultaneous interest, concern and caution. I entirely agreed with him. It was one thing to report tumor stimulation by DPPE, an unknown drug under development to help chemotherapy kill cancer cells. It was another to suggest that commercially-available drugs, prescribed to millions of people for the treatment of depression, might share this tumor-stimulating property with DPPE. "I'm going to call Rob Warrington and ask him to test the drugs in his lab," I told my colleague. Arnold thought that to be an excellent idea. If an independent laboratory could reproduce our findings, it would add significant credibility to the observation. Given the stakes, it was also the responsible thing to do.

I called Rob that afternoon. When I told him about my obser-vations in the three patients and the results of the two "latency" experiments with amitriptyline and fluoxetine, he immediately agreed to test the two antidepressants in his lab. His longtime assistant, Wei Fang, would inject melanoma cells under the skin of mice and then treat them for two to three weeks to observe any effects on the growth and size of the tumors. I suggested that we send him our drug preparations so that both labs would be testing exactly the same formulations.

The summer months went by quickly. Each week, Pat and Cheryl would record the number and size of any breast tumors in each coded group of rats and bring the data sheet to my office for me to keep. That way, they would not have any measurements to which to refer the next week, and I could track the consistency of their observations. By the beginning of August, it was clearly apparent that, as in our earlier tests, the antidepressant-treated rats were pulling way out in front of the placebo group.

When we finally called it quits after an additional six weeks, the breast tumors were five-times bigger than controls in the rats that were treated with fluoxetine, and nine-times bigger than controls in the rats that were treated with amitriptyline. I think we were all shocked by the magnitude of the effect. In support of these findings, Randi, who quickly got the hang of the labeled thymidine experiments, determined that both amitriptyline and fluoxetine increased the amount of radioactive DNA in the MCF-7 breast cancer cells, suggesting that, like DPPE, they were stimulating them to divide.

Interestingly, this effect was only seen at certain "low to middle" concentrations of each drug. Below or above these levels, the stimulation fell off. Therefore, rather than a "straight-line" effect, the stimulation followed a "bell-shaped curve", akin to tracing a line that goes up and down a hill. I showed Randi's data to Frank. He was not surprised. I didn't know it, but many years previously he described this type of curve in another biological system involving chemicals called "peptides". On learning of this, I was impressed, even more so when he told me that other researchers who later published work on that same system, referred to the bell phenomenon as "a LaBella curve"! The Lord continued to work in mysterious ways.

When Rob called soon after to say that he had also found a marked degree of melanoma growth-stimulation by the two antidepressant drugs, it was the nail in the coffin. We now both believed that this effect must be real....scary, but real. A very careful approach would need to be taken when writing up the findings as they were bound to cause a stir. Not for the first time, I felt very nervous about how this news would be received. "Don't shoot the messenger!" I said to no one in particular.

CHAPTER THIRTY-ONE :

The Review

Our paper reporting chemotherapy potentiation and bone marrow protection by DPPE and histidinol was finally published in *JNCI* in the late summer. However, I did not have the luxury of enjoying the moment, as my time was now taken up preparing for an external review that the University had requested. Marion had recently stepped down as research VP, to be replaced by Dr. Terry Hogan, a psychology professor. He wanted a critique of my research on DPPE, and an assessment of the clinical potential of the pilot study that had now been underway for nine months.

At issue was whether the University should continue to fund the ever-increasing patent costs for the drug. Although the prospect made me nervous, I did not think that this review was unreasonable. I'm sure I might have done the same if I were in Terry's shoes. I was reassured by the fact that Lyonel, who remained very supportive, would have a major say in the final decision.

A few months earlier, Terry and I had gotten off to a bit of a rocky start. There was need for an urgent filing of a "defensive" patent to help protect DPPE before publishing our findings that amitriptyline and fluoxetine were "DPPE-like" drugs. By naming these, and other likely "antagonists of intracellular histamine binding" in a new filing, hopefully we could prop up our DPPE patents by preventing others from filing use patents for these other agents as possible chemopotentiators. Landis Henry, who had just replaced Morris in the technology transfer office, strongly agreed with this strategy. I had discussed it with Michael Stewart, who also felt it would be a worthwhile thing to do. However, Terry had just taken up his new position and was not up to speed on my file. He would need time to review it, but could not say when he would get back to me. The trouble was, there was a looming deadline that, if missed, would greatly weaken our position.

I tried to explain this, but when Terry continued to hesitate, I told him right then and there that, if necessary, I would undertake the filing myself and pay the costs. That was my right under the agreement I had signed with the University. I realized I had set off a firecracker under his chair, but I knew what I was talking about. He had to trust me. After a long silence, he said, icily, "Go ahead.... this *one* time." I could feel his seething anger right through the phone. I thanked him and quickly hung up the receiver.[52]

A month later, Terry came to the Cancer Foundation to talk with Lyonel about various matters. I wanted to smooth things over and sought him out after the meeting. We went into the boardroom and sat down, face to face. He started the conversation: "Lorne, Lyonel and I discussed your program as part of the agenda this morning. He thinks very highly of you, as do various people at the University. I'm sure that, in time, I will too. But I'm telling you right now, *you are never again to put me in that position!*" His face was starting to turn purple as he emphasized this point, but he controlled himself.

"Terry, I am truly sorry we had to start off this way but, honestly, I really had to do what I did," I replied.

52　Years later, Janet Scholz recounted the story from her end. "Who is this guy Brandes, anyway?" he thundered after he hung up the phone. Janet just laughed.

"I understand that now. Just don't sneak up on me again, because I won't be so accommodating the next time," he responded. I nodded. We shook hands and then smiled. I decided I liked him because he told it like it was. Perhaps he felt the same about me. From then on, Terry and I enjoyed a happy and mutually-supportive relationship.

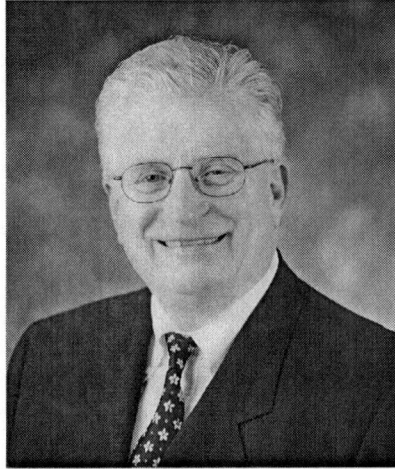

Terry Hogan (Photo courtesy of Terry Hogan)

The review took place at the end of September. Dr. Ronald Feld, an oncologist from the Princess Margaret Hospital in Toronto, was the external reviewer. Lyonel, Terry and Landis were with him in the small conference room as I presented an overview of my research. Lucky for me, it was once again funded by the NCIC. In addition, I tabled the reprint of the just-published paper in the *Journal of the National Cancer Institute*. For once, timing was on my side.

I then brought everyone up to date on the clinical study. Susie and I had now treated upwards of twenty patients. In addition to our own records, Kerry McDonald had kept detailed files on their blood counts and any side effects. We had continued to observe that the lower doses of DPPE were virtually free of side effects and appeared to protect against nausea, whereas the higher doses added some nausea and vomiting on top of the doxorubicin. It appeared to us that the patients were suffering from a form of motion sickness brought on by those higher DPPE doses. We again documented an apparent increased benefit of longer DPPE treatment times: five patients treated this way had documented shrinkage of their tumors by at least fifty percent. Four of them had breast cancer and one had thyroid cancer. Two of the patients with breast cancer had complete disappearance of all their tumors and were in what is called a complete remission.

I was not surprised that most of the responses occurred in patients with breast cancer. Doxorubicin is a tried and true drug in this disease, and can also be effective in thyroid cancer. On the other hand, it is not normally effective in colon cancer or many of the other tumors that were present in our group of patients. One of the reasons for including them in this first study was to determine whether DPPE might make doxorubicin more active against such stubborn cancers. It didn't seem to have that particular effect, but the number tested was small.

In concluding my presentation, I proposed that we move forward with a new, more structured, study combining DPPE with a chemotherapy drug that was proven effective[53] for any particular cancer we would treat. The drug would differ from patient to patient, depending on the type of tumor. Moreover, it would already have had to be used to treat the patient, and either failed to shrink the cancer, or stopped working after initially being effective. I also proposed a change in how we administered DPPE, as I felt that we were straining our resources with the seventy-two hour treatment.

When designing any type of therapy, there are often trade-offs. To succeed in the real world, we would have to make the administration of the drug simpler and prevent as many side effects as possible. From our experiments in mice, it appeared we could best

---

53   A chemotherapy drug is ordinarily considered "effective" if it shrinks cancer in at least twenty percent of patients, a value that reflects how very difficult many tumors are to treat.

succeed in shrinking tumors using the highest tolerated dose of DPPE. I planned to seek approval from Dr. Klein and our ethics committee to use the six milligrams per kilogram dose, giving it over eighty minutes, instead of one hour, as a way of taming any side effects. In addition we would add medication to prevent motion sickness and, based on Ranjan Bose's experiments, inject a short-acting Valium-type drug, called lorazepam, to prevent muscle twitching (or worse).

My presentation over, the review ended. I nervously waited for a verdict. It came quickly. Although there remained many uncertainties about the outcome, Dr. Feld and the others appeared to recognize the potential merit of what I was trying to do. It remained a chancy venture, but the University would continue to fund the patents.

CHAPTER THIRTY-TWO:

News, Views and Wall Street Blues

Even while designing the new DPPE study, the observation that amitriptyline and fluoxetine stimulated tumors continued to weigh heavily on my mind. However, before writing up the results, I decided to present the data to my colleagues. Their feedback would be important, given the implications. With everyone assembled in a conference room, I reviewed the histories and findings in the three patients that I had seen in the clinic, followed by the results of the laboratory studies that these clinical observations had engendered.

The effect on those present was obvious; all agreed that the rodent data were robust and concerning. No objections were raised over my intention of submitting a paper for publication, but Lyonel, Frank and Harvey Chochinov, a psychiatrist who primarily treated anxious and depressed cancer patients, argued against any inclusion of the anecdotal case reports in the manuscript. They suggested I write up only the rodent study and submit to a basic science journal. I had wanted to send the paper to the prestigious *New England Journal of Medicine*, because its editors often published papers that combined clinical and basic science aspects of important subjects. Carl agreed with that view. Differences of opinion notwithstanding, the group as a whole felt that human epidemiological studies[54] would be required to determine whether antidepressants might pose a similar risk to humans with cancer. I had my doubts about how such studies could be designed to test the question at hand.

To be perfectly honest, I did not anticipate a negative reaction to the inclusion in the paper of the three case reports. After all, I would not have carried out the lab studies were it not for them. Anecdotal observations in humans have led to important discoveries in the past. I went to see Georgie Hogg and Dr. Ian Morrow for their opinions. Ian, a professor of radiology, had good insight and, like Georgie, his views were worth hearing.

Both were highly supportive of including the case reports in the paper. Ian, in particular, was impressed that a clinical observation had led to the study. "That's what science is all about: you make an observation, you formulate an hypothesis and then you test it, which is exactly what you did," he mused. Georgie had the same take. I went back to Lyonel to tell him what Ian and Georgie had to say. He remained convinced that I should leave out the "human element" and write up only the rodent findings. In the end, after consulting with my two senior co-authors, Frank and Rob Warrington, I followed my intuition, included the case reports and submitted the manuscript to the *New England Journal of Medicine*. It was accompanied by a covering letter indicating why we thought it should be published there.

Three weeks later, the manuscript was returned along with a letter of rejection saying, among other things, that the paper was not judged to have wide-enough appeal to the readership. It had not even been sent out for review. Stunned, I immediately wrote a strongly worded letter to the editor, questioning the motive for

---

54 Epidemiology is the study of human populations to determine potential causes of disease and other health-related events, with the hope that any findings may be applied to prevent illness.

a blanket rejection of such potentially important findings. Did the fact that the journal carried a large amount of drug advertising play any role here? That prompted an outraged letter of response within a week. "I take great exception...." the editor scolded . The tone was so angry, I thought the letter would spontaneously combust in my hands. "It must have hit a nerve," I decided.

Undeterred, I sent the same manuscript and covering letter to *The Lancet*, a London-based publication. Next to the *New England Journal*, it is the most widely-read international journal of clinical medicine. After six weeks without a reply, I suspected that the paper had gone out for review at the very least, and was even starting to believe that I might receive a favorable response. Unfortunately, my optimism was dashed two weeks later upon receipt of a kind letter of rejection to the British tune of, "So sorry. Too many good manuscripts and too little room to publish them all." I just shook my head in disbelief, truly believing that both journals were afraid to publish the paper. "Too hot to handle," I concluded.

By chance, I saw Harvey Chochinov in the hospital corridor that afternoon and filled him in on what had transpired. In his gentlemanly way, he refrained from saying, "I told you so," but took the opportunity to once again give me his advice. "The data deserve to be published, but take out those case reports and send it to a basic research journal. I understand that they led you to do the studies, but they get in the way. Including them could even suggest that you may have a bias in interpreting your results," he counseled. I hadn't considered the latter point, but the results were so obvious that, in my opinion, they left little room for bias, mine or anyone else's. I promised him I would reconsider. There was no point in further discussion with Lyonel, as he had already made his opinion clear.

The following week, I temporarily put my frustrations aside. Jill and I flew to sunny and warm Torremolinos for our second annual European Histamine Research Society meeting. Walter Schunack and I were each to give a major lecture named in honor of the late British histamine researcher, Dr. Geoffrey West, the founder of the society.

That year was the 500th anniversary of the discovery of the New World by Christopher Columbus. To commemorate the event, and as a gesture of thanks to Manuel Garcia-Caballero and my other Spanish hosts, I had asked Patty, who hailed from Santiago, Chile, to translate my opening remarks into Spanish. I practiced the words phonetically for weeks. The laughter and applause that greeted my surprise opening undoubtedly resulted more from my fractured pronunciation of that beautiful romantic tongue than any humor in the remarks themselves. Nonetheless, the old adage, "You can fool some of the people some of the time…" proved true, as the other unilingual English-speaking attendees at the meeting were mightily impressed. Madeleine Ennis, a colleague from Belfast, wrote in the official meeting report, "In an attempt to prove that people from North America are not illiterate, he began his talk in what sounded like fluent Spanish!"

Wishing a further chance to obtain critical feedback from my scientific peers, I took the opportunity during my thirty minutes to present the antidepressant data, sans case reports, with emphasis on the correlation between the ability of the two drugs to compete for the binding of DPPE and histamine in the microsomes and nuclei, and to accelerate tumor growth. Much discussion ensued after the presentation. Pier Mannaioni, Börje Uvnäs, Wilfried Lorenz and Manuel, all physician/researchers, and Henk Timmerman, an expert on drug chemistry and pharmacology, shared my concerns about the findings and were eager to know when and where the work would be published. I told them that I hoped to have that issue sorted out soon, but spared the gory details of my two recent disastrous attempts with the *New England Journal of Medicine* and *The Lancet*.

Science aside, the meeting was punctuated by wonderful excursions to the caves of Nerja and the Alhambra Palace, planned by our hosts, and the eating of fresh seafood at little open-air restaurants lining the beach. The most memorable moment came, once again, at the final banquet. Anita Sydbom, the Swedish member who penned those new verses for the official *Polly Wolly Doodle* song and led the singing, had to leave the meeting early for family reasons and could not attend the banquet. Nonetheless, she dutifully faxed Pier a copy of her latest yearly addition to the anthem. Come time for the song, the piano player was poised and ready to play. However, without Anita, Pier was at a loss as to what to do until someone yelled out that Jill had a great voice. She took the copy from a relieved Pier, went to the microphone and led the group in the song. From that time on, Pier conscripted her for the yearly sing-along. Such is the price of talent.

As soon as we arrived back in Winnipeg, I pressed into action to get our paper published. I knew it was time to quit fighting City Hall about including the case reports, but worried that such potentially important findings could be "buried" in a purely research journal. I strongly believed that epidemiologists, regulatory authorities and doctors in clinical practice needed to know about this issue. To that end, I devised a three-part plan of action.

First, I rewrote the paper, concentrating purely on the science, and sent it to *Cancer Research*, requesting that it be considered for *Advances in Brief*, a journal category reserved for accelerated review and publication of papers reporting important new findings. I personally called Margaret (Marge) Foti, the managing editor with whom I was long-acquainted, to tell her that it was coming her way. She agreed to an expedited review. To my great relief, within a few short weeks the paper was accepted without the need for revision. It would appear in the July 1, 1992, issue.

With that problem solved, I wrote a letter to the editor of the widely-read *American Journal of Epidemiology*. In it, I outlined the historical studies that had raised a possible link between depression and cancer, and referenced our research results with the two antidepressant drugs. I ended by suggesting that epidemiology studies be initiated to determine whether the actual link with cancer incidence or growth might be the taking of antidepressant medication. Within a few weeks I received notice that the letter was accepted for publication. I was especially pleased by this, believing that the results now would be noticed by an important group of researchers who, hopefully, would heed my request.

Finally, I contacted Agnes in Ottawa, telling her of my concerns and then sending her a copy of the *Cancer Research* manuscript. I asked her to feel free to share the information, on a confidential basis, with her colleagues in the Bureau and in the FDA. My thinking was that federal regulators should know about the impending publication so that they could examine the data and be in a position to comment, if asked. All too often I had witnessed TV interviews of health officials who stumbled when trying to answer questions about a new development of which they were unaware. I did not want that to happen in this case. Agnes was grateful for the advance notice and assured me that she would review the paper and discuss the findings with regulators on both sides of the border.

True to her word, she brought the data to the attention of Dr. Gregory Burke, a former pediatric cancer specialist and head of the FDA's oncology division in Bethesda. Ironically, for bureaucratic reasons, his section was also responsible for the regulation of antihistamines. Dr. Burke called me at home shortly thereafter. We were quickly on a first name basis. He shared with me his longtime concern about the possible implications for humans of liver and other tumors that often developed in mice and rats chronically dosed with various pharmaceuticals, including antihistamines. These tests for carcinogenicity were now routinely mandated as part of the preclinical toxicology assessment of all new drugs.

Tumor development had been such a common "low-level" phenomenon over the years that many regulators did not get concerned unless the incidence with any given drug was significantly higher than the usual "background noise". The general consensus was that many of the observed tumors were specific to mice and rats and not representative of the human situation. Greg was not so sure that this was a wise position and felt that our binding studies and other tests might form a basis on which to evaluate drugs in a different way, to see whether they might stimulate tumor growth even though not themselves carcinogens.

"Would you be willing to meet with some of our people at the FDA and give a talk?" he inquired.

"Of course," I replied.

Taking the "Frank walk" to report on these latest developments, I arrived to find him in his usual mode, sitting at the desk reading the latest issue of *Science*. In addition to the biological sciences, the magazine usually included papers on physics or mathematics, or the latest findings on tectonic movements and other geological and astrophysical phenomena. None of the latter were particularly interesting to us. However, we both liked a popular section called *News and Views*, where medical or science journalists reported on hot new developments or issues of general interest. Their stories were written in everyday language for the edification of non-experts in the field. This day, I noted that Frank was reading a *News and Views* story about the genetic control of metabolism.

Suddenly, I had an idea. "What would you think if I called *Science* to see if they would be interested in writing a story about the findings in our *Cancer Research* paper?" I asked. Frank thought it would be worth trying. I went back to my office with one of his copies of a recent issue of the magazine. One of the editors of the *News and Views* section was Jean Marx. I had read many of her reports and found them to be well-written and, often, illuminating. I took a chance and called the number for the editorial department listed in the journal.

As luck would have it, she was in. I introduced myself and told her my reason for calling. She appeared interested. "What journal did you say is publishing your paper?" she asked.

"*Cancer Research*," I replied.

"Never heard of it. Is it peer-reviewed?" *Wow. That one really came out of left field. At Science, it's like "New York and the rest of the world".*

"Yes. It's the official journal of the American Association for Cancer Research. It's widely read by people in the field," I answered nonchalantly, as if hers were an everyday question.

Satisfied, she asked for details. "I'll speak to my editor and get back to you," she promised.

Jean called the next day while I was in my clinic. Could I send a copy of the galley proof for them to read? I faxed her the paper. Two days later she called for more background, and to tell me that she was writing up our findings for *News and Views*. It would appear in *Science* on July 3, two days after the *Cancer Research* paper was published. I was delighted and Frank was impressed. However, I was not prepared for what happened next.

The night before our paper was to appear in print, Jill and I were at Lyonel's house for dinner. A visiting professor had come to town and was being entertained. Esther Israels, herself an internationally-recognized expert in blood coagulation, had made her favorite lasagna recipe and was just taking the food out of the oven when the phone rang. Lyonel answered it. A moment later he motioned for me to come over. Covering the receiver with his hand, he said softly, "It's for you....the *Wall Street Journal*." I turned white.

All eyes were on me as I listened to the person at the other end. He identified himself as Thomas Burton, a reporter. He apologized for interrupting my evening, but had called my home and was told where to reach me. Having just read Jean Marx' article, entitled, "*Do Antidepressants Promote Tumors?*" in a pre-released copy of *Science*[55], he wanted to ask me some questions.

---

55   It is not unusual for prominent medical and scientific journals to give the press an early look at the next issue so that any interesting paper or story can be quickly researched and reported by the media. It's also good for circulation and "impact rating", a measure of a journal's influence on other scientists who read its contents and then refer to the papers when writing their own manuscripts for publication. An embargo is almost always imposed on reporters by the journals so that no story can be released to the public until the evening before, or day of, publication.

"What are the trade names for fluoxetine and amitriptyline?" Burton inquired. I knew immediately where this story was going.

"Can you confirm the following facts about your study?" he asked, quoting several statements that Ms. Marx had written in her report.

"Yes, that is all correct," I answered. Finished with his questions, he thanked me for my time and told me it was quite a story. *Oh, my. Oh, my.* And I had once fretted that, if the study was published in a basic science journal, it would be invisible?

Once off the phone, Jill and the others peppered me with their own questions about what had just transpired. "I have a strong feeling that this will hit the fan tomorrow," I lamented.

"You simply published what you found," Jill said reassuringly. Esther and the others agreed. Lyonel just smiled and nodded. He understood that the findings were entirely consistent with what I had observed with DPPE. I think he was proud of his protégé.

C H A P T E R   T H I R T Y - T H R E E :

Aftermath

Coming on the heels of our *Cancer Research* paper, Jean Marx'
Science story had a powerful impact and, based on the number of
phone messages and letters I received for the next several months,
a wide audience. The depth of her reporting was impressive. She
had even gone so far as to interview Agnes Klein, who said that
our work was "interesting" and "well done", and Greg Burke, who
was quoted as agreeing that "he too was interested" and "had
invited [Brandes] to FDA headquarters to discuss his results".
From their comments, it appeared that, in this instance, giving the
drug regulators a "heads-up" was a good idea.

_____DRUG REGULATION_____

Do Antidepressants Promote Tumors?

As if cancer patients don't already have enough to worry about, a new animal study conducted by a team of Canadian researchers has raised a disturbing possibility. The study, which is published in the 1 July issue of *Cancer Research*, shows that two widely used antidepressants, Elavil and Prozac, act as "tumor promoters" in rats and mice. That means that the drugs, although they are not carcinogens by themselves, accelerate the growth of existing tumors in those animals.

While there's currently no evidence that the antidepressants promote tumor growth in humans, the new results are troublesome because cancer patients are more likely to suffer from depression—and thus to be prescribed antidepressant drugs—than members of the general population. Says oncologist Lorne Brandes of the Manitoba Institute of Cell Biology in Winnipeg, the leader of the team that did the work: "I think that the antidepressants are valuable drugs. But the message is disturbing, and there's no way around that."

Indeed, officials at both Canada's Health Protection Branch and the U.S. Food and Drug Administration (FDA) are taking a look at the Brandes group's results. Agnes Klein, chief of the Health Protection Branch's

Oncology Division, characterizes the work as "interesting" and "well done," although she declined to comment on what action, if any, her agency is considering. And Gregory Burke, director of the FDA's Division of Oncology and Pulmonary Drug Products, says he too is interested, because the Brandes team's results bear on the wider issues of how tumor promoters work and how to assess the cancer risks of such compounds. At present, for example, carcinogen screens aren't set up to detect promoters. "The agency and the whole world are trying to design better tests," says Burke, who has invited Brandes to FDA headquarters to discuss his results.

Brandes and his colleagues decided to undertake the animal studies as an outgrowth of their research on an intracellular receptor known as the "anti-estrogen binding site" (AEBS), which was identified by Robert Sutherland and his colleagues at the Ludwig Institute in Sydney, Australia, on the basis of its ability to bind Tamoxifen, the anti-estrogen drug used to treat breast cancer. The Manitoba group wanted to pin down the role the AEBS plays in the cell, and to do this they needed a compound that would bind specifically to the receptor and tweak its activity. Tamoxifen itself wasn't suitable be-

cause it also binds to the estrogen receptor and has other cellular effects as well. But the researchers thought that by tinkering with Tamoxifen's structure they might be able to come up with a specific AEBS binder. They eventually hit on a compound called DPPE that seemed to fit the bill.

DPPE proved to have several effects on cell growth, including stimulation of tumor growth in rats and mice. And Brandes noticed something else as well: DPPE is structurally similar to the antihistamines, which led the researcher to suggest that all or part of the AEBS might be a novel type of histamine receptor, an idea supported by further work. Previously discovered histamine receptors mediate allergic reactions, among other things, but not cell growth.

But the antihistamines aren't the only compounds that DPPE resembles. It is also structurally similar to antidepressants, including Elavil and Prozac. And since DPPE proved to have tumor-promoting activity in rodents, the question then was, might the antidepressants have similar activity. The answer, according to the current study, is yes. The researchers found, for example, that when they used the chemical carcinogen known as DMBA to induce mammary tumors in rats, animals treated with either antidepressant, in doses comparable to those given to human patients, developed the cancers both more rapidly and in greater numbers than controls. That led Brandes to ask one of the paper's co-authors, cell biologist Robert Warrington of the University of Saskatchewan in Saskatoon, to test the drugs in another cancer model in which melanoma cells are transplanted into mice; they also stimulated the growth of those cells. Brandes suggests the drugs are promoting tumor growth by virtue of their ability to bind to the intracellular histamine receptor.

What everyone agrees are needed now are more studies. "It would be interesting to see if the [intracellular histamine] receptor has the activity in human cells," says FDA's Burke. If it does, the information might be helpful in designing better screening tests.

It would also heighten concerns about antidepressants. Brandes calls for epidemiological studies aimed at determining how the fates of cancer patients who take the antidepressants compare to those of patients who don't. Although some previous studies have indicated that depressed individuals are at higher risk of developing cancer than people who aren't depressed, other studies haven't shown any differences between the two groups. Brandes says, however, that none of these studies appeared to take antidepressant use into account. And then there's the question of whether any of the antihistamines might themselves be tumor promoters. As Burke says, "[Brandes] has a lot of interesting experiments to do."

–Jean Marx

Jean Marx' Science story reporting our findings with amitriptyline and fluoxetine

Not unexpectedly, the *Wall Street Journal* article was somewhat more narrowly focused on the implications for the pharmaceutical industry. Emphasizing the results with fluoxetine, to which he then continually referred as Prozac, Tom Burton's story, entitled, "*Tumor Growth In Mice Linked With 2 Drugs*", obviously got under the skin of the powers-that-be at Eli Lilly. He quoted a Lilly vice-president as saying, disparagingly, that our study was "not predictive of anything". This was followed by the comment, "We don't know what these studies are good for." Perhaps they didn't, but several market analysts in New York had an inkling. They called, wanting my opinion about the impact of the study on market share for Prozac and other antidepressants. I told all of them that I was a scientist and had no intention of "going there".

Harvey Chochinov was among the first of my colleagues to contact me, saying how pleased he was to see the paper published at last. At a recent international meeting, he had shared his own concerns about the data with some fellow psychiatrists who specialized in treating depressed cancer patients. Among them was the pioneering Dr. Jimmie Holland of the Memorial Sloan-Kettering Cancer Center in New York. She called me soon after. "How does it feel to be in the eye of the storm?" she asked.

"The eye is always calm, as am I," I replied. Appearing to enjoy my answer, Dr. Holland assured me that the findings were being taken seriously and would be followed up. I felt better for her call.

Soon, stories and editorials reporting on our work were popping up in various psychiatric publications. I went out of my way in interviews to explain that I had no hidden agenda, that I believed that antidepressant drugs were valuable in the treatment of depression, but that this potential downside had to be explored. I was relieved that, apart from the expected defensive statements from drug companies, the response of the scientific and medical community was overwhelmingly one of concern and support. "Keep doing those studies," was the comment I heard most often from doctors and the public alike.

In September, I made my long-anticipated visit to the FDA, meeting with Greg Burke and Dr. Joe DeGeorge, the agency's associate director of pharmacology and toxicology. One topic discussed at length was the "bell-shaped" dose response for DNA synthesis we had described with amitriptyline and fluoxetine. The finding suggested the possibility that low to middle doses of the drugs might have a stimulatory effect on cancer growth, while doses above or below might have no effect or, in the case of very high doses, an inhibitory effect. This would possibly make it difficult to detect an overall detrimental effect of a drug in people who might be prescribed different doses of the same drug, or whose metabolism might differ significantly (faster or slower) such that the same drug dose might be high for one person, but low for another.

We all agreed that the bell phenomenon was most likely indicative of a "biphasic dose response", meaning that a substance has opposing effects at different concentrations or doses. Historical examples are the female hormones, estrogen and progesterone: low doses of each, as are given with hormone replacement therapy (HRT), stimulate breast cancer growth, while high doses inhibit, or even kill, breast cancer cells. Indeed, for many years before the discovery of tamoxifen, diethylstilbesterol (DES), a synthetic estrogen, was used in high doses by oncologists to treat women with advanced breast cancer that had spread (metastasized). High doses of a progesterone derivative, megestrol acetate (Megace), are still sometimes prescribed in similar circumstances. Greg himself had found multiple reports of biphasic effects of drugs and substances on cancer growth in the scientific literature.[56] Thus, it appeared that our "non-linear" dose response with the antidepressant drugs were consistent with what had been observed for many other compounds.

Greg had also set up a meeting with the epidemiologists at the FDA. That proved a very interesting exercise. I made it clear

---

56   In the months that followed, he would fax me a copy of a paper each time he found another example.

to those assembled that we did not think that either drug was a carcinogen, that is, neither caused cancer to develop. Although amitriptyline came along at a time when drugs were not routinely tested for carcinogenicity, fluoxetine had been tested and declared a non-carcinogen. What I was concerned about was the "DPPE issue", the possibility that these, and other chemically-similar drugs, might stimulate underlying cancer to grow faster.

A roundtable discussion ensued as to how this hypothesis could be tested on humans. One of the epidemiology team had an idea. "We identify depressed cancer patients and ask them to enter a trial comparing treatment with an antidepressant or a placebo," he suggested.

"That would be unethical," interjected another. "You cannot morally withhold an antidepressant from a depressed patient."

"If patients don't know whether they are taking the active drug or placebo, that is not immoral. After all, we know that placebos are effective in approximately one-third of people who take them, whether for depression, blood pressure control or almost any other condition," opined yet another.[57]

From that point on, the discussion appeared to go around in circles. Greg got in the last word (or words) when he asked, "And what would the consent form for any proposed study say?" It was obviously a rhetorical question, as he quickly answered it himself: "You have been diagnosed with cancer and depression. The purpose of this study is to determine whether, as compared to a placebo, your cancer will grow or spread faster if you are prescribed an antidepressant drug." He then paused and asked the group, "Who would want to participate in a study like that? And what ethics committee would approve it?" Sobered by his assessment, all the participants agreed that further thought would have to be given on how to proceed. Rather than a forward-looking study, perhaps a large retrospective chart review of thousands of

---

57 Often, drugs are only a few percent more effective than a placebo. However, if enough patients are tested, small differences can be statistically significant....enough to win regulatory approval.

patients with cancer, looking at the drugs they were taking, could be mounted. Thanking them, I left the room with Greg.

"After hearing that discussion, I am very pessimistic that epidemiological studies will ever be able to test the question of tumor stimulation," I lamented. I also knew that a so-called retrospective chart review was one of the weakest methods of looking for a cause and effect in any disease, let alone what we had described. "I tend to agree with you," Greg said, adding, "it may be impossible to separate out a tumor-accelerating effect of a specific drug when so many people are taking other medications at the same time."[58]

The end of the afternoon was taken up with the talk I had prepared. The FDA lecture room was quite large. This time the crowd numbered in the several hundreds. I had no idea whether there was always a full room for visiting lecturers, or whether it was because of the "controversial nature" of my topic. All having assembled, Greg introduced me by saying that I and my subject needed little introduction. I was very discomfited by this apparent "notoriety", especially as Greg had candidly told me in earlier phone conversations that there would be a lot of skeptics in the room. Even more candidly, he had informed me that his worry about the occurrence of tumors in rodents chronically dosed with drugs was not shared by many in the FDA. In other words, he was an outrider. "Join the club," I had told him.

Over the allotted hour, I detailed the results of our histamine research, emphasizing the effects of DPPE on tumor growth that had led us to examine this same phenomenon in amitriptyline and fluoxetine, but steered clear of the human case reports that initiated my interest in the first place. I was still smarting from the rejection by the two clinical journals and didn't want to antagonize this crowd if I could help it. "Just stick to the laboratory facts," Lyonel had counseled me before my visit. This time, I took his sage advice.

---

58   The concern that human epidemiology studies would not specifically address the issue in question (stimulation of existing cancer) was borne out in the studies that followed.

Scanning the audience during my presentation, I detected cynical looks and what can only be described as a lack of involvement in what I had to say. Save for the sounds of chairs moving back and people getting up, the atmosphere remained muted as everyone filed out after my presentation. Few, if any questions, had been asked. As Greg might have predicted, my data did not seem to have much of an impact on those present. The FDA regulators appeared unimpressed. Once again I was swimming against the tide. "Another alarmist heard from," I said to myself as I shuffled together all my overhead transparencies and put them back into my small business suitcase.

A week or so after I returned to Winnipeg, a little certificate arrived in the mail. Mounted in a leatherette folder embossed on the front with the official seal of the FDA, it commemorated the date of my visit and the title of my presentation. Greg had kindly sent it to me as a gesture of his appreciation. He and I continued to stay in close touch thereafter.

We both suspected it would not be the last the FDA heard from this "alarmist". I had told him that our lab had begun testing some common allergy-fighting antihistamines and I was not happy with what I was observing. Soon it would be time to call Rob Warrington......

CHAPTER THIRTY-FOUR:
The Premier Saves The Day

Over the next few months, it was a constant juggling act: overseeing the new tumor studies with antihistamines, collaborating with Frank on the P450 enzymes, making ever more DPPE and gearing up for the second clinical study. The first trial ended after we had treated twenty-five patients. It was now time to move forward. I had my approval from Agnes and Ivo to use the six milligrams per kilogram dose of DPPE over eighty minutes, followed by the chemotherapy drug over the last twenty minutes of the DPPE infusion. The patients would be pre-medicated with ondansetron, a very effective drug to prevent nausea. They would also receive lorazepam, based on Ranjan's experiments in mice. Once again, Susie would oversee treatment in the chemotherapy room. She would monitor and fine-tune the intravenous drug administration as we gained experience with each new patient.

Sadly, John Maclean died suddenly of a heart attack before the new protocol cleared his ethics committee. He was only sixty-four and had been suffering from severe coronary artery disease that was not amenable to bypass surgery. I soon met with his replacement, Dr. Gordon Grahame, a gastrointestinal specialist in the medical faculty, and brought him up to speed on what had been going on for the past two years. Gordon, not normally given to hyperbole, let alone small talk, was amazed. The idea that a cancer drug was being developed locally really caught his fancy. After reviewing the application, he approved the trial on the condition that I combine DPPE only with approved chemotherapy drugs and not exceed their usual dose range. "No problem," I assured him.

Everything was in place to start in July, 1992. The first patient was Arnold Brown, a well-respected former politician in the province's governing Progressive Conservative (Tory) party, and mentor to its leader, Premier Gary Filmon. A fine organist who once owned a music store, Arnold had represented the riding of Rhineland, which included his home town of Winkler. This predominantly Mennonite community, south-west of Winnipeg, is well-known for its close family ties and entrepreneurial spirit. Arnold had advanced colon cancer. After a year of therapy with two commonly-used drugs, 5-fluorouracil (5-FU) and leucovorin (a vitamin-like substance), the disease spread to his liver, causing pain and jaundice. We would now substitute DPPE for the leucovorin and continue the 5-FU.

Much to our relief, the eighty-minute treatment went well. There was no nausea or vomiting as Arnold, drowsy from the intravenous lorazepam, slept for an hour or two. When he awoke, he felt slightly drunk and had some muscle incoordination. However, within another two hours he had recovered sufficiently that his wife, Katie, was able to take him home by car. He called the next day to report that he went to bed as soon as he got home and woke up that morning feeling fine. Within a week, repeat blood tests showed that his liver function tests were better and his jaundice resolved. A "tumor marker"[59] test called CEA, which stands

---

59   Tumor markers are chemicals produced by cancerous tumors that can be monitored in the blood to detect tumor growth or shrinkage. Another example of a tumor marker is the PSA test in prostate cancer.

for "carcinoembryonic antigen", had decreased significantly. His white blood cell count was fine. He was a happy camper, ready for his second treatment.

With my busy oncology practice continuously generating new cases, over the ensuing months we quickly accumulated patients into the new study. Amazingly, Arnold continued to respond to his treatment, which we were now administering to him three out of every four weeks. His quality of life remarkably improved, he was once again a regular visitor to his party's caucus room in the legislature. But Arnold was not the only one doing well. By my reckoning, two-thirds of the patients were responding with shrinkage of their tumors or stabilization of their disease. Given that they had previously worsened on the same chemotherapy drugs without DPPE, I was becoming optimistic that what we had observed in mice was happening in humans. Susie got busier and busier, but she loved the challenge. The patients' charts were getting thicker and thicker, always a good sign.

Susie was soon a firm believer that a lot of people were benefiting from the treatment. In addition to her own assessments, many of her subjects had told her of their improved symptoms. This was important, because experience suggests that patients are often much more candid with nursing staff than their physicians about how they are faring. The other chemotherapy nurses, led by Nancy Johnson, also cheered us on. They too believed that something good was happening. I told Nancy repeatedly that I did not want her staff to be wasting their time; they had enough to do with all the standard treatments they were administering. "Keep going. We'll be the first to tell you if we don't think DPPE is working out," Nancy assured me in response to my constant ruminating. Her support meant a lot to me. Nobody knew the landscape better than Nancy and her staff.

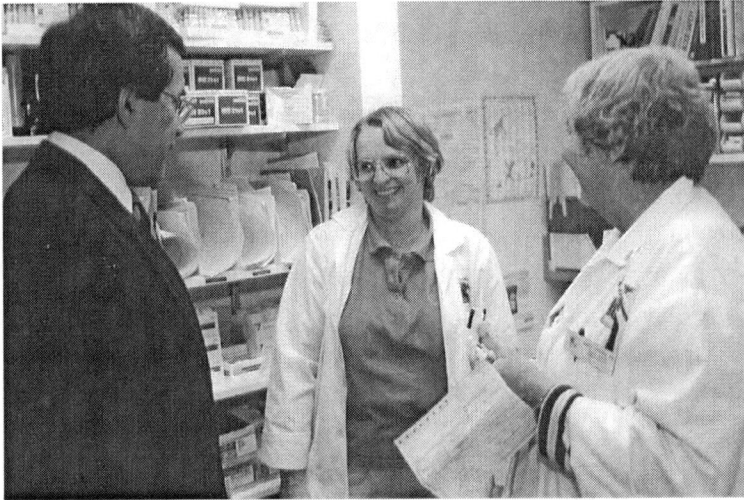

Premier Gary Filmon, Susie Bracken (centre) and Nancy Johnson (CancerCare Manitoba Archive)

As an added benefit, the side effects of the chemotherapy drugs that we combined with DPPE, such as low blood counts and hair loss, appeared to be much less than we would normally have anticipated with the drugs alone. This was all the more impressive because we were treating many patients for up to three weeks in a row, rather than the more usual schedule of once every three weeks! Since many of the chemo drugs had a much shorter half-life[60] in the blood than doxorubicin, I reasoned that DPPE was now more effective to protect the normal cells. In other words, it was a matter of DPPE "outlasting" a particular chemotherapy drug; if that happened, the toxic effects on the bone marrow and hair follicles should be diminished.

---

60 The half-life means the time it takes for fifty percent of the drug to disappear from the bloodstream. This usually occurs as a result of metabolism by the liver and excretion by the kidneys. Doxorubicin has a half-life of over twenty-four hours. We subsequently determined that the half-life of DPPE was eleven hours. That could explain why DPPE was less effective to prevent falling blood counts and hair loss in our first pilot study.

Everything was proceeding smoothly until one day I was asked to meet with our new CEO, Dr. Brent Schacter. After over twenty years at the helm, Lyonel had recently stepped down, but continued his research and writing. Brent, a longtime colleague in the department, strongly supported the DPPE project but was having fiscal problems. This was a time of ballooning federal and provincial deficits. Budget cutbacks were deemed a major part of the solution. As a result, the Canadian universal medicare system, so widely admired at home and abroad, was becoming seriously underfunded. Health administrators were forced to rationalize institutional spending in an attempt to pare down the red ink. My program was experimental and the government had a policy of not funding such therapies. It was all they could manage to pay for approved treatments. Moreover, some of the hospital bean counters were not at all supportive of the DPPE study, believing that it sapped scarce resources.

Luckily, board chairman Arnold Portigal had an idea with which Brent readily agreed. Arnold had direct access to Gary Filmon and set up a meeting with him in his office at the legislature to discuss our dilemma. As it turned out, the premier did not need to be swayed. He knew only too well about DPPE from Arnold Brown and thought that the turnaround in his mentor's condition had been miraculous. Like everyone, he knew that the improvement would not last forever, but it was all about buying good-quality time and Arnold clearly fit that bill. The premier also had first-hand knowledge of how cancer affects families. His wife, Janice, was herself a very public breast cancer survivor.

"Leave it with me," he assured Mr. Portigal. Shortly after, a letter arrived on Brent's desk from the Deputy Minister of Health. In a move unprecedented in the country's history, the Manitoba government had approved funding for DPPE, an experimental treatment, to the tune of a quarter of a million dollars over three years! In addition to taking care of all the additional costs, such as pharmacy preparation of the DPPE powder, it would also pay for Susie's salary. She could now devote full time to treating the patients on the study. Another nurse would be hired to take her place to administer regular chemotherapy treatments.

Years later, after leaving office, Gary told me that he had absolutely no qualms about using taxpayers' dollars to support my study. He had tapped discretionary monies for the financing and acted swiftly, believing that I was striving for the good of cancer patients in the province, offering some hope where none existed. Always a "big picture" politician, he was also delighted by the prospect that, if DPPE was ultimately successful, patients far beyond Manitoba's borders would benefit from a drug developed here. I cannot emphasize strongly enough that, had he not come up with the money, the clinical development of DPPE would not have moved forward. The government's top bureaucrat had saved the day.....big time.

CHAPTER THIRTY-FIVE:

Going It Alone

Between being busy in the lab and the clinic, the weeks and months passed in a flash. Before I knew it, 1993 was winding down. It was hard to ignore Mother Nature's signs that this was so. The days were getting shorter as the wispy white clouds of late summer quickly gave way to the roiling grey-black skies of October. Autumn is a short season in this part of the world. The wind soon develops a frigid nip all too predictive of the snow that usually comes by early November. That prospect always makes most prairie kids happy, as they excitedly sharpen their skate blades and wrap fresh black tape around their sticks in readiness for the next hockey season. Having grown up in southern Ontario, where the weather is usually much milder, I never shared their enthusiasm for winter temperatures that can stay below zero for days or even weeks at a time. Every January, Jill and I took comfort in visiting my folks at their condo in south Florida, where I relished telling people that spring comes to Winnipeg when the snow finally wears out, rather than melts.

That fall, I had little time to fret about the impending inclement weather as Susie and I poured over the numbers of our second study. In addition to the usual clinic charts containing my documentation of each visit, she kept her own meticulous flow sheets and graphs outlining the details of every treatment, side effect and blood count. Incredibly, in the preceding eighteen months we had treated forty-eight patients in this second trial. Not only that, but Keith Simons, a co-author of the histamine paper in *Science*, had lent his expertise by measuring DPPE levels in the blood at various times during the treatment.[61]

Based on Keith's findings, Rob Warrington was then able to show that, at the specific level achieved in the patients' blood, DPPE increased, by almost ten times, the cancer killing effect of two different chemotherapy drugs, even in tumor cells that had developed gene mutations that made them resistant to the drugs. This was a very important observation, because cancer cells all too frequently become resistant to chemotherapy. The term for them is "MDR+" (multiple drug resistant). As a result of one common mutation, the abnormal DNA sends out signals to increase the production of a cell protein called the P-glycoprotein (P-gp) pump.

The P-gp pump is really a sophisticated, energized "pore", or tiny hole, in the cell wall that acts as an ejection device to quickly rid the cell of chemicals and drugs. When resistant cells make many more of these pumps, the chemotherapy drugs are rapidly expelled before they can damage or kill the cells. However, the clinker in Rob's data was that, although DPPE helped chemotherapy to kill these MDR+ cancer cells, it didn't seem to do so by taming the P-gp pumps. There appeared to be some unknown mechanism at work here.

Science aside, the most impressive aspect of the study was the number of patients who were still alive, including Arnold Brown. Although the "DPPE miracle", as he called it, had finally come to an end that July, almost exactly one year after he was first treated,

---

61   The scientific term for this is "pharmacokinetics".

he remained active. He was now slowly failing, but determined to keep going as long as he could. In addition to Arnold, several other patients with colon cancer also responded to the combination of DPPE and 5-fluorouracil. The most significant tumor shrinkage was again seen in women with breast cancer who received DPPE combined with a variety of single chemotherapy drugs. We also numbered among the responders, patients with hard to treat melanoma, advanced ovarian cancer and a form of inner chest wall cancer called mesothelioma. It was hard to argue with those kind of findings.

After tabulating hundreds of blood counts, it was also apparent that, despite the intensity of our treatments, the infection-fighting white cells were generally higher than would be expected. However, this was only a phase two study that did not have a control group of patients treated with the same chemo drugs but not DPPE. A phase 3 study that has this type of control group would be needed to know for sure.

One peculiar side effect of DPPE we observed was a type of "drug trip" experienced by ten patients. They reported seeing people who appeared to be cartoon characters, or hearing family members talk to them despite the fact that none were present. We had a preview of this phenomenon in our first study, where one of the patients thought he heard a non-existent radio playing. For some reason, this side effect, which was regarded as harmless or even humorous by most who experienced it, usually only occurred with the first DPPE treatment. Unfortunately, the term that describes this phenomenon is "hallucination", one with negative connotations for doctors and regulators alike. We would have to go out of our way to reassure them about the mild hallucinatory experiences with DPPE.

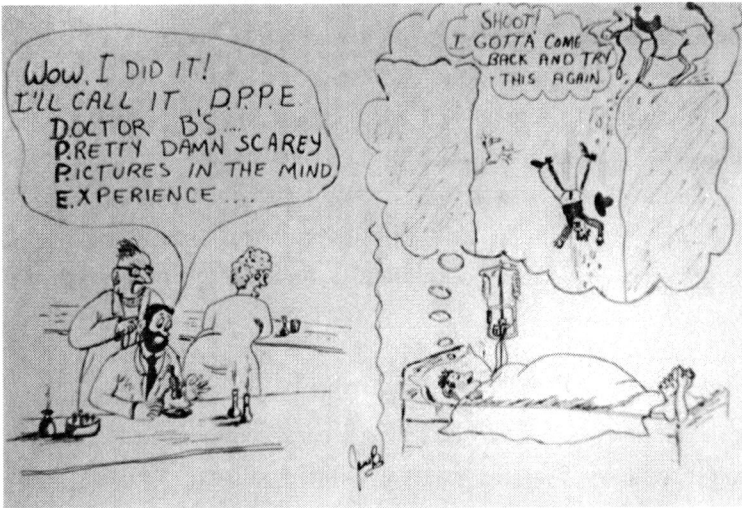

A patient's wife presented me with this clever cartoon that she had drawn
(Personal photo collection)

After reviewing the results, I decided to go for broke and submit the report of the study to the *Journal of Clinical Oncology* (*JCO*), the publication most widely read by doctors who treat cancer. My co-authors included Susie, Keith and Rob. While all three had made highly important contributions to the trial, I was especially delighted to have Rob on the "masthead" of this clinical paper, given his pioneering work with L-histidinol.

Much to my chagrin, a few weeks later the manuscript was returned, accompanied by five pages of criticism. The long and short of it was that the paper was perceived to have so many flaws that it was rejected "in its current form". Nonetheless, perhaps out of respect for what we were trying to accomplish without any drug company or clinical trials group support, the editor left the door open to a revision if we could satisfactorily address the myriad of concerns raised by the two referees....a daunting chore by any measure.

Somewhat depressed by the Herculean effort that would be required, I spent the next weekend combing over every point of contention. As hard as it was for me to read the litany of comments, they were all fair ball. After several false starts at answering them, I put down my pencil. I just didn't know where to begin and was about to give up in despair. "Do you want this paper published in *JCO*?" an inner voice suddenly asked.

"You bet I do," I answered.

"Then get down to it and make every change requested," came the inner command. Two days and a cramped left hand later, the rewriting was done.

In addition to the revised paper, part of the process required a formal letter of reply from me, addressing each criticism and indicating the remedy taken in the revised manuscript. "The letter could be longer than the original paper," I told my secretary. I was joking. In this case it wasn't. "Having carefully reviewed the criticisms of the referees, I agree with all of them and have made every change requested. As a result, I believe that the revision is much better than the original paper," I wrote. Actually, I now really did believe that. It *was* much better. A few weeks later, I had my answer. I think that the editor and reviewers were all in shock at the magnitude of the improvement. "We agree with Dr. Brandes that the paper is significantly improved," was the general consensus. It had been accepted!

Elated by this turn of events, I decided to call Dr. Lee Schacter, director of clinical research at Bristol-Myers. We had met a few months earlier in Winnipeg when I gave a seminar on DPPE in the pharmacology department. He had been visiting on business and took in my talk. Afterwards, he came up to me to say that the work was very interesting. "Your company certainly doesn't think so," I retorted. He was taken aback by the poorly disguised anger in my voice. Although my statement was true, I quickly regretted the tone of my reply as he had not been a party to what had happened previously and seemed a genuinely nice guy. In part, I was now calling to apologize to him for my curtness.

"Lee, I wonder whether Bristol-Myers might take another look at DPPE," I said after my opening mea culpa. It was obvious that

Julius Vida had no clinical information to go on when he nixed the file; drug companies constantly re-examine potential business propositions. Telling Lee that I now had some potentially exciting clinical results, I offered to send him a copy of the *JCO* manuscript. He said he would be pleased to read it and get back to me.

A week or two later, Lee called back. "I truly wish I could help you but there is not yet sufficient interest from the company in your data," he reported. Then he quickly added, "If it is of any consolation, I personally remain very interested in your concept and would be happy to keep in touch." Then, unexpectedly, he gave me the name of a new oncology-oriented drug company, called Sparta Pharmaceuticals, that I might contact. It was based in the Research Triangle Park area outside Raleigh-Durham, close to where Lyonel and I had visited Burroughs Wellcome. I had never heard of Sparta, but I thanked him for the lead.

Nuts! I was still on my own. But Lee's response was genuine, indicating that he could be a potential conduit to Bristol-Myers. To ultimately succeed with that pharmaceutical company, or any other for that matter, I clearly needed to generate results of "strategic interest", to use industry parlance. After giving the situation some thought, a new approach took hold in my mind. There were several possibilities, but I decided to focus on two specific and common tumors: breast and prostate cancer.

The first choice was easy, as we had accumulated evidence in the first two studies that DPPE appeared to be adding something significant to chemotherapy in women whose breast tumors had metastasized. In our new study, we would once again combine it with our old friend, doxorubicin, one of the most powerful breast cancer-fighting agents available. However, this time, we would test only women who had never been treated with the drug. Such an approach would likely result in a much higher rate of tumor shrinkage than would be expected if doxorubicin had already been given before. It was also problematical to retreat patient with doxorubicin, as too much exposure to that drug increases the risk of a nasty side effect called "cardiomyopathy", a severe weakening of the heart muscle that can sometimes be fatal.

The second choice was more of a high-flyer. Other than radiation, the treatment of advanced prostate cancer at that time was based almost entirely on using drugs that block testosterone, the male hormone that drives the growth of this disease (similar to estrogen in breast cancer). Once the tumor became resistant to this approach, as was almost always the case, there was little else to offer. Over the years, various chemotherapy drugs had been tried. The results were not encouraging, although a review article on this subject published in *JCO* revealed that cyclophosphamide, an "oldie" developed in the late 1950's, showed "some" activity.

That fact caught my attention. I quickly searched out two small published studies in which patients with late-stage prostate cancer were treated with very high doses of the drug. While they required daily injections of a white blood cell-stimulator, called "granulocyte colony stimulating factor (G-CSF)", to help overcome the effects of the high-dose treatment on the bone marrow, there appeared to be some definite responses, with shrinkage of tumors and a drop in the PSA test. I had combined DPPE with more conventional doses of cyclophosphamide in my just-completed trial and was impressed that we had seen some excellent results in patients with a variety of progressive tumors where the cyclophosphamide alone had stopped working. Moreover, with DPPE, the bone marrow side effects of cyclophosphamide seemed to be negligible.

"Maybe DPPE could make cyclophosphamide much stronger against prostate cancer cells without the need for special bone marrow protection," I thought. If so, it might convert a so-so drug into a potent killer. I discussed the idea with Ernie Ramsey, who was involved in many clinical trials of hormone blockers in patients with prostate cancer. Agreeing that we needed to explore new alternatives, Ernie offered to collaborate by sending potential candidates my way. I was delighted that the two of us were "back in the saddle again" and promised that this time things would turn out better than the skin transplants in the mice. As usual, we had a good laugh remembering that packed suitcase for Stockholm.

Gordon Grahame made it easy to get started on the new trials. From his point of view as ethics board chairman, both studies were a logical extension of the previous trial. He did not see the need for a lot of new paper work. Luckily for me, the bureaucratic shuffle was not his dance. He simply reiterated his rule that we combine DPPE with non-experimental chemotherapy agents and use only approved dosages. The last piece fell into place when a fax arrived from Agnes and Ivo stating that they had no objection to my proceeding. It was time to make more DPPE...a lot more!

CHAPTER THIRTY-SIX:

A Guy's Gotta Do What
A Guy's Gotta Do

One floor above the clinic, my lab assistants were being kept busy. As Greg Burke and Agnes Klein knew, we had spent much of 1993 assessing several common H_1 antihistamines, similar in structure to DPPE, for their effect on tumor growth in mice. Among the scores of allergy-fighters, we decided to test two old "war horses", hydroxyzine (Atarax) and doxylamine (present in many over-the-counter sleep and cough remedies), and three of the newer class of non-sedating antihistamines: cetirizine (Zyrtec; Reactine), a relative of hydroxyzine; loratadine (Claritin); and astemizole (Hismanal).

Loratadine was of special interest because it is chemically very similar to tricyclic antidepressants such as amitriptyline[62], and was about to be marketed as a low-dose (10 milligram) formulation. Our concern about tumor stimulation by amitriptyline had

---

62 Tricyclics, and related antipsychotic drugs called phenothiazines, have been known for years to possess potent H_1 antihistamine properties.

recently been reinforced by a Japanese study, also published in *Cancer Research*; the authors reported that low doses of a related tricyclic antidepressant, called desipramine, stimulated DNA synthesis and the growth of colon cancer induced by a carcinogen in rats. Their model was similar to the one we used in our study of antidepressants, where we gave rats "DMBA" to cause breast cancer.

Hydroxyzine and doxylamine were off-patent and therefore available as pure powders, purchased from a chemical supply house. Luckily, pure astemizole had been supplied to us a few years earlier by the manufacturer, Janssen Pharmaceuticals, for binding experiments. However, as commercially-available loratadine and cetirizine contained additional ingredients beside the active drug, it remained for us to obtain them in a form that we could test. Although I expected to be turned down, I wrote Pfizer and Schering-Plough, asking if they could send me a sample of pure cetirizine and loratadine, respectively, "to assess binding to a new intracellular histamine receptor".

I received only one reply, a polite non-committal letter from the Canadian branch of Schering-Plough, saying that my request was being forwarded to the American head office in New Jersey. I suspected that it would end up on Allen Barnett's desk. I heard nothing further until November when Allen wrote, saying he remembered me from Henk Timmerman's meeting in 1990. "I am not sure what type of study you are planning with loratadine. We would like to hear more about it and to share some of our information on loratadine with you," he wrote. He suggested that I visit him and his colleagues in New Jersey and present a seminar.

I decided to call. As we exchanged pleasantries, I sensed that Allen was decidedly nervous about my interest in his antihistamine. The antidepressant paper in *Cancer Research* had definitely caused shock waves throughout the industry, and Jean Marx' *Science* story had alluded to our newly-turned attention to antihistamines. Recently, he had other reasons to be nervous about loratadine. An increase in liver tumors had been observed in the company's chronic dosing studies in rats. Apparently, there were "regulatory concerns" about this because drugs and chemicals that induce (increase) the level of a certain P450 enzyme, called "2B1", have long been linked to the chemical promotion of liver tumors in rats (an example is phenobarbital, a barbiturate still used in the treatment of some patients with epilepsy). As a result, the company had sponsored a study to determine loratadine's effect on the level of 2B1 and other P450 enzymes in the liver.

Allen took the opportunity to tell me that those experiments had just been completed and were reassuring about the safety of the antihistamine.[63] Nonetheless, I could only imagine what was going through his mind as we spoke, something like, *"this is the last guy from whom I need to hear!"* Still, he maintained his gentle-manly composure and again suggested that I come to New Jersey to "share information" with company scientists. I told him I would consider his offer. He promised to get back to me shortly with an itinerary for a visit.

After hanging up the phone, I decided that a meeting would be a waste of everyone's time. I wanted to test loratadine on tumors and there was no way Allen and his company would ever willingly give it to me. I could just envision our discussion at the proposed meeting:

Brandes: "So, in conclusion, I want to test loratadine to deter-mine whether, as I suspect may be the case, it stimulates the growth of existing cancer in mice and rats."

Barnett and colleagues: "What a wonderful idea. Why didn't any of us think of this?"

Brandes: "Well, you can't be expected to think of everything."

Barnett and colleagues: "Quite right. How much loratadine do you need?"

---

63   The study, carried out at the University of Kansas, and published in 1994, showed that loratadine increased 2B1 activity by 700 - 800% in rat and mouse livers. Nonetheless, the increase was only about one-quarter to one-third of that seen with phenobarbital. Was this a reassuring result? Not in my opinion.

Brandes: "Five hundred milligrams should be enough."

Barnett and colleagues: "Here's a thousand....and keep the change."

I needn't have fretted. As luck would have it, I soon received a visit from Henk Timmerman. He had flown in from Amsterdam to plot strategy for a histamine research symposium that I was organizing in Manitoba the following summer. It was to be a "satellite meeting", part of a larger international pharmacology conference scheduled to be held in Montréal. After discussing our plans for the symposium, we had lunch and then took a leisurely walk down a scenic path that meanders through the grounds of the legislature and along the banks of the Assiniboine River, past its junction with the Red.

The antihistamine issue surfaced soon after we began to talk science. Henk told me that his lab had samples of pure loratadine and cetirizine. He was very aware of the previous antidepressant data, was concerned about the tumor issue in general, felt that the tests needed to be done, and would send the two drugs to me. His only request was that his role in providing them not be divulged in any paper that might be published. It could complicate his relationships within the pharmaceutical industry.[64] A short time later, he sent me the drugs.

After having their chemical structures verified by Kirk Marat in the analytical lab, I called Allen Barnett. There was no point in continuing our pretense about a meeting. Without beating around the bush, I informed him that I had obtained loratadine and would be testing the drug, along with four other antihistamines, to see whether it had any effect on tumor growth, stimulatory or otherwise. I could hear a pin drop at the other end of the line. His potential multi-billion dollar drug had been launched only recently with an expensive television, newspaper and magazine advertising campaign. Any adverse news linking loratadine with cancer growth would be his company's worst PR nightmare.

---

64   As the paper was published in 1994, and Henk has been retired for years, I am divulging his identity in this book.

"Did I tell you that the 2B1 study was reassuring?" he inquired after a few seconds of tense silence.

"Yes, Allen, you did," I replied. "However, as you know, our experiments involve a different approach, looking at whether drugs may accelerate existing cancer."

"Well, I guess a guy's gotta do what a guy's gotta do," he sighed. "Is there anything you can share with me at this time?"

"No," I replied, assuring him that he would be given the courtesy of a heads-up at an appropriate time some months down the road.

I truly felt sorry for Allen's predicament, but I believed that we had a duty to do these tests and report any findings in the appropriate forum of a peer-reviewed scientific journal. My resolve on this issue had recently hardened after *Cancer Research* published a paper by scientists at Eli Lilly that was intended as a direct rebuttal to ours. The company took the unusual step of presenting all of the preclinical "carcinogenicity" studies pertaining to fluoxetine.[65] The development of all malignant or benign tumors in mice and rats receiving chronic doses of the drug for up to two years was documented and tabulated in the publication.

Using a "Z statistic" test to detect a "straight-line" dose response effect (meaning that, if the drug stimulates the growth of tumors, the number of tumors should increase in tandem with the dose), the paper's authors noted that there was no evidence of any significant increase in tumors in fluoxetine-treated animals as compared to controls that received saline (placebo). In fact, pituitary and breast tumors were decreased with fluoxetine. Furthermore, tumors did not develop sooner in fluoxetine-treated rodents than in the controls. In short, our findings were not borne out by their chronic dosing studies.

While their study looked at a very different issue than ours (new tumor development rather than the stimulation of existing

---

65   Drug companies are under no obligation to publish their toxicology data and usually do not. However, they must furnish all such test results to regulatory agencies such as the FDA.

tumors), some findings in the paper immediately caught my eye. Bell-shaped or biphasic curves showed up for tumors of the lung, adrenal gland and immune system. For example, compared to nineteen control mice that developed lung tumors, twenty-six receiving a low dose of fluoxetine, and twenty-nine receiving an average (middle) dose, developed lung tumors. In contrast, at the top dose of fluoxetine (up to four times higher than most people would take), only eight mice developed lung tumors. In other words, at low to average doses of the drug, corresponding to what is taken by most patients, fluoxetine increased the number of lung tumors by about fifty percent, while at the highest dose, it decreased their numbers by the same amount.

I was intrigued by the possibility that this lung tumor data was of potential relevance to humans because it had been found in a recent epidemiology study that depressed smokers developed significantly more lung cancer than non-depressed smokers. Was this because depressed smokers consumed more cigarettes, or because they smoked and took an antidepressant? The increase in immune system tumors was also an eye-catcher because, in our published study, the ability of fluoxetine to inhibit the stimulation of normal immune cells was very obvious. Correlating with that, several reports had just come out that fluoxetine re-activated herpes virus infection in patients taking the drug for depression. When the drug was stopped, the infection resolved; when the drug was restarted, the infection came back, a sign of immune suppression. It has long been known that chronic impairment of the immune system increases the risk of cancers such as non-Hodgkin's lymphoma. Could the mice be alerting us to human cancer risks from taking fluoxetine?

Bringing along my "numbers" from the Eli Lilly study, the curves we observed for increased DNA synthesis with amitriptyline and fluoxetine, and copies of several of the many published examples of biphasic effects of drugs and other substances on cancer growth, I went to see our statistician, Mary Cheang, to seek her input. After spending many hours of review, Mary then applied a non-linear statistical test, called the "Poisson Exact Test", to compare the number of tumors that were observed in rodents receiving each dose of fluoxetine or saline. According to that analysis, the differences I had detected in the three types of tumors were statistically significant.

So here was the conundrum. The usual statistical test employed by pharmaceutical companies and regulatory agencies dictated a positive result only if the number of tumors went up in a straight line (a "linear response") as the dose of drug increased. By that criteria, fluoxetine had no significant effect on tumor development. On the other hand, if the actual dose response was bell-shaped or biphasic rather than linear, a different type of analysis showed that fluoxetine *did* have a significant effect to increase (or decrease) tumors at certain doses. Who was right here? I believed it was us. In fact, Frank and I were not alone in questioning the validity of the "linear rule".

Over two decades earlier, Dr. S. H. Kon, a chemist at Mount Sinai Hospital in New York, published a paper that made minced-meat of the notion of a straight-line dose response.[66] He felt that scientists did not pay attention to the "non-linearity" exhibited in most physical and chemical reactions, and went so far as to state that the continued adherence by regulatory agencies to straight-line dose responses "may constitute a public health hazard". I now thought that this admonition was both correct and, it appeared, totally ignored.

Hopefully, our tests of antihistamines would shed new light on this very important issue.[67]

Along with the question of dose effect, we decided to see whether any potential of the antihistamines to stimulate tumor

---

66   Kon SH. Underestimation of chronic toxicities of food additives and
      chemicals: the bias of a phantom rule. Medical Hypotheses 1978;
      4: 324-339.

67   As will be told, Ed Calabrese, at the U. of Massachusetts, recently
      reopened, in a big way, the whole issue of non-linear responses of
      cancer growth to drugs and chemicals.

growth correlated with how strongly each performed in certain of our lab tests that measured a drug's ability to block histamine binding in liver microsomes and to affect the growth of normal and malignant cells in culture. In addition, based on Frank's hypothesis on the relationship among the AEBS, intracellular histamine "receptor" and P450 enzymes, we would employ a sophisticated detector to measure the binding of the antihistamines to P450 enzymes and determine their ability to interfere with the activity of a specific P450, called "aminopyrine demethylase".[68]

While we would focus on the suitability of these five tests as possible screening tools, the very fact that we were using them to assess common antihistamine drugs, used by millions of people, would be cause for concern, no doubt about that. Since it continued to be vitally important that we demonstrate reproducibility of the results in two separate laboratories, we again asked Rob Warrington and Wei Fang to test the drugs in their melanoma model while we looked at them in the mouse sarcoma model. Along with Patty, Tong, and Cheryl, Randi, who had come back to the lab to spend the summer after completing her second year of medical school, rounded out my team, while Gary and Doug worked with Frank on the P450 enzyme tests. With loratadine and cetirizine now in hand, it was full steam ahead to finish our experiments.

---

68 This P450 enzyme (actually several P450s working together) removes a carbon and three hydrogen atoms from a chemical, called aminopyrine, to form formaldehyde, commonly used as embalming fluid. Its distinctive smell is well known to anyone who has ever taken a biology course.

CHAPTER THIRTY-SEVEN:

On A High

The new breast and prostate cancer trials were now up and running. Ernie had so many patients who had failed hormone therapy that within the first four months we enrolled ten of them for treatment with DPPE and cyclophosphamide. Their average age approached seventy. Many had additional medical problems such as high blood pressure, heart disease and diabetes. This was not an unusual mix of patients, as prostate cancer is most often diagnosed later in life, when other common diseases are also prevalent; our subjects were typical in this regard. Given their other infirmities, the big question was how they would tolerate the treatment.

All had symptoms of their cancer. Most had bone pain that was severe enough to require morphine and related narcotic drugs. That was also par for the course, as prostate cancer most commonly spreads to the skeleton, where the constant discomfort can wreak havoc with the quality of life of many of its victims. The main goal of the trial was to see whether the combination of DPPE and cyclophosphamide was effective in decreasing bone pain to a point where the patients could significantly reduce their narcotics. We also assessed the level of PSA in the blood as an indicator of whether the treatment caused tumor shrinkage.

Some of the patients were in such severe pain that we first brought them into hospital to get this distressing symptom under control before starting them on the trial. Several needed around-the-clock morphine, delivered directly into their veins. These men were completely bedridden and would ordinarily never be accept-able candidates for a clinical trial.[69] A host of previous clinical studies showed that the chance of a response to any treatment was much lower in such individuals. I decided to disregard the rules and, with their permission, treat them. As far as the patients and I were concerned, they were doomed if nothing was done. There was little to lose by trying. I was most fortunate that Marilyn Bruce, a hospital-based chemotherapy nurse with years of experi-ence, agreed to give the treatment on the ward after learning the ropes on administering DPPE from Susie.

In contrast to the men, the women on treatment with DPPE and doxorubicin in the breast cancer study averaged almost ten years younger and, despite their malignancy, tended to be healthier overall. I was soon struck by the number of cases where treatment caused rapid shrinkage of tumors in vital places such as the lungs and liver. Several complete remissions were soon docu-mented. I was becoming very excited by what I was seeing; the number of dramatic responses seemed much higher than I nor-mally observed using doxorubicin alone, or combined with other drugs. "Something impressive is happening," everyone agreed.

---

69   The term to describe the amount of daily activity that can be under-taken by a patient is "performance status", to which a numerical score can be assigned. A performance status score of zero means that a person has no limitation of daily activity, while a score of four means that the person is completely bed-ridden. The cut-off for most studies is a score of two, meaning the patient has some limitation of physical activity, but is able to be up and around for at least half the number of waking hours in a day.

There was more. Soon it was evident that we were also seeing dramatic responses in many of the men with prostate cancer, including some whose pain went down so drastically that they were able to get off their intravenous morphine and leave the hospital. It was truly amazing to see this. Ernie was as impressed as I, especially as most of these patients also had a steep drop in the PSA test, suggesting that the pain was improving because the tumor in their bones was shrinking. Just as important was the observation that most of the men, despite being elderly, could tolerate the DPPE and cyclophosphamide treatment for up to four weeks in a row without suffering from low white blood cell counts. Many also kept their hair. The addition of DPPE appeared to make cyclophosphamide act as though it were given at a very high dose but without the toxicity! With Terry Hogan's blessing, a new use patent for DPPE in prostate cancer was quickly filed by Michael Stewart.

On a high, I decided to follow Lee Schacter's lead and contacted Sparta Pharmaceuticals. I was put through to the company's vice-president and medical director, Dr. Bill McCulloch, an oncologist by training. By his brogue, it was obvious that he was a Scot...and a very pleasant one at that. I learned from him that the company was fairly new, oncology-oriented, and founded by William Sullivan, who had previously been CEO of Burroughs Wellcome. Obviously, I was amused by that bit of news. Sullivan had been at the helm of the company during the development of AZT, the first effective drug for HIV-AIDS.

I told Bill a little bit about the history of DPPE and my belief that it was now showing promise in making chemotherapy more effective, often with lower side effects. Was he interested? You bet he was. It appeared to fit exactly the type of drug that Sparta was looking to acquire and develop. When he asked about publications, I suggested that I fax him the earlier *JNCI* paper showing the histidinol-like effects of DPPE in mice, and the just-published human study in *JCO*. He thanked me warmly and said he would call me back as soon as he had reviewed them.

The following morning he was on the phone. Bill was definitely excited by what he had read, and recommended to the other Bill (Sullivan) that DPPE go to the top of the company's agenda. He wanted to sign a confidentiality agreement as soon as possible and come to Winnipeg with John McBride, the company's licensing director, to meet with us. During our discussion, Bill mentioned that Dr. Joe Bertino, formerly of Yale, and now at the Memorial Sloan-Kettering Cancer Center, was one of the company's scientific advisors. That was a good omen. Joe, a renowned pharmacologist and oncologist, had served with Lyonel on a National Cancer Institute panel some years earlier. The two remained quite close. Joe visited our group in Winnipeg and I often bumped into him at scientific meetings.

When I told Lyonel about this development, he immediately called Bertino to get his take on the company. Shortly after, he reported to me that Joe spoke very highly of Bill Sullivan. In addition, the company's other scientific and clinical advisors included Nobel laureate, Sir John Vane; New York University oncologist, Franco Muggia; Johns Hopkins scientist, Mike Colvin; Chester Beatty chemist, Tom Connors; and University of Indiana oncologist, Lawrence Einhorn. With a cast like that, Lyonel believed we should definitely give Sparta a hard look. Brent Schacter agreed with him. Board chairman, Arnold Portigal, an experienced businessman, was asked to play a major role in any negotiations. Arnold loved the "art of the deal" and was pleased with the opportunity to do what he could.

Within a week, we all sat around the infamous boardroom table as Bill and John each made their pitch on behalf of Sparta. In a refreshing way, there was no posturing. Speaking on behalf of Bill Sullivan, both made it clear that Sparta would like the opportunity to help us develop the drug. Admittedly, they were a small company, but with good contacts in the industry. Their approach would be to finance clinical trials of DPPE, all the while exploring licensing partnerships with major drug companies. We were all pleased with Sparta's enthusiasm, but any final decision would

have to be made by the boards of the Cancer Foundation and
University of Manitoba as well as by the provincial government.[70]

Bill and John left later that afternoon to report to their boss.
Soon after, Bill again contacted us, suggesting a return visit; this
time it would be the two Bills. William (Bill) Sullivan, a Harvard-
trained lawyer, wanted to see us first hand. He liked what he heard
from his two colleagues, but wanted to put his own imprimatur on
any potential negotiations. A meeting was soon arranged among
all the parties, including Brent, Lyonel and Arnold representing
the Cancer Foundation, and Landis Henry and Terry Hogan representing the University.

I learned afterward from Bill McCulloch that, prior to coming
to Winnipeg, Sullivan had consulted both Franco Muggia who,
unknown to me, had followed my work for some time and was
very intrigued by my research, and Sir John Vane, discoverer of
the very prostaglandin that was greatly increased by DPPE in
Gary Glavin's rat ulcer experiments. Undoubtedly, Lyonel's discussion with Joe Bertino had not hurt either. Bill Sullivan was
obviously getting good vibes from his advisors. By following up
so quickly after the first contact, he made it clear that he wanted
to do business.

With Bill McCulloch looking on, Sullivan did all the talking,
explaining how his company would approach a potential licensing deal. Sparta itself had limited funds and would not be able to
make any up-front payment in cash. The issuance of stock war-
rants was proposed as an alternative method of payment. Sullivan
was preparing an IPO in conjunction with a major Wall Street
broker to raise the cash he would need to move acquisitions, such
as DPPE, forward. Compared to hard money from an established
drug company such an approach was "dicey" and depended on
difficult-to-predict market conditions. Yet there was overall agreement on our side to proceed with negotiations.

---

70 Both the University and Manitoba Cancer Foundation are Crown
    Corporations that require provincial government approval to undertake
    ventures such as licensing agreements.

To that end, several months of due diligence would be required to examine all the issues such as patents. Everyone agreed to expedite the process in any way possible to move us forward. After the rest of us left the room, Bill Sullivan and Arnold Portigal remained behind in discussion. Both were astute entrepreneurs and talked the same language. They obviously established a rapport with one another and believed that they could broker a deal. We were all pleased at the prospect, realizing that, although Sparta was just a small player, good people were involved and positive things might result.

CHAPTER THIRTY-EIGHT:

A Water Cooler Story

As these events were unfolding, so were our findings. The results were almost identical in both laboratories: Rob and Wei found that loratadine and astemizole significantly stimulated the growth of melanoma in their mice, while we found stimulation of sarcoma tumors in ours. Each lab also tested astemizole at three different doses and found a bell-shaped dose response for the two types of tumors.[71] We were also in complete agreement that doxylamine and cetirizine did not appear to have an effect on tumor growth. The one disparate finding involved hydroxyzine: Rob found that it stimulated melanoma, whereas we did not find a significant effect on sarcoma.

Importantly, the battery of five lab tests seemed highly predictive of what we found in the mice. Loratadine and astemizole scored identically at the top of the scale, followed by hydroxyzine, while doxylamine and cetirizine both ranked equally, at the bottom. Frank, Rob and I each poured over the data and came

---

71   This suggested that my concerns about the fluoxetine "curves" were probably valid.

to the same conclusion: certain antihistamines had the potential to accelerate tumor growth and this property appeared to be predicted by the combo of screening tests. We wrote up the findings and submitted the paper to *JNCI*. "Here we go again," I thought to myself.

During the inevitably long wait for the reviews and editorial decision, Frank and I kept busy with our collaborative research on the P450 enzymes. It had become increasingly clear during the antihistamine study that Frank was almost certainly bang on about the true nature of the "AEBS" and "H_{IC}". The radioligand binding test "numbers" had matched the P450 test "numbers", meaning that histamine and the drugs were all interacting on these enzymes. The stronger a drug competed for labeled histamine binding to "H_{IC}" in microsomes, the stronger it blocked histamine binding to P450 and inhibited formaldehyde production by the "aminopyrine demethylase" P450.

Backing up these findings, a test called "spectral analysis" honed in to a specific pocket, called "the substrate site", on certain P450s. The "AEBS" *was* that pocket…the actual site of attachment of DPPE and tamoxifen to these enzymes! The same test found that "H_{IC}" represented the attachment of histamine to a different site on the enzymes, comprising an iron molecule surrounded by four five-sided rings.[72] Since this iron-containing structure was vital for the enzymes to carry out their metabolizing function, perhaps histamine modulated the entire process.

A theory took shape: as a result of binding to the "AEBS" on P450 enzymes, DPPE, tamoxifen and other drugs (including certain antihistamines and antidepressants) interfered with the ability of histamine to latch on to the iron molecule, thereby

---

72   The iron-ring structure is called "heme". Heme groups also form part of the red pigment, called hemoglobin, in our red blood cells. Hemoglobin carries the oxygen that the red cells deliver to the tissues. P450s are "heme enzymes", meaning that, like hemoglobin, heme forms part of the overall P450 enzyme structure. The "COX" enzymes are also "heme enzymes".

blocking the enzyme. While we still did not know the nature of the binding sites for DPPE and histamine in the DNA-containing nucleus, it was now clear that Frank was absolutely right in his initial caution that an intracellular histamine receptor, in the true sense of that word, might not exist in the microsomes. Yet, the discovery that histamine interacted with an all-important cell-regulatory enzyme system, as ancient as life itself, had exciting connotations.

Among the P450s to which DPPE and histamine bound, one, called "CYP3A4"[73], stood out. In addition to being responsible for the metabolism of a host of drugs, including many chemotherapy agents, this particular P450 also metabolizes estrogen and testosterone, and a molecule called arachidonic acid that is a building block for many cell-regulatory molecules such as prostaglandins. By attaching to CYP3A4, drugs such as DPPE and tamoxifen could alter the metabolism of these substances, thus changing their normal levels in cells and affecting cell behavior, including growth. This likely accounted for how and why DPPE markedly increased the prostaglandins that protect the gut and that promote both inflammation and cell division. Now, it made sense that this same interaction applied to other "DPPE-like" drugs, such as certain antihistamines and antidepressants.

A few weeks into 1994, we received word from *JNCI* that what made sense to us also made sense to the reviewers. The manuscript was accepted. It would be published in the spring, accompanied by an editorial. I was both happy and apprehensive. I kept thinking of Jimmie Holland's question of two years earlier: "How does it feel to be in the eye of a storm?" The answer now was, as they say, "Been there, done that."

My first duty was to inform Agnes and Greg of the paper's acceptance and send them a confidential copy of the manuscript. Soon after, Greg put me in touch with Dr. Charles Grieshaber, who ran the FDA's toxicology laboratory in Bethesda. He had

---

73   The term "CYP" stands for "cytochrome P[450]", while, like a ZIP or
     postal code, "3A4" denotes a specific P450 of the many that exist.

received his PhD at the National Cancer Institute under Dr. Vincent DeVita, famous for developing the first highly-effective chemotherapy treatment for Hodgkin's lymphoma that often strikes young adults. Dr. Grieshaber's co-investigator in the FDA lab was Dr. Ralph Parchment. Together, the two had started their own studies to assess tumor growth-stimulation by various drugs and requested that Rob Warrington and I supply them with the actual melanoma and fibrosarcoma cells that we had used in our experiments. We were both happy to do so, pleased that our work was being taken seriously by the FDA and confident that our experiments would be replicated.

As promised earlier, I now called Allen Barnett on his direct office line.

"Hello?"

"Hi, Allen. It's Lorne Brandes. I wanted to get back to you on our findings with loratadine." Other than a quiet "Yes?", all I could hear was his breathing on the other end. I knew he was tense. Who could blame the poor man?

I continued, "The bad news is that loratadine behaves like amitriptyline and fluoxetine. It appears to stimulate tumor growth. A paper describing our findings has just been accepted for publication in a major journal. The good news, if it can be called that, is that two of your competitors' antihistamines do the same. We are not singling out loratadine here."

I could feel his consternation at the other end.

"You know, Lorne, all you need is one negative report out there, and no matter how many good ones, the bad one always keeps going around and around."

"I understand, Allen. But I believe that this is too important an issue. If there is a potential problem, the public needs to know. Nobody wants to unintentionally harm people with underlying cancer."

He agreed with that premise but was obviously distressed. "When can we see a copy of the paper?"

"I will fax you a copy in the late afternoon the day before publication. Hopefully that will give you and your colleagues time to go over the data before the phone starts ringing," I promised. *The phone....following publication, he and I would have something in common on that front.* Thanking me, he hung up. Oh to be a fly on the wall of their corporate boardroom that afternoon!

JNCI was known to provide embargoed copies of each issue to the media a few days before publication. Once again, our findings would be widely reported. This time, I hoped the publicity would result in the issue of tumor growth-stimulation being placed firmly on the regulatory agenda. However, given the millions of people taking antihistamines, I was very worried about what alarming "spin" might be applied by various journalists and discussed this concern with Rob, Frank, Lyonel, Brent Schacter, Arnold Portigal, and our own media relations staff. Everyone agreed that we had to be prepared to deal with the press and public when the story broke.

To that end, I contacted Julianne Chappell at *JNCI*. She was responsible for all scientific publications emanating from the National Cancer Institute. Julianne confirmed that our paper would be highlighted in a press release from her office that accompanied the embargoed journal copy. The "package" would be sent out on May 10, one week before publication date, set for May 17th. During the prepublication week, we were allowed to speak with the press as long as we first stressed that the embargo date be respected. In response to my request, she and Don Holt, the senior editor who handled our paper, sent me the fax numbers of all the print and broadcast journalists on *JNCI's* list.

On the evening of May 10, I sent each of those on the list a fax, headlined on each page with the words "*Subject to JNCI Embargo Until 6:00 PM EDT, May 17, 1994*". I included a four page double-spaced summary of the antihistamine study, a review of our work on DPPE and the previously-published findings on amitriptyline and fluoxetine that led to the current study, the reasons for our concern about what we had found, and several specific requests we were making of federal regulators; I would be available by telephone to answer any remaining questions. Rob Warrington would also make himself available for interviews. "We'll be under a microscope," I warned my Saskatchewan colleague.

On publication day, the University arranged a press conference in the medical school amphitheatre so that Frank and I could discuss our findings with local and national Canadian media. The two of us met early to go over the opening statement that I had prepared. Frank thought it was fine. After spending two hours writing it, I had slept fitfully through the night, knowing that today and the days to come likely would be stressful. The press has a vital duty to report the news, but the intrusion on privacy can be daunting. Moreover, I expected a brisk negative response from the drug makers and was unsure of the response of the regulatory agencies.

Flashbulbs went off as a photographer arrived to take some pictures of the two of us. At the appointed hour, we walked in and sat at a table at the front of the large auditorium. Looking over the room, I was not prepared for the number of reporters and TV cameras trained on us. The University media people had obviously banged the drum loudly.

As Frank looked on, I read the statement enumerating our perspective of the issues raised by our antihistamine study: the stimulation of existing tumors in rodents, *not* causing cancer; the importance that other laboratories replicate our studies; and public awareness not to take antihistamines or, for that matter, any drug, including over-the-counter medications, indiscriminately.

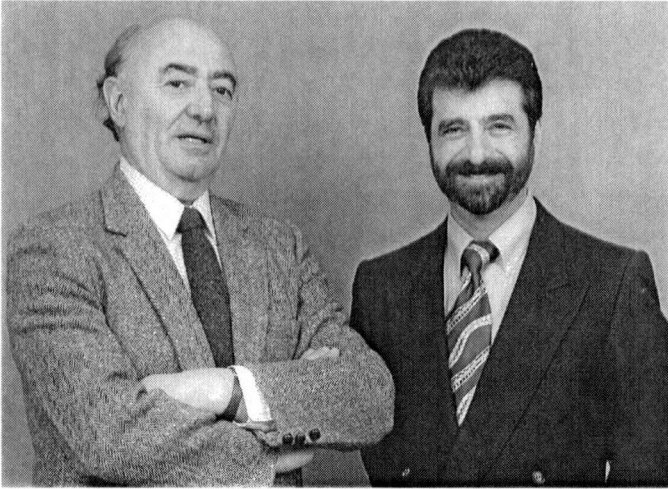

Frank LaBella and me just before the news conference (U.of Manitoba Archive)

I continued. We were also requesting that federal regulatory agencies should consider mandating studies of tumor growth-stimulation by drugs; should reassess toxicology data for various drugs already in clinical use to determine whether, in light of our findings, evidence existed in rodents for bell-shaped or biphasic effects on tumor growth at clinically-relevant doses; review their policy on over-the-counter sale of specific antihistamines where rodent studies demonstrate stimulation of tumor growth; and require manufacturers to include "stimulation of growth of experimental tumors has been observed in laboratory rodents" in the product monograph (the information insert that comes inside the package) of the drugs that had tested positive in our studies.[74]

Frank and I answered questions for almost one hour. During that time, one of the reporters informed us that the FDA had just issued an official statement. It was taking our findings seriously and would be carrying out experiments to see whether they could be validated. I just sat there, nodding my head. I was sure

---

74   The increase in liver tumors (benign and malignant) in rodents adminis-
     tered high doses of loratadine is already in the product monograph.

that Greg Burke had been active behind the scene. Our credibility had ratcheted up several notches and the drug companies had been put on notice. Little did I know that soon CNN would be broadcasting that FDA statement, accompanied by a clip of our news conference, around the world for the next twenty-four hour news cycle.[75]

After the news conference ended, I stopped at the hospital newsstand to buy the *Globe and Mail*, a Toronto-based national newspaper; its medical reporter had interviewed me at length the afternoon before and the story would be in that day's paper. The rack was empty. "I suspect we sold out because of you, Dr. Brandes," said the lady behind the counter. She had finished reading her own copy and offered it to me. Thanking her profusely, I took it back to my office to read the report. Just then the phone rang. The switchboard operator told me it was the *Globe and Mail*. "That's strange," I thought as I asked her to put the call through.

This time it was a different reporter. She wanted to do a followup that would appear the next day. Everyone in the editorial office was talking about it....truly a "water cooler" story, she said.

Question: "Do you suffer from allergies?"

Answer: "No."

Question: "What advice do you have for people with allergies who have to take antihistamines?"

Answer: "First off, I would tell them not to panic...."

The minute I said that, I regretted it. What a hackneyed reply! Every time some sort of health-related study with negative connotations comes out, two things are said by those who have carried out the research: "Don't panic," and "More research is needed." No one ever has the guts to simply say, "Yeah, I think our findings

---

75 A week later, Asher Begleiter, who had attended a scientific conference in Singapore, told me of viewing the CNN news clip over and over on his hotel TV. "Can't I go anywhere without seeing you?" he joked.

suggest that there could be a problem here." Now I was at the top of that list of offenders.[76]

In truth, my answer was not totally without merit. I was less worried about consumption of antihistamines than antidepressants. The reason was simple. Antidepressants are usually prescribed for prolonged periods of time, often years, whereas antihistamines are most often taken sporadically, or for short stretches during hay fever season. A long exposure might have more consequences for tumor growth than sporadic or intermittent exposure. However, one concern was that various antihistamines are still commonly prescribed for nausea control in patients with cancer. Could some of them be adversely affected by such medication? Who could tell?

Soon after I hung up, the phone rang again. "I have CNN on the line wanting to speak with you, Dr. Brandes," the switchboard operator told me, her voice filled with awe.

"Put them through, Gerry," I replied.

A producer's assistant from Atlanta said that CNN wanted to interview me "live" the next morning. Would I be willing to fly at my own expense to their nearest regional studio in Minneapolis? *Was she kidding? I should pay my way for them to interview me? Did some people really pay out of their own pocket for the privilege of being on CNN?*

"No thanks," I replied.

"Are you sure?" she asked, almost incredulously.

"Absolutely sure," I responded, thanking her for her easy-to-refuse offer.

After hanging up, I again turned my attention to the newspaper. The phone soon interrupted me once more. "Yes?"

---

76   Sure enough, the followup story pointed out that I personally did not suffer from allergies, and quoted my admonition to users of antihistamines "not to panic". The next day a CTV commentator, Valerie Pringle, herself an allergy sufferer, commented on her nationally-broadcast show, "Sure. The guy tells people not to panic. That's easy for him to say!" Right on, Valerie. Mea culpa.

It was the lady from CNN calling back. The network really wanted to do this live interview and would settle for a phone link with me the next morning.

I demurred. "I really don't think so. It's already being reported widely on CNN and everywhere else today." *Honestly…what else was there for me to say about this matter?*

"Well, of course, it's your decision, Dr. Brandes. But you should know that Dr. Weed has already agreed to the interview." With that comment, she had me on the hook.

Dr. Douglas Weed, chief epidemiologist at the Preventive Oncology Branch of the National Cancer Institute, had written the editorial that accompanied our paper in *JNCI*. Entitled *"Between Science and Technology: the Case of Antihistamines and Cancer"*, it was a cautious, well-crafted piece. Based on an overview of our results and other available human and rodent data, Weed counseled "… no change in current practice or policy regarding the use of the five antihistamines or the in vitro tests reported here."

Likely intended by the journal as a counterpoint to any potential public alarm generated by our paper, there was little in Dr. Weed's editorial that I did not expect. As a result of my previous dealings with the FDA and Canadian regulators, I did not believe for one moment that our study would lead to a sudden change in policy without a long period of gathering additional laboratory and human data. My mission was to ensure that our concerns were seriously considered by them.

"Given that information, I guess I'll do it," I replied after a few seconds of thought. *What choice did I now have?*

"Good. It will be a five minute piece starting just after eight o'clock Eastern time tomorrow morning….that's seven your time. Just give me the phone number where we can reach you. An operator will call to connect you about five minutes before air time."

The morning of the interview I awoke at six-thirty, made a pot of strong black coffee and then, still in my pajamas and bathrobe, sat down on the sofa in our den with the TV tuned to CNN. "What minefield am I getting myself into?" I wondered nervously as I watched the minutes tick by on the clock. Jill could read my expression.

"Just relax. I know you'll do fine," she said, hugging me.

Right on time, the phone on the coffee table next to me rang. I quickly exhaled as I put the receiver to my ear. It was someone in the studio. "Dr. Brandes? Good morning. Nice to have you with us. We will be starting right after the station break at the top of the hour. If you have your TV on, just make sure the sound isn't up too loud."

Thanking him, I gazed glassy-eyed at what seemed like a never-ending series of commercials. Time stood still as I waited and waited.

Suddenly, a voice on the other end of the line cued me to stand by. As I could see on the screen, *Daybreak* was back on the air. The host, Brian Christie, gave his lead-in. "We told you about a new medical study linking three allergy drugs to accelerated cancer growth in laboratory mice. Now we would like to flesh out those findings and find out exactly what it means to allergy sufferers."

He first introduced Douglas Weed who, formal in suit and tie, was sitting on a set in a Washington studio. *Boy, it's a good thing no one could see how I was dressed for this auspicious occasion!* Suddenly a map of Canada, highlighted by Manitoba, with a red dot over Winnipeg, appeared on the screen. A picture of me, apparently taken at the previous day's news conference, appeared to the left of the map. "...and Dr. Lorne Brandes...the author of this study...joins us on the phone from Winnipeg, Canada..."

Christie: "Dr. Brandes, let's start with you on the phone. [This] study is obviously going to scare a lot of people. Give us the three drugs so that people are aware of which drugs we are talking about." As I enumerated them, a graphic naming the three antihistamines that had stimulated tumors appeared on the screen.

Christie: "Do these antihistamines promote cancer?"

Brandes: "In our studies they very definitely do."

Christie: "Is this cause for concern?"

Brandes: "To me, as a researcher, it is, because these are studies done in mice and rats. The same mice and rats are used by the pharmaceutical companies to screen various chemicals for carcinogenesis, that is, the ability to cause cancer, before they are released to the public. In our studies, we don't believe that these agents cause cancer, but the same mice and rats tell us that in the presence of tumors the drugs promote, or accelerate, the growth of cancer. But we do have to be careful in the extrapolation [to humans], I agree with that."

Christie: (to Dr. Weed) "Your assessment, sir?"

Weed: "This study is an important one because it brings an important question to the table: What should be done when the results of biological research suggest links to medical practice? Those are difficult, complex decisions. They're part science. They're part ethics. We currently believe that what is known about these drugs shows that their benefits outweigh the risks. But we are aware of the uncertainties, and we believe that we need more research, specifically research on human beings, to ascertain the effects of these antihistamines on human cancer."

Christie: "So, Dr. Weed, is this study too premature to act at this point?"

Weed: "That is correct."

Christie: "Dr. Brandes, should people stop using these antihistamines right away?"

Brandes: "Well, my answer is very simple. If you need an antihistamine to control serious medical symptoms, there is no question that you should take the antihistamine. I do not believe you should take an antihistamine for any trivial symptoms, and if you do have to be on antihistamines, I believe you should get off them as quickly as possible. Having said that, it's a good paradigm for any drug."

Christie: "All right. Dr. Weed?"

Weed: "I agree with that assessment."

Christie: (to Dr. Brandes) "....would it help to change the label here?"

Brandes: ".... your question is an important one. I personally believe that, since there is already labeling that indicates that certain antihistamines, for example, Claritin, cause an increase in liver tumors in mice and rats at higher than human-equivalent doses...this is already on the labeling in the United States...I believe our finding that, at human-equivalent doses this antihistamine accelerates cancer growth, is also worthy of being put into the small print. I think labeling is an important factor here. This is really what we would like to see happen. We agree with Dr. Weed that, from the standpoint of epidemiological studies, this is what needs to be done. But, on the other hand, I think consumers like to be aware of various findings. So, since toxicology findings are labeled in the inserts for these medications, I believe that when new findings come along showing something like tumor growth acceleration, this could at least be put into the small print and then the consumer can make his or her own decision."

Christie: "Dr Weed, some antihistamines [are] obviously risky, some are not. Why allow the risky ones on the market?"

Weed: "As I mentioned before, we would like to get the assessment of these antihistamines in human studies. We cannot make a decision, a good decision, about human health without that information."

Christie: "Dr. Douglas Weed....Dr. Lorne Brandes...thank you very much."

As I hung up the phone, my overriding emotion was thankfulness that I had survived the ordeal. Jill, who had been listening to the TV in the bedroom, came into the den to find me still meditating on the sofa. "You were wonderful. I'm very proud of you," she said as we kissed. I knew if I had been otherwise, in her diplomatic way she would have told me that too. Just then, the phone rang. It was Arnold Portigal. He had also watched and was laudatory in his comments. I was relieved to hear them. Arnold was a tough critic who did not mince words when aroused. As board chairman, his first concern was that the Manitoba Cancer Treatment and Research Foundation always be well represented

in public; nothing could have been more public than what had
just transpired.

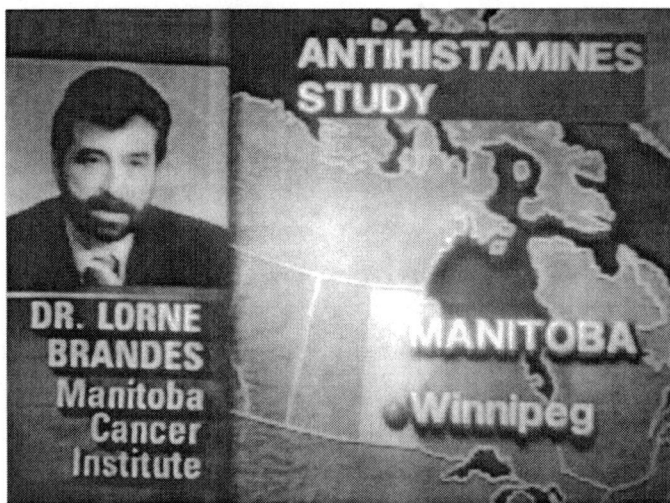

Screen capture of my "appearance" on CNN (Personal photo collection)

A few hours later, I called Douglas Weed. We had not previously met; our first contact was during the morning's interview.
He had shared my nervousness about being interviewed and the
relief, now, that neither of us had misspoken.

"I only consented after they told me you had already agreed to
it," I confided.

"What? They told me that you had already agreed to it,"
he replied.

We both laughed...a couple of pawns in the game that
was CNN.

We then briefly discussed the epidemiology studies that might
be designed to test our hypothesis. Largely influenced by my previous meeting at the FDA, I told him of my pessimism that such
studies could adequately assess the stimulation of existing cancer.
Weed appeared optimistic that it could be done. Time would tell.

Later that morning, Brent Schacter left a copy of a *Wall Street
Journal* story on my desk. He had circled the final paragraph. The

article, entitled *"Allergy-Drug Study Raises Concerns On Tumors, But Methods Are Questioned"*, had been written by Michael Miller. In addition to interviewing me, Miller had spoken with Dr. Robert Temple, director of the Office of Drug Evaluation at the FDA. On reading the story I decided that either the writer had an attitude or his words were simply reflecting what he had been told by Temple. Referring to my views on tumor growth-stimulation by antihistamines as "maverick", Miller also interpreted my pre-publication fax to journalists as "an aggressive public-relations campaign to generate media interest". *Live by the sword, die by the sword.*

That aside, in the circled paragraph that caught Brent's attention, Dr. Temple questioned the validity of the bell-curve approach. Referring to me, Temple was quoted as follows: "He's saying if you see a high rate in any group, you should be inclined to believe it. But you have a huge false-positive rate, so you drown in misinformation. If you start putting in the label of every drug that it caused increased tumors in mice and rats, pretty soon the information is degraded."[77] *What on earth was he talking about? Drowning in misinformation? Information degraded? Was the "huge false-positive rate" he quoted the same as the "background noise" to which Greg Burke had referred when he described the occurrence of tumors in rodents given chronic doses of antihistamines and other drugs? Who was he to say that an increase in tumors at certain doses is a false positive?*

I immediately picked up the phone and called Greg. He too had read Miller's story.

"Does anyone there believe our findings?" I asked.

---

77   In a subsequent (May 26, 1995) letter to me, Dr. Temple said the following:... "Based on available data to date, we believe your suggested mechanisms of tumor promotion and carcinogenicity are generally unsupported. The putative "bell-shaped" curves in the fluoxetine data are the sorts of spontaneous variability typical of animal carcinogenicity studies which involve multiple tests for differences and require statistical adjustments for multiplicity." *Of course. How stupid could I have been? Uhh...what did he actually say?*

"A few," he answered. I assumed Greg to be among them. Although, by his own words, Dr. Temple appeared to be firmly in the other camp, Greg assured me that he (Temple) had met with his staff that very morning and instructed them to "leave no stone unturned to get to the bottom of this matter". Dr. Grieshaber's lab was now hard at work with the tumor cells Rob and I had sent him.

Thanking Greg, I called Rob Warrington to apprise him of Dr. Temple's statement. "Rob, do you have any doubt about what you observed with the antidepressants and antihistamines?" I asked.

"Absolutely none," my friend offered without hesitation. "If they carry out the experiments exactly as we did, they should find the same thing."

I agreed with him but was starting to feel nervous by what I had read in the *Wall Street Journal*. Having very publicly forced the issue with the federal regulators, we were in their face and my impression was that they did not like it one bit. Drug companies were likely pouring on the pressure to quickly resolve this thorny issue. We had upset the equilibrium in regulatory offices and corporate boardrooms. Who were we to tell the experts how to test drugs for safety? The tepid response to my seminar at the FDA the year before lingered in my mind. No matter. The ball was now in their court. All we could do from this point on was to sit tight.

CHAPTER THIRTY-NINE:

From Water Cooler To Cold Water

We did not have very long to wait, four months to be exact. In late August, Dr. Brian Gillespie contacted me to set up a September 8th meeting with us and the FDA on our "home turf", in Ottawa. Brian, a former family practitioner, was responsible for regulating antihistamines within Canada's Bureau of Non-prescription Drugs (BNPD). As a result of differences in regulatory policy, many of the allergy drugs that were available only by prescription in the United States were sold over the counter in Canada, therefore coming under the supervision of BNPD. Greg Burke, Charles Grieshaber and Ralph Parchment were representing the FDA. Brian suggested that Rob and Frank accompany me.

At the appointed hour, we all assembled in a conference room in the Scott Street building that housed BNPD. Dr. Claire Franklin, representing the Health Protection Branch, appeared briefly to open the meeting, saying that federal regulators were taking our findings extremely seriously and therefore had arranged for the day's "exchange of information". She then turned the chair over to Dr. Gillespie and left. He asked me to start the proceedings by presenting an overview of our work and any other data that I considered pertinent.

For the next thirty minutes, I did just that. In preparation, Frank and I carried out a literature search on the effect of various drugs and other substances on tumor growth in the test tube or in animals; many of the examples we found were the same ones that had been faxed to me over the preceding months by Greg. There were so many published reports of bell-shaped curves and biphasic responses (stimulation at low doses and inhibition at high doses) that I presented only a representative portion of them. I concluded my talk by suggesting that what we had observed with the antidepressants and antihistamines had also been reported by others for a litany of drugs, chemicals and natural substances. There really didn't seem to be any doubt about the existence of this phenomenon.

Without commenting on the data I had just reviewed, Drs. Grieshaber and Parchment then presented their findings. In short, using our cell lines, *they had been unable to verify any of our cell-culture or rodent data!!* Both expressed their amazement that this had been the case. Dr. Parchment went so far as to say that, before undertaking the experiments, he had expected to find the stimulation that we had reported. Nonetheless, slide after slide of negative results was put up on the screen for us to view.

I sat speechless through all of this, not believing what I was hearing. The whole reason for involving Rob from the very beginning was to make absolutely sure that what we had observed in our lab could be reproduced independently in another. The concordance of findings in both our labs had been quite striking. Moreover, the NCI, like my own laboratory, had shown tumor stimulation by DPPE in rodents. Multiple other examples in the research literature suggested that our findings with the antidepressants and antihistamines were by no means unique. What was going on here??? Rob and I stared incredulously at one another. Frank wore his poker face.

During the discussion that followed, Rob did not conceal his skepticism. A very meticulous investigator who would never put his name on a publication if he had any doubt about the data, Rob remained resolutely convinced that the growth-stimulation of melanoma that had been seen with the drugs was both real and reproducible. He was also adamant that there were certain significant differences in how some of the tests had been carried out at the FDA. Frank agreed, pointing out that seemingly minor differences in methods could lead different laboratories to report opposing results when researching the same topic, and provided some examples from his own long experience.[78] I continued to sit silently, letting my two colleagues do the talking.

In response, Dr. Grieshaber suggested that we send our lab assistants to the FDA to work with his people to see whether this might lead to a different outcome. While believing his offer was genuine, I also knew that it was not remotely possible. We could not ask our people to leave their families (often including young children) to spend many weeks or, more likely, months, away from home. Moreover, our own research programs would be forced to grind to a halt without them.

The meeting ended in impasse just before noon. No minds were changed. We believed our results and they stood by theirs. As everyone gathered up their papers and slides, Greg and I talked privately for a short time. I thought he was in a difficult position. All too aware of the multitude of examples of tumor stimulation by low doses of substances in the scientific literature, Greg did not necessarily believe that the FDA results were definitive. All we could now do was wait for further studies to come along from other laboratories that might shed additional light on the

78 Former U. of Manitoba pharmacology head Clive Greenway corroborated Frank's view when he later wrote me, "The negative finding of the FDA reminds me of when I read a paper publishing work diametrically opposite to our own unpublished findings and how dumbfounded I was. I never did resolve why their results from Australia were the opposite of ours - perhaps it had something to do with the cats [see P. 70] walking upside-down."

subject. Would human epidemiology studies still be conducted in light of this negative development? Based on the results of today's meeting, not by the FDA. They would have to be done by others. Even if studies went ahead, grave doubts remained that they could resolve the question of stimulation of existing tumors.[79]

As Greg headed for the door, we shook hands warmly. We would continue to stay in close touch. I did not know it then, but I would not see him again. Only a few months later, he resigned his position at the FDA and joined the oncology division of pharmaceutical giant Ciba-Geigy (now known as Novartis) in their Zurich office. My only supporter, a person with great insight who, by his own admission, was often an outrider, had jumped ship. The regulator now worked for the regulated.

---

79 In an interview he had just given to medical writer Alex Robinson in the *Canadian Medical Association Journal*, Greg said, "….it is very difficult to get good epidemiological data….people take drugs for years and years, on and off, and they use an antihistamine, and they smoke, and they drink, and they eat all kinds of fats—-and they get a lot of cancer. How do you know what caused it? It's very difficult….[Discussing the biphasic response and epidemiological studies assessing drugs and cancer risk]: "…without regard to dose you could have an effect at the low dose that's bad and an effect at the high dose that's good and…overall there's no effect at all. You know? It's really complex." He had hit all the nails squarely on the head.

CHAPTER FORTY:

Pulling the Rug

While my confidence may have been shaken on one front, it continued to build over DPPE. The new clinical trials were accruing rapidly, now aided by referrals from other oncologists and urologists, in major part because the responses remained impressive in both studies. Having evaluated the first twenty patients with prostate cancer, Ernie Ramsey and I had just submitted our findings to the *Journal of Clinical Oncology*. Ernie, who had been involved in many drug company-sponsored clinical trials in prostate cancer, was particularly impressed by the quality and duration of the responses in these late-stage cases. "I think the results are gre-e-yat," he said in that unmistakable Ulster accent of his. I loved his pronunciation of that word to the point that if something caught my fancy, I would mimic Ernie with some degree of embellishment, proclaiming it "gr-e-e-e-e-yat!"

Negotiations with Sparta were also on a fast track. The due diligence process had been completed to Bill Sullivan's satisfaction. He and Arnold Portigal worked well together and the first draft of a potential licensing agreement was circulating within the bureaucracy by autumn of 1994. Three months earlier, I had presented a review of my laboratory studies to several members of the Sparta board of scientific advisors, including Franco Muggia and Mike Colvin. Bill McCulloch booked one of the many conference rooms at the Airport Hilton in Chicago so that everyone could fly in and out the same day. The meeting had been arranged in the hope that, after hearing what I had to say, Bill Sullivan's scientific team would support his quest to license DPPE. Apparently the session had gone well and they did.

Finally, in early December, after several rounds with the lawyers representing the Cancer Foundation and the University, a final draft of an agreement with Sparta was hammered out. Arnold Portigal was proud and delighted by the success of his negotiations. Although the document would still need to be sent to the Manitoba legislature for cabinet approval, it was essentially a "done deal", as everyone in government, from Premier Filmon on down, was totally supportive.

My attorney, Gerry Arron, had Jill and I meet with him in his downtown office to sign a separate consulting agreement with Sparta and to adjust our wills to include disbursement of any potential royalties to our descendants. As we put our signatures to paper, there were hugs all around. "In addition to famous, one day you may be rich as well," my longtime friend and counselor (and father of Randi) beamed. He then pulled a piece of paper out of his wallet. He had saved it for a month. I instantly recognized that it was a from a fortune cookie.

"Here, read this out loud," he instructed.

"Your experience will help a friend make it to the top." *IF ONLY.* "From my lips to God's ear," I added.

To celebrate his pending acquisition, Bill Sullivan planned a gala weekend event in New York. Jill and I were invited as Sparta's "special" guests for the two-day event in mid-December. We were thrilled. A frequent traveler to New York, Sullivan had booked his usual Manhattan hotel, the Kimberly, a small but exclusive place on East 50th, for all of us to stay. Knowing that the "Big Apple" was Jill's hometown, Bill McCulloch was thoughtful enough to suggest we come a day early to enjoy New York's magical festive season. Taking him up on his offer, we lost no time shopping at Sak's Fifth Avenue, admiring the world-famous mechanical Santa, reindeer and elves in Macy's windows, and walking through Rockefeller Center to watch the skaters on the rink below the huge Christmas tree. A beautiful star was perched on its top. Thousands of lights twinkled on its fir branches. Mel Tormé's recording of *The Christmas Song* played over the speakers. Although the weather was generally mild, even a few snow flakes fell for the occasion. It just didn't get any better than that.

As they left a private meeting of Sparta's scientific advisory board on Saturday morning, I bumped into Tom Connors and Sir John Vane in the hotel lobby. They had flown in together from London. Tom, a chemist, was long associated with the Chester Beatty Institute. Having known one another from my year at the Royal Marsden, we reminisced about "old times" and eagerly compared notes on colleagues-in-common. Both he and Sir John congratulated me on my work with which, by this time, they were well-acquainted.

Professor Vane was especially intrigued by our studies showing the effect of DPPE to increase prostacyclin; the discovery of this precise prostaglandin had netted him a share of the coveted Nobel Prize in Medicine in 1982. He was also the first to show that the common aspirin worked by inhibiting prostaglandin production by the COX enzymes. My ego was soaring as I basked in the knowledge that scientists of the stature of Vane and Connors were giving Bill Sullivan the thumbs-up on our histamine research and DPPE.

That night, one of Sullivan's most-frequented restaurants, "The Leopard", catered a private dinner on their premises. Owned by a rather portly gentleman from Louisiana, it proudly offered specialties derived from the likes of alligator and rhinoceros. Most of us opted for more conventional dishes. Throughout the dinner, expensive Bordeaux wines were poured and various toasts made.

The food and drinks were wonderful and our feelings inside even more so.

Following a Sunday morning breakfast, their business finished, Tom Connors and Sir John Vane said their goodbyes and bade good wishes to everyone as they left for the airport. The rest of us then walked several blocks to a Park Avenue office building where a boardroom had been procured by Bill Sullivan from one of his financier friends. I was to present a review of the prostate cancer study to several prominent clinicians. The morning's invitees included Joe Bertino; Robert Pinedo, a prominent oncologist from Amsterdam; and Lawrence Einhorn who, some years previously, had developed a highly effective life-saving chemotherapy regimen for testicular cancer that made him internationally famous.[80]

Before turning the proceedings over to Bill McCulloch, Sullivan announced to all present that, pending the formality of cabinet approval, Sparta and the University of Manitoba had successfully concluded a licensing agreement for DPPE. After the polite clapping stopped, Bill McCulloch told the group that Sparta was especially interested in pursuing further studies in prostate cancer, based on the results of a study that had just been submitted to *JCO* that I would now present.

Since I assumed that those present were hearing about this for the first time, I explained that we had combined DPPE with cyclophosphamide, a drug generally regarded as showing a low degree of activity in that disease. Then it was on to the slides of the data we had compiled in our twenty patients. All but two of the thirteen men with severe bone pain had major improvements in this symptom. A drop in the PSA of greater than fifty percent was observed in half of the patients. There was major tumor shrinkage in five of seven patients where, in addition to the bones, the disease had spread to vital organs or tissues. All this was achieved with remarkably low toxicity to boot. Many subjects had a very

---

80   The treatment was universally called "the Einhorn regimen". It saved cyclist Lance Armstrong's life.

poor performance status and therefore would never have been accepted into a conventional trial. I ended the presentation by showing slides of various X-rays and bone scans.[81] One scan in particular, that had lit up everywhere with metastases, dramatically returned to normal in a patient after treatment.

My talk now over, Bill McCulloch invited comments. Lawrence Einhorn immediately offered his opinion. It was highly negative. From his point of view, all he had heard that morning was a "series of anecdotes".

Silence.

"Uh, would you care to elaborate on that, Larry?" a stunned Bill McCulloch asked. I saw Bill Sullivan looking somewhat startled, while Joe Bertino just shook his head slightly from side to side.

Einhorn then enumerated his criticisms: most chemotherapy drugs are useless for prostate cancer; it's a terrible disease in which to assess responses; x-rays and bone scans are often impossible to interpret in these cases; the patients are usually in very bad shape; you need to have large, properly-designed randomized studies to know whether DPPE added anything to cyclophosphamide.

"Dr. Einhorn, I don't wish to appear argumentative, but rather than a 'series of anecdotes', don't you think it would be fair to categorize this as a small, phase one/two study of DPPE and cyclophosphamide? I am not making exaggerated claims here, but the results do appear encouraging and that is why we submitted them to *JCO*. In fact, as you have observed, given the lack of effective chemotherapy available to men at this late stage of their disease, I think this treatment is very promising," I countered.

He just shrugged and remained silent.

The others seemed to agree with my version.

After a further half-hour of discussion, the proceedings ended and coffee and pastry were served. I immediately went over to Dr.

---

81   A radioactive isotope is injected into the vein, resulting in an outline of
      the skeleton that is often used to assess spread of cancer to the bones.
      Abnormal areas of bone show up as dark spots that usually stick out
      from the less-intense outline of normal bone.

Einhorn in the hope of smoothing things over. He was friendly enough, assuring me that nothing personal was intended by his remarks. We shook hands and he left, seemingly in a hurry. "That's just Larry. He has very strong opinions and sometimes I find his ideas a bit peculiar," Bill reassured me after Einhorn had departed. Our wonderful weekend in New York had ended on a slightly down note.

Back in my office the next morning, I found a large envelope carrying the *JCO* logo among the mail in my inbox. At most, it had been ten days since I had submitted our paper. My heart sank. Could this be the returned manuscript...a quick rejection? The address on the corner of the envelope indicated that it had been sent from the University of Indiana. Quickly opening it, I found exactly what I had feared, accompanied by a letter from none other than Dr. Lawrence Einhorn. He was a senior editor of the journal!! *Oh, no!!!*

According to Einhorn, our paper had been "... reviewed by an expert in the field who had serious concerns...not rated highly enough to merit publication...being returned...thank you for the opportunity of reviewing your work... " I quickly looked for the referee report outlining the "expert's" concerns. None was included. "Well, that certainly explains a lot about yesterday," I thought, as I quickly dialed Bill McCulloch.

"What kind of clinical advisors do you have at Sparta?" I asked him rhetorically, and then read him Dr. Einhorn's letter. Bill was dumfounded. Putting the pieces together, we now both assumed that, as he was sitting through my presentation, Larry Einhorn suddenly realized that he had just read my manuscript, hated it and turned it down. From my comment that it was under review by *JCO*, he knew that I had not yet received his letter of rejection. Feeling uncomfortable, he may have decided that a verbal critique after my talk was necessary to explain his action. It now became painfully clear that Einhorn himself was the "expert in the field" who had "serious concerns".

"What are you going to do?" Bill asked.

"I'm going to call *JCO*," I replied.

I soon reached Dr. Robert Young's office. He was editor-in-chief of the journal. His assistant took my call and asked for details. "That's just it, there are no details," I told her. "Dr. Einhorn wrote that the paper had been reviewed by an expert in the field who had concerns, but no critique was sent. We believe we have a right to see the reasons our paper was turned down."

"This is all very strange. There must be a mistake. Perhaps he forgot to include the referee's comments. I'll look into it immediately and get back to you promptly," she promised.

The journal assistant called later that day. "Dr. Brandes, apparently there is no critique. We apologize. Although senior editors have the right to reject a paper without sending it for review, it seems that in this case things were not handled properly. Dr. Young has instructed me to inform you that he personally will be the editor responsible for your paper and will send it out to two new referees. We are even assigning your submission a new file number to clear the slate." I thanked her. The world could be a fair place after all. I called Bill and gave him the good news. Satisfied by this development, we then took the opportunity to tell each other how much we looked forward to our pending collaboration. Onward and upward.

On Thursday, December 22, 1994, I attended the pharmacology department's annual Christmas party. In addition to wonderful Indian cuisine prepared by Ratna Bose, and the usual large turkey with stuffing, expertly carved, as always, by Dr. Ian Rollo, we were treated to Frank's murder of the Italian warhorse, *Torna A Surriento* (Return to Sorrento). Carl, who tried to accompany him on the lute, and couldn't, added to the groans. "Why does every Sicilian with a tenor voice think he can sing?" I asked myself, wincing when an intended high C fell significantly short of the mark. "Keep your day jobs," I jokingly told the two over a plate heaped with delicious food. The conversation quickly turned to the good news about Sparta. They were both very excited for me.

"This kid's going places," Frank quipped.

Just as Carl started to speak, my pager went off, indicating an outside call. Excusing myself, I walked into the secretary's office down the hall and dialed the hospital operator. "Mr. Portigal is on the line," she said.

"Arnold?"

"Hi, Lorne."

I could sense from a certain flatness in his voice that he was down about something.

"Is something wrong?" I asked.

"You bet there is. Are you sitting down? Because if not, you'd better!" His speech was becoming a staccato. I immediately sat down on the desk, heart pounding with concern.

"Okay, what's the matter?"

"I'll tell you what's the matter. The Sparta deal is off," he replied tersely. *What????* "You heard me. I just got off the line with Bill Sullivan. He literally called me from a phone booth at the airport. 'Arnold,' he said, 'I have bad news. We can't close the deal.'

" 'Bill,' I said, 'don't fool around with me.'

"And he said, 'Arnold, I'm not kidding.' Lorne, I tell you, the guy was actually in tears....."

And by this time, so was I.

Then, for what seemed like an eternity, I sat in stunned silence as Arnold methodically recounted the gory details. Right after the weekend meeting, Bill Sullivan had presented the monetary aspects of the deal to his company's board of financial directors. Their verdict was a harsh one. IPO or no IPO, the company just did not have the resources to do everything that Sullivan had promised Arnold and the University. The board would not approve the deal and pulled the rug out from under him. He left the meeting a broken man.

I spent quite a while commiserating with Arnold. As sorry as I felt for myself, at that moment I felt even sorrier for him. I could tell by his voice that he felt personally humiliated by what had happened. After all, he had put his own good reputation on the line and had spent countless hours brokering a deal with Bill

Sullivan, never thinking that, at the end of the day, Sparta would not be able to carry out its end of the bargain. I thanked Arnold for all his efforts and hoped that he would carry the torch in the future should the opportunity arise.[82] Still badly shaken by this totally unexpected news, I went back to the party to tell Frank and Carl of the calamity that had just unfolded and then left for home to tell Jill the same. Another drug company deal down the tubes. *What a lousy break!!!*

---

82   It did and he did.

CHAPTER FORTY-ONE:

Not All Bad

New Year's Eve that year was a quiet affair. Two weeks previously we had been in New York, toasting our looming success in style; now, we were at the home of friends in Winnipeg, solemnly watching Times Square on television as midnight approached. The crowd waved and cheered as the countdown proceeded and the lit ball slowly descended down the mast at the top of one of the skyscrapers. I just didn't feel up to celebrating and was quietly glad that 1994 was coming to an end. To say the year had turned out to be a dud was a gross understatement. Between the FDA and Sparta fiascos, it was my version of what Queen Elizabeth had once called her "annus horribilis".

I had spoken to Bill McCulloch immediately after learning that the deal fell through. Understandably, there was no trace of the ebullience in his voice to which I had become accustomed. Like all of us, he had been totally unprepared for what happened and was as heartbroken as I that we would not get to work together. He was also very candid in his assessment that Sparta probably would not survive the loss of DPPE[83] and soon he might have to look for a new job. It was a very unhappy situation all around.

Since Arnold's call, I had also spent innumerable hours, on the phone or in person, telling my close friends and colleagues the sad story. The first was Lyonel, who kept shaking his head at the news. He really felt badly. Brent and Janet were very supportive, saying that the Cancer Foundation and University would continue to help develop DPPE in any way they could. Astonished by the sudden turn of events, Frank uttered his usual, "The Lord works in mysterious ways." Georgie counseled in her kind way that when one door closes, another opens. Ernie just gave me a big hug. He still thought DPPE was "gr-e-e-e-yat!" In all that time, I broke down only once, when I phoned Gerry Arron to thank him for all his hard work on my behalf. While negotiations were under way with Sparta, my friend of many years was always there for me, conscientiously representing my interests during meetings with the other parties.

As my wife and friends watched the midnight festivities, I sat quietly, reviewing for the umpteenth time in my mind all that had happened that year. After all, not everything had been bad. There had been the plaudits for my histamine meeting, and a major news story on our research was in the works by a prominent U.S. national news magazine....

That July, I had hosted the international histamine research symposium at the Elkhorn ranch in Riding Mountain National Park, a geographical gem stretching over three thousand square miles in western Manitoba. One hundred researchers from eleven countries, including many of my colleagues from the European Histamine Research Society, attended. With Frank as co-chairman, the meeting was an unqualified success. At its conclusion,

---

83   A year or two later, Sparta was bought out by another company and effectively disappeared. Along with his wife, also a physician, Bill McCulloch now runs his own medical consulting company in North Carolina. Bill Sullivan is still active in the industry; he lives in Nantucket, MA.

Walter Schunack, Wilfried Lorenz, Pier Mannaioni and Henk Timmerman led the others in a round of applause in appreciation for all the effort we expended to assure that everyone had a good time.

Putting the event together had been a real "mom and pop" affair. Jill was the major force behind the arrangements, writing letters, booking rooms, arranging bus transportation to and from the site, and making sure that the cuisine was up to snuff. "Feed them well and they will be happy," we reasoned. Jason had the onerous responsibility of projecting each speaker's slides (our Japanese guests took to calling him "Mr. Jason"). Only Carolyn was missing. She was spending the year in England.

On the first day of the meeting we took everyone on a tour of the park. Our guide had the bus stop in the middle of a huge field so that everyone could get out and take pictures. I wasn't sure why he had picked such an ordinary spot. As the doors opened, our guests rushed down the steps and ran into the wild grass, oohing and aahing, their cameras furiously snapping photographs of the small prairie flowers, and of lichen growing on rocks. All the while, Pier gazed upward as he turned in every direction. "It's the big sky, Lornie," he repeated to me over and over (with his Italian accent, my name always came out "Lornie"). Such a vast horizon was hard to come by in Florence, Copenhagen and Sendai. So there it was: people from other countries pointing out wonders of nature that we, in this part of the world, so often take for granted.

One of the invited speakers was Michel Dy, a researcher from Paris. Michel and his group had published a series of papers implicating intracellular histamine in the production of white blood cells by the bone marrow. Given Rob Warrington's findings that histidinol and DPPE protected the bone marrow in mice, and my observation in patients that DPPE appeared to shield the white cells from being knocked down by many chemotherapy drugs, I had taken a keen interest in Michel's work. He had recently conducted experiments with DPPE that convinced him I was correct in my hypothesis that there was some sort of intracellular "receptor" for histamine. I was delighted that he thought so since, from my point of view, he was a highly cautious scientist whose research was by far the most exciting in the whole histamine field.

During his stay, Michel told me that the research director at the Nêcker Hospital, where he conducted his experiments, was pressuring him to turn his attention away from histamine to other areas of study. It all had to do with attracting more money to fund the lab. Apparently intracellular histamine was not considered "sexy" by his director or, apparently, by France's leading scientific funding agency, INSERM. *Hmm. Where had I heard that one before??* Michel, who was a PhD, had little choice but to capitulate or jeopardize his career.

I was shaken to hear this and told Michel so. If he was forced to quit this line of research, vital new clues about histamine and growth would be left in the dust.[84] He was quick to agree, his tone melancholy as he spoke. Here was the most flagrant example of someone having to abandon important work because of the short-sightedness of others with dollar (or franc) signs in their eyes. At that moment I realized more than ever how lucky I had been to have Lyonel Israels for a boss. He loved all good science and never, ever interfered with the direction of research carried out by his staff.

Three months later, I received a call from Susan Brink, a senior medical writer for the Washington-based weekly magazine, *U.S. News and World Report*. She had talked with her editor and wanted to write a story about our research, specifically the studies on the effect of antihistamines and antidepressants on tumor growth. It was to be part of a cover story on the potential hazards of medications. She also told me that because of its likely impact on readers, she had already discussed the proposed story with University of Pennsylvania ethicist, Dr. Arthur Caplan. His view was that it was

---

84 Shortly after, Michel's research shifted direction away from histamine. Eventually, he became the lab's director and was able to return to studying the substance. Nonetheless, almost ten years had been lost.

potentially important for people to know about this issue and she should write it.

I was initially very leery about her proposal. Having just gone through the pain of that Ottawa meeting a month earlier, I was not anxious to relive the agony, and immediately told her of the inability of the FDA to reproduce our findings. Somehow, that thunderbolt did not seem to deter her. "Do you believe your results?" she asked. I replied in the affirmative. She assured me that she planned on speaking with people in the FDA and then told me that other knowledgeable scientists outside the FDA, to whom she had already talked, shared many of my concerns about the potential of drugs to affect tumors. She intended to write a balanced account of the story, pro and con.

While mollified by this, I had a lingering concern about her. At the time our *JNCI* paper on antihistamines was published, Susan had called me for details. She edited a column in the magazine that reported on health-related news and wanted to include a short précis of the findings. I spent considerable time with her, going over the potential clinical importance of our data, only to read a rather flippant statement in her piece, to the effect of, "Don't worry about this if you're not a rodent".

I now told her of my pique over her dismissive tone but was disarmed by her immediate apology that, on hearing me recount what was written, she agreed the inclusion of the sentence had been "tacky", the wrong thing to say; the fact that she now intended to write a major story signaled her true feelings about the potential importance of this research. How could I not like and respect someone who immediately owned up to a mistake? Moreover, as she was clearly going ahead with her story irrespective of what I thought of its merits, there were two choices open to me: don't co-operate and whatever happens, happens; or, co-operate in the hope that a good and factually-accurate story will result.

I opted for the latter, but struck a bargain in return for an agreement to make myself available for "background". Since complex science and controversial findings were involved, we would need to work together to ensure the accuracy of those particular aspects of the story. This would also mean interviewing Frank and going over any text relating to our work before publication. She agreed, a rare concession for any writer to make. Moreover, as the story contained an inherently worrisome message, I requested that a "positive" be included in the article: the promising early clinical trials with DPPE and chemotherapy. Susan promised to accommodate me if she could interview a patient.

For the next few weeks, we spent long periods on the phone. Her questions were always intelligent and penetrating. I would sometimes criticize a certain word or phrase that she had written. "What you are saying could be scientifically misconstrued," or, "I don't think that is an entirely accurate description of the experiment," I would comment. She was always willing to listen and to revise. As time went on, Susan and I became increasingly comfortable with each other and our mutual trust grew. As promised, I asked one of my patients, a lady named Irene Powroznik, if she would be willing to be interviewed for the story. Irene was one of the originals on my second study, having started DPPE and 5-fluorouracil treatment for advanced colon cancer shortly after Arnold Brown.[85] Irene was still going strong eighteen months later. Her painful liver metastases had shrunk on treatment and had remained stable. She was pain-free, active and enjoying life. Hopefully her story would be an inspiration to others.

In late November, Susan called to say that Scott Goldsmith, a photographer who freelanced for the magazine, would be coming to Winnipeg for a "shoot" the day after traveling to Irene's small town to take her picture. "I have a great idea," I said to her. "What about having him take a group picture of all of us for the story?

---

85   Arnold had finally succumbed to his cancer a few months earlier, almost one and one-half years following his first treatment with DPPE and 5-fluorouracil. In my opinion, he gained at least a year of good-quality life from the treatment. I was an honorary pallbearer at his funeral, as were Gary and Janice Filmon. The Premier and his wife drove me to the funeral at the Mennonite church in Winkler. The whole town turned out.

Everyone has worked very hard on this research. It's been a real team effort."

"Well, you can speak to the photographer, but I have to tell you we don't usually publish pictures like that," Susan sighed. *Oh, right. I forgot. Pictures have to convey interest. Anyone can take a group picture at a Sunday picnic, and millions do. They end up in photo albums, not in U.S. News and World Report.*

A few days later, Scott arrived with his array of lenses, cameras and lights. It quickly became obvious that he had great creativity, with the panache to frame scenes out of the seemingly mundane, an ability that clearly distinguishes the professional from the amateur. When I asked him about the possibility of taking a group picture, he did not hesitate. "That sounds like a great idea!" *Gee. Wasn't that what I had said to Susan? Maybe I had what it takes to be a Hollywood director after all.* "Let's see how we can do it. We need some space to get all of you in the photo. What's that large room over there?" he asked, pointing to the boardroom of my nightmares. As soon as Scott saw the large oak table in the center, it all came together....a nifty portrait took shape in his fertile mind. "If we can move all those chairs out of sight, I think it would be kind of neat for all of you to actually sit on the table."

I quickly called the others to report to the boardroom. They were thrilled and excited at the prospect of their picture being in the magazine. All that is, but Frank.

"No way," he barked.

"Why not?" I asked, amazed that he would refuse. He had already been interviewed by Susan. From going over the text with her, I knew that Frank's insights and comments on technical matters pertaining to the research were prominently featured in her story. "I have no intention of being lumped in with the others in a group picture over a caption that reads, something like, 'Dr. Brandes and his team," he said vehemently, immediately reaching for a Rolaids, his upper lip sweating. Those were definitely his "I'm upset" signals. From past experience, I knew them only too well.

I was totally unprepared for his response. I considered him my closest collaborator and a good friend. We were, as they say in Sicily, *alla familia*. Without his wisdom and insight, we would not be where we were. There was no way it would not be "LaBella and Brandes" or "Brandes and LaBella" in any caption. That was how it always was when we published our papers together. Trying to lower his rising blood pressure, I told Frank I would personally speak to Susan Brink about his concern. She would make sure that there was no slight. Frank just shook his head. He wasn't going to put his pride "in the hands of some *bleeping* editor." *Oy vay!! Mama mea!!* Although I really thought he had gone overboard and was being excessively thin-skinned, even paranoid, his ego in a knot, I quickly backed off. I had no intention of allowing this incident to have a negative impact on our relationship. Frank assured me it would not as long as I didn't persist in asking him to be in that *bleeping* picture!

Not long after, the editors reviewed all the different photographs Scott had taken that day (finishing up with "artsy" lab shots at almost ten o'clock in the evening). They were unanimous in their verdict. "I am almost embarrassed to tell you this, but everyone here loved the photo of all of you on that table. That's the one we are going with," Susan reported.

"Next time, don't argue with a pro," I cajoled.

Wishing each other season's greetings and good luck with the story, we agreed to talk again once it was published in early January.

"....three, two, one....HAPPY NEW YEAR EVERYONE," shouted the TV announcer as the large ball hit bottom and pandemonium erupted in Times Square. Interrupted by the noise, my "absence" having lasted but a few seconds, I now returned to the real world and joined in a drink of champagne as we all toasted the arrival of 1995.

Are you okay?" Jill asked with concern. She had been watching me stare vacantly into space.

"Sure I am, as long as I have you. To good health and better times," I proposed to my lovely wife amid a long hug and kiss.

CHAPTER FORTY-TWO:

Creating A Stir

The January 9, 1995 issue of *U.S. News and World Report* hit the stands for only a short time before all available copies were snapped up in Winnipeg. Gerry Arron personally cleaned out one downtown news vendor. After all, it was not every day that his daughter Randi's picture was in a national newsmagazine.[86] The cover title itself probably ensured brisk sales: *"Drug Alert! What your doctor may not know: The undisclosed side effects of some prescription drugs could hurt or even kill you"*. Inside were thirteen pages of a "U.S. News Investigative Report", devoted to the issue of "dangerous drugs". Susan Brink's contribution was a four-page story entitled, *"A different kind of cancer risk"*. I quickly winced at the sub-heading, *"If researcher Lorne Brandes is right, a number of drugs are to cancer as gasoline is to fire"*. Although accurately stating the possibility that concerned me, I immediately felt that the wording was way over the top, more suited to the *National Enquirer*. It was very upsetting. However, after reading the actual

---

86 Gerry had the group picture professionally matted and framed as a gift. What a friend!! It has hung on the wall of our family room ever since.

story, I calmed down. There were few surprises, just one very well-written piece.

The article covered all the bases. Should people who require medication for depression be told that the treatment might pose a cancer risk? What about patients with cancer who need to be prescribed an antidepressant drug? The story addressed the non-linearity issue based on our bell-shaped curves for tumor growth-stimulation, and even included a remarkable artist's rendering, based on Frank's hypothesis, of how we believed histamine interacts with P450 enzymes in a way that could alter hormone metabolism to perturb the already-damaged DNA in cancer cells, resulting in even faster cell division.

Several experts were quoted. While complimenting our experiments, Douglas Weed reiterated his remarks, made on CNN, that the benefits of the drugs were proven, while any theoretical cancer risk required further assessment in laboratory and human studies. David Rall, former director of the National Toxicology Program, believed that in addition to testing pharmaceuticals as potential carcinogens, the FDA should seriously consider testing them for tumor-promoting properties. Devra Davis, an epidemiologist who advised the U.S. Department of Health and Human Services, believed that our findings could provide a clue to explain the continued rise in cancer rates that could not be entirely explained by smoking or exposure to other known carcinogens.[87]

Susan also managed to obtain interviews with Robert O'Neill, acting FDA epidemiology director, who stated that within twelve months the agency expected to know whether our hypothesis was worth pursuing "big time", and Joe DeGeorge, who said that if our results could be validated by the FDA, they might consider adding the battery of predictive tests we reported in our paper. Their statements caught me by surprise since both must have known by then what Charles Grieshaber and Ralph Parchment believed

---

87   This was not the issue our studies had raised. My concern that epidemiology studies would focus on increased cancer incidence, rather than possible stimulation of growth of existing tumors, proved correct.

they had not found. Could it be that somehow neither had heard? In Joe DeGeorge's case that was highly unlikely, as Greg definitely would have told him following the Ottawa meeting. Maybe at the time of the interview there had been no official decision to "blow the whistle". I just didn't know.

Then there were the two pictures. The larger showed six of us, sans Frank, sitting on the boardroom table. Scott's lighting technique lent a slight "glow" to our faces, while the oak of the table beneath and the wood-paneling of the wall behind, imparted a warm honey-brown coloration to the scene. There I sat, front and centre, hands clasped in front and knees scissor-crossed beneath me; Patty and Randi, backs slightly bent forward, arms around their knees, sat immediately behind and to each side of me; Tong and Cheryl, backs straight to give them height over the other two, sat close behind and slightly to the right; finally came Gary, who was actually on his knees to give his head and shoulders good visibility in the centre at the back.

Despite being a group picture, the effect was to create a striking, very intimate portrait of each of us, none dominating the other. It was a masterpiece. No wonder the editors loved it. And the caption? "*The research team led by Lorne Brandes...*" Was Frank correct to absent himself, worried that he would be merely among the "led"? We'll never know, but I truly doubt it.

The second, no less remarkable photo, showed Irene Powroznik in her home. It was a beautiful shot of her sitting in her dining room, a cup of coffee in her hands, looking wistfully sideways. As promised, Susan had linked the negative story about antidepressants and antihistamines to the positive story of DPPE and the hope it held out for patients like Irene. I thought she had struck just the right balance.

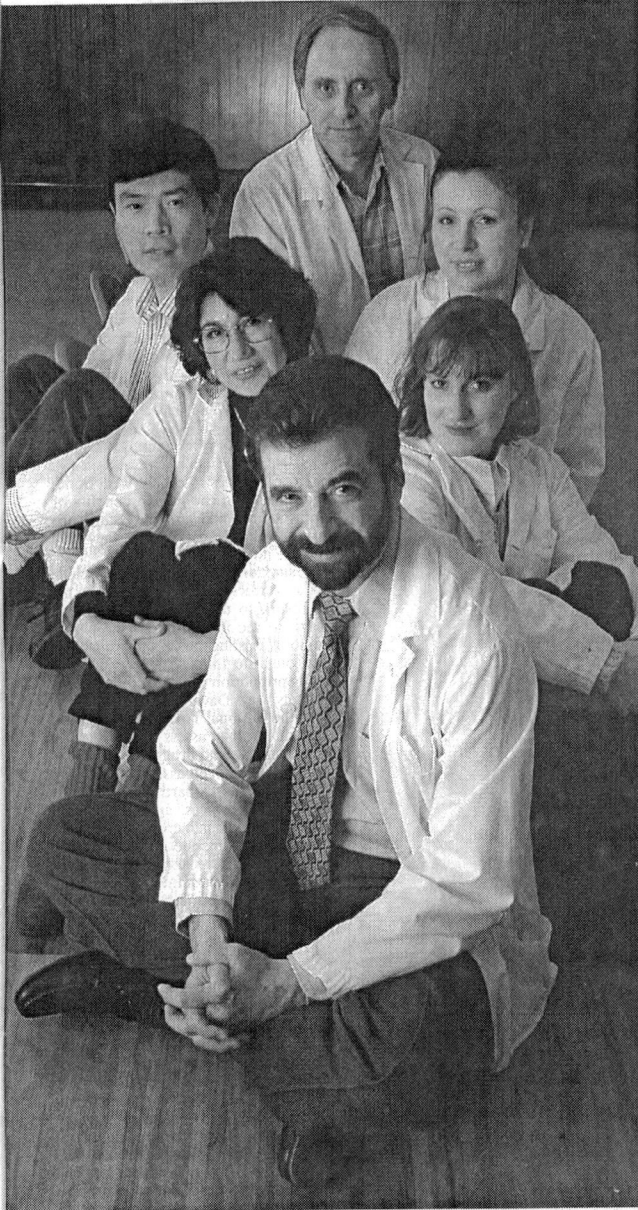

inside the body's cells, histamine binds to an enzyme, cytochrome P450, that plays a role in regulating cell growth.

LaBella and Brandes believe that because some antihistamines and antidepressants resemble histamine's structure, they bind to the same enzyme, making it harder for histamine to find a place. In Brandes's study, Reactine and doxylamine did not promote tumor growth and were also found to be the least effective of the five antihistamines at binding to P450. In the presence of cancer, say the researchers, some doses of drugs that effectively block out histamine from its enzyme nook may throw the cell's growth further out of kilter (diagram, Page 60). But very high doses may actually kill the cancer cells—thus explaining the bell-shaped response.

High-dose cure. Brandes's study of antihistamines and antidepressants began after years of research on a cancer drug called DPPE. He had found that in test tubes and lab rodents, DPPE made cancer grow faster at low and medium doses—but killed malignant cells at high doses. He then gave large doses of DPPE along with chemotherapy to 48 cancer patients, all with a poor prognosis after chemotherapy alone had failed. The results, reported last June in the *Journal of Clinical Oncology*, showed that 16 patients continued to worsen, but 12 stabilized, 12 improved, 7 had partial remissions and one had a complete remission.

Brandes's DPPE study may help explain a puzzle noted by many oncologists: Aggressive cancers sometimes respond better to treatment than do those that grow more slowly. Brandes's theory about DPPE's success with some patients is that the drug made the malignant cells divide faster, making tumors easier targets for cancer drugs. His early work with laboratory rodents led him to wonder about other chemicals that might make tumors grow faster. Since DPPE's chemical structure is similar to that of many antidepressants and antihistamines, Brandes began testing those drugs in rodents, even as he was taking his DPPE research to human trials.

The makers of the drugs Brandes tested point out that no one knows whether rodent results apply to humans and that human studies are needed. Brandes agrees, as does the Food and Drug Administration—but FDA regulators were intrigued enough by the findings to begin their own rodent studies last fall and to embark on plans for a study of medical records of cancer patients who have taken antihistamines or antidepressants.

Responding directly to Brandes's work, Eli Lilly & Co., which makes Prozac, published results of its own ongoing

The group photo, sans Frank LaBella, in U.S. News and World Report
(Credit: Scott@ScottGoldsmith.com)

As a result of Susan's article, I quickly learned two important lessons about magazines. Firstly, reporters must spend a lot of time reading each others' stories. Additional articles about our findings soon appeared in *Science News*, *Scientific American* and *Macleans*, a widely-read Canadian weekly. Secondly, each issue has a long shelf-life, ending up for who knows how long in places like doctors' and dentists' waiting rooms where thousands of people read them. I know because I began to receive scores of letters, e-mails and phone calls from ordinary citizens, many of whom told me they read the story while waiting for their appointments. It became obvious that the topic had resonated and people took note.

Most wanted to tell me of a personal experience, where they thought taking an antidepressant or antihistamine might be linked to their cancer diagnosis, sudden growth of a lump or spread to distant parts of the body. Based on what I had originally observed in my clinic that had led me to carry out the rodent studies, many of their stories sounded plausible. Nonetheless, as Larry Einhorn would say, they were all anecdotes. Then, unaccountably, the mother of all anecdotes occurred. After reading a newspaper account of our research, one of my own patients stopped taking a daily dose of an antihistamine-containing decongestant and her tumor disappeared shortly thereafter!

It is often said that fact is stranger than fiction. Here are the facts. The woman had a malignant tumor removed from her large bowel and surrounding tissue by a surgeon. After she recovered, I treated her with what is called "adjuvant" chemotherapy. Oncologists often prescribe this type of treatment after an apparently successful operation to try to decrease the risk of the cancer returning or spreading. Unfortunately, the chemotherapy was not effective in her case and the tumor recurred in a few months.

The first sign that there was something wrong was signaled by a routine blood test. It showed that the level of CEA, a "tumor marker" for her cancer, had skyrocketed from its previous normal value. A CT scan now showed a large tumor deep in the pelvis.

Using a long thin needle attached to a syringe, the radiologist was able to locate the suspect tissue and literally suck up some of it for the pathologist to examine. Colon cancer cells were seen under the microscope. Although it was potentially possible to operate and remove the cancer, my patient, who was seventy-four, decided against any further surgery or chemotherapy but agreed to have regular blood tests to monitor the CEA and her liver chemistries.

Her first followup lab result arrived by fax eight weeks later while I was away on vacation. Linda Friesen (no relation to Henry), my clinic nurse at that time, noted a precipitous drop in the CEA test. In the absence of any treatment, why would that be? Being highly attuned to my research, Linda called the lady to ask some questions. How was she feeling? Fine. Had she made any change to a medication? Yes. Which one? She had stopped an antihistamine/decongestant preparation that she had taken every day for the last twelve years for "rhinitis" (a chronic inflammation of the membrane lining inside the nose that may be due to allergies). Why did she stop it? She had read a story about her doctor's research on antihistamines and cancer in the local paper. If Dr. Brandes thought there could be a problem, that was good enough for her. She threw the bottle away. Linda was agog.

"You probably won't believe this," she said as she told me the story on my return. She was right. I was very skeptical.

"It was probably a lab error or they mixed up her sample with someone else. Let's get a repeat CEA test," I suggested.

The next day, the fax machine spewed forth yet another normal CEA test report. Her value had dropped from a level of almost one hundred three months previously, to a normal level of two! I immediately ordered a repeat CT scan. Where a proven tumor had previously been evident, only a thin scar remained! *Incredible!* How to explain this?

Some cancers can simply vanish on their own. It is a distinctly rare event, but cases of so-called spontaneous remission have been well documented in published reports. However, this phenomenon, which may involve the immune system rejecting the cancer as it would a foreign tissue, occurs mainly with melanoma (skin cancer arising from a mole) and renal cell (kidney) cancer. No one knows exactly why. I immediately reviewed the medical literature over the previous ten years. While finding the usual reports of spontaneous shrinkage of melanoma and kidney cancers, I could not find a single report in patients with colon cancer. I presented the case to my colleagues. None of them, including Lyonel, the "old man" in our group, had ever seen, or heard of, colon cancer disappearing on its own. This appeared to be the first recorded case in medical history!

So there we were. A patient stopped the chronic ingestion of an over-the-counter decongestant containing an antihistamine, in this case, an "oldie" called chlorpheniramine, and her tumor seemingly vanished. Was it a coincidence? Who could say? Would it stay away? Who could tell? Should she go back on the decongestant to see whether the tumor would start to grow again? Sure.... if she was a mouse or rat. But a human? Not on your life. That would be unethical.

"Are you going to report this?" asked Linda.

"I really need some time to think about it," I told my very brilliant nurse.

As things turned out, I didn't have that luxury. Like manna from heaven, a second mother-of-all-anecdotes almost immediately landed at my clinic door.

The wife of a medical colleague had been taking lithium for many years to control symptoms of severe manic-depression (bipolar disorder). Now, she had suddenly developed a very red, raised "splotch" over the center of her forehead. It bled easily and the skin around it started to swell to the point that both her eyes were very puffy, almost slit-like. A biopsy of the reddened skin showed a rare type of vascular cancer called "angiosarcoma" (the term "angio" derives from the Greek "angeion", meaning "blood vessel"). An MRI scan showed that the tumor's blood vessels were also spreading from the forehead to her eyes and upper nose. Angiosarcoma responds very poorly to chemotherapy or other treatment and often spreads rapidly to other organs such as the lungs and liver. This was definitely a bad-news situation.

Primed by my previous "anecdote" and realizing that there were few, if any, effective therapeutic options, I made a brash recommendation to the patient and her doctor husband. I wanted to try stopping the lithium to see whether the tumor on her face might shrink. "I'm serious," I said to her husband, who felt she needed the lithium and was skeptical that it could be stopped. Nonetheless, he was both scared and broadminded enough to say he would go along with the premise if her psychiatrist, Dr. William (Bill) Bebchuk, head of the psychiatry department at the University, agreed. I called Bill to explain the dilemma, summarizing the reasons for my proposed modus operandi and buttressing the argument with some additional provocative information from the medical literature.

For many years, it had been known that lithium stimulates the bone marrow to increase the number of white blood cells. Some published reports had even linked the drug to leukemia. If lithium could affect the growth of normal and abnormal white cells, could it also affect the growth of abnormal blood vessels through which they traveled? After discussions back and forth, all were in agreement that we try discontinuing the lithium. The patient remained on her two other drugs (estrogen for menopausal hot flashes and thyroxin, a hormonal replacement to offset low thyroid function, another side effect of lithium).

With Linda in attendance, I anxiously followed the woman in my clinic. Within two weeks, her forehead looked less angry. The areas that had been moist and bled easily were now drying and crusting over. However, her eyelids were still quite inflamed. She was having trouble seeing through the swelling. I decided to prescribe a low dose of a steroid pill called dexamethasone. It worked rapidly to take down her eyelid swelling. She and her husband were becoming hopeful that the future might be less dark than originally feared.

After six weeks off lithium, the improvement in her forehead was obvious and dramatic. Most of the red "splotch" was gone and the skin over the area was now dry and scabbed. That was the good news. The bad news was that she was becoming increasingly paranoid and irrational. The message was clear. She couldn't live with lithium and she couldn't live without it.

I immediately called Bill Bebchuk for advice. He knew her skin was much better, but felt that the addition of the steroid clouded the issue of how much the cancer had improved off lithium. Perhaps the drug should be restarted. I agreed that the steroid was very effective to suppress the inflammation associated with the tumor but argued that removing the lithium appeared to be working in the two weeks before starting the steroid. I now thought the two maneuvres might be complementary in causing her improvement. Whatever was going on, she had improved physically but now was worsening mentally. Something had to be done, but I wondered whether there was an alternative to lithium.

"Carbamazepine (Tegretol) can be an effective substitute in these circumstances," my colleague counseled. *Oh, no.*

"Carbamazepine is a tricyclic, like amitriptyline," I replied, immediately concerned that, like its close cousin, this drug had the potential to enhance tumor growth. I had just come across an eight-year-old issue of *The Lancet*; a patient with non-Hodgkin's lymphoma went into remission after carbamazepine was stopped. The authors thought there was a temporal link between these two events.[88] The story was reminiscent of the first lady with the colon cancer who stopped her decongestant.

"Have you tested carbamazepine for tumor stimulation in your lab?" he asked. I had not. "Then, in the absence of any data on that front, I recommend we substitute it for lithium. After all, we have to do something, *boychik*."

"I agree, but I'm really nervous about this," I confessed.

---

88   Schlaifer D, Arlet P, Ollier S et al. Carbamazepine (CBZ) can participate in the induction of an unusual but serious side-effect: non-Hodgkin lymphoma. [letter] *Lancet* 1989, 2: 981.

"Welcome to the real world," my professor friend replied with a trace of exasperation in his voice. *The real world? I didn't know about the real world? Gimme a break!*

Just six days after starting the carbamazepine, my patient's thinking improved dramatically, but the bottom fell out of her tumor. Her face exploded. As Linda and I examined her in the clinic, we could only shake our heads. The forehead "splotch" was again bright red and oozing blood. Several new angry red lumps had quickly appeared on her nose and cheeks. Her eyes were surrounded by a new sea of red skin. In desperation, I increased the dexamethasone dosage. It made absolutely no difference, suggesting that any benefit of the steroid on her tumor had been greatly overestimated. I could only conclude that the timing suggested a link between stopping lithium and regression of her cancer, and starting the carbamazepine and a rapid worsening of her cancer.

Despite heroic radiotherapy, chemotherapy and a drug called interferon that can shrink blood vessels, the angiosarcoma continued its relentless course and the poor woman rapidly went downhill in two weeks. The tumor spread to her lungs where it caused massive internal bleeding that killed her. Watching all of this unfold, I felt especially sorry for her poor husband. He had always been there for her during her long years of struggle and seemed totally lost.

I now firmly believed that common medications could influence the behaviour of cancer in humans. It was not really such a leap of faith. Medical science has long accepted that drugs intended to help one disease may be bad for another. Why not cancer? Our case reports needed to be published. As Linda had "dug the dirt" on the first patient, I asked her to be my co-author. "Since they have published a previous letter on carbamazepine, we'll send our report to *The Lancet*," I suggested. She readily agreed. In a letter accompanying our paper, I pointed out the previous report in that journal linking carbamazepine to lymphoma. Hopefully this information would help our case. It didn't. Three weeks later we had our rejection. One reason given was that the link between

carbamazepine and lymphoma had already been published! *Duh!*
Once again the editors had been squeamish when Dr. Brandes
came knocking with his scary anecdotal observations. I decided
to call someone who possessed a backbone. Dr. Bruce Squires,
editor of the *Canadian Medical Association Journal (CMAJ)*, had
taught me in medical school at Western. We had recently renewed
our acquaintance at my twenty-fifth year class reunion.

I was impressed by the job Bruce had done since taking over
the *CMAJ*, once a very learned journal that, in recent years, had
fallen on hard times. He had made it learned and relevant once
again. Bruce had previously commissioned Alex Robinson to
write an in-depth report about antihistamines and tumor stimulation in the *CMAJ*, where he had interviewed Greg Burke. After a
breezy conversation about people and things we had in common,
I hit him with my request.

"Bruce, would you be willing to have a look at two case reports
that were just rejected by *The Lancet*?" I asked, explaining the
background to him. He was at once receptive, suggesting that I
send him both the manuscript and the correspondence with *The
Lancet*. He would go over it himself and get back to me. I sent
everything he requested and added reprints of our rodent studies
and Susan Brink's story for good measure. Within a few days, I
received a fax saying that he had read the paper with interest, was
impressed by the unusual case reports, and was sending them out
for peer review.

A few weeks later, Bruce again contacted me. The reviews
were positive and he would publish the case reports. Then he surprised me, asking that I flesh out the manuscript. In my attempt
to be as non-controversial as possible with *The Lancet*, I had
kept the discussion of the two case reports very short, not going
overboard in discussing our previous studies or other supporting material. Bruce wanted me to go into detail about them and
also reference any other studies implicating an effect of medications on cancer growth in the test tube or in people. He was also

commissioning a major editorial to accompany the paper. I told you he had backbone.

Three months later the paper was published under the title, *"Can the clinical course of cancer be influenced by non-antineoplastic drugs?"* Somewhat unusually, the editorial, entitled, *"The Brandes-Friesen case reports: how should we interpret the news?"* was written by two individuals, rather than one: Dr. David Roy, an ethicist at the University of Montréal, and Dr. Neil MacDonald, an oncologist and director of the ethics program at McGill University. Their commentary was scholarly. With well-chosen words, they illuminated the issues surrounding drugs and tumor stimulation. At the same time, their recommendations were very cautious, not all that different from those in the *JNCI* editorial by Douglas Weed. Roy and MacDonald also took aim at that inflammatory and injudicious "...gasoline is to fire" headline in *US News and World Report* that had so upset me, saying, "...Such language can provoke unconsidered action in clinical situations—-situations that require the most careful and prudent deliberation people can muster." *Amen.*

I was especially pleased that the editorial concluded with the following comments and advice: "Brandes and Friesen have alerted us to begin taking stock of what could possibly be happening to people who have detected or undetected tumors and who are taking antidepressants or antihistamines. Their concern that some patients with a high risk of cancer or a history of the disease could be affected adversely by antidepressants and several other classes of commonly-used drugs should be neither ignored or downplayed.

"However, taking stock rationally means taking things step by step. The first step is to alert physicians so that they can report any similar cases that they encounter. If and when such case reports begin to accumulate the next step will be to conduct systematic epidemiologic and controlled studies. Meanwhile, balance in interpretation, prudence in clinical counsel and transparency in discussion with patients should guide clinical practice and research."

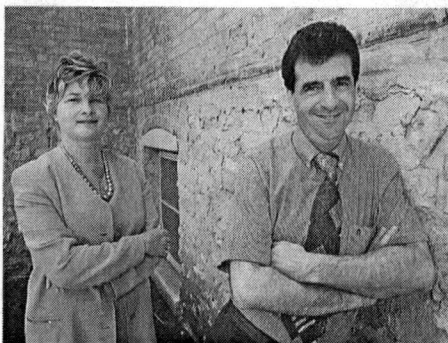

HEALTH

Sounding an alarm

Can some medications promote cancer?

Lorne Brandes is a man with a mission. A physician and researcher at the Manitoba Cancer Treatment and Research Foundation in Winnipeg, Brandes has long suspected that some widely used drugs may have the unintended side-effect of stimulating tumor growth. In 1992, he and other researchers published a study showing that two popular antidepressants, Prozac and Elavil, seemed to promote cancer growth in laboratory animals. Two years later, Brandes published the results of another investigation, which showed that three commonly used antihistamines also appeared to promote tumor growth in mice. Now, in an article published in the latest issue of the *Canadian Medical Association Journal*, Brandes describes two fascinating cases in which drugs being used for unrelated conditions had a striking effect on tumor growth. As an editorial in the *Journal* notes, the cases by themselves prove nothing about the safety of the two drugs involved—the antidepressant lithium and a widely used antihistamine that is not identified in the article. But the editorial suggests that the cases should cause physicians to "begin taking stock of what could possibly be happening to people

who have detected or undetected tumors and who are taking antidepressants or antihistamines."

Both cases occurred last year and involved patients of Brandes. One was a 63-year-old woman who developed cancer that affected her forehead, upper eyelids and the bridge of her nose. The woman was taking daily doses of lithium carbonate—a substance that has been linked to some forms of cancer in the past—to treat her manic-depressive illness. When, at Brandes's suggestion, she stopped taking lithium, the cancer showed signs of subsiding. But when her mental state deteriorated and she was put on another antidepressant drug—and eventually back on lithium—the tumor grew rapidly and killed her.

In the other case, a 74-year-old woman who had previously been operated on for colon cancer was found to be suffering from a recurrence of the disease. The woman decided against further surgery, and received no more treatment. But she was aware of Brandes's earlier study involving antihistamines. As the woman later explained to Brandes's nurse, Linda Friesen, she decided to stop using an over-the-counter decongestant, which she had been taking for 12 years and which contained an antihistamine. Within 60 days, her cancer—a type that rarely, if ever, undergoes spontaneous remission—had vanished. So far, her cancer has remained in remission.

Brandes predicted that medical authorities would dismiss his observations. "They'll probably say, 'Don't worry about Dr. Brandes—he's overreacting.'" But some cancer researchers said that Brandes's paper was potentially significant. "It's important that doctors know about these cases, in the event that they come across the same thing in their own practices," said Dr. David Hedley, a cancer researcher at Toronto's Princess Margaret Hospital. "But if no other cases come out of the woodwork, then I think we will be able to conclude that what Dr. Brandes saw were simply coincidences." Until that question is resolved, some patients and their doctors may become more cautious about using the medications singled out in Brandes's disturbing study.

MARK NICHOLS

Brandes (right) with Friesen: fascinating and disturbing cases

Linda Friesen and me in Macleans magazine

At just that time, I received a call from James Mathews, a science reporter with *JNCI*. Like *Science*, *JNCI* also had a section, in this instance called, simply, *News*, that reported developments in basic and clinical cancer research. He had already spoken with Dr. Grieshaber and now wanted to interview me about the failure of the FDA to reproduce our results. Word got around after both Grieshaber and I had been invited to present our findings at a meeting of the American Society for Clinical Pharmacology and Therapeutics that March in San Diego.

Now, with Mathews' first question, I knew what was coming. Given the failure of the FDA to confirm our study, did I still believe there might be a link between drugs and cancer growth? "I must ask myself, based on what I and others have seen, is it possible that human beings are being affected by these pharmaceuticals, and my answer, intuitively, is yes," I answered, our just-published human observations once again making ripples on television and the Canadian newswires. *Yes, yes, a thousand times yes.* I believed we were correct in what we reported. Confirmation or no confirmation by the FDA, I was not about to back down. *How could this guy possibly appreciate the series of events that led me to this conclusion?*

When Mathews' story finally appeared in *JNCI*, I was struck by the tabloid-like headline: *"Concern over Prozac-Induced Tumor Growth May Dwindle Following FDA Study"*. No matter what other drugs were involved, the infamous fluoxetine always seemed to "sell more newspapers". In the article, Dr. Grieshaber now appeared to be speaking for senior FDA officials when he stated that earlier animal studies suggesting a link between antidepressants and tumor growth may have been premature and "created a stir where a stir should not have been created."

Mathews continued: "The [1994 *JNCI*] article piqued the interest of FDA regulators and scientists who set out to replicate Brandes' findings. A large-scale epidemiologic study examining the records of thousands of patients would have likely followed any replication. But Grieshaber, to his admitted surprise, discovered no discernible link between antidepressants/antihistamines and tumor growth in rodents. 'The whole basis for our study was to gain a sound scientific basis on which to jump into epidemiological and mechanistic studies and have the FDA make some kind of regulatory statement. Now our regulatory people don't feel they can make any immediate regulations based on non-reproducible data....Had we been able to duplicate or come close to duplicating or even seen a hint [of tumor growth] activity that Brandes suggested, it would have stimulated additional studies to find the mechanism, not only in FDA labs, but across the country. But you can't look for a mechanism if the *effect* isn't there,' Grieshaber added."

No matter that the same *effect* was found in two independent laboratories separated by hundreds of miles; no matter that researchers in Japan had reported the same *effect* with another antidepressant; no matter that bell-shaped and biphasic curves of this *effect* had been published for scores of other drugs and substances, including, by my analysis, fluoxetine; no matter that I and others had observed that certain medications may have an adverse *effect* on cancer in humans; no matter anything....we had just been discredited by the FDA in a news report in *JNCI*...the very same journal that, a few months earlier, had published our study! The "*effect*" was now officially declared a non-effect.

But had we not earlier used a similar approach with Jean Marx' *News and Views* report in *Science* to disseminate our viewpoint? From my perspective, it was apples and oranges. We already had our paper peer-reviewed and published in *Cancer Research* when she wrote her story. Where was the peer-reviewed paper behind the news report in this case? Normally, scientific data, whether positive or negative, should be published in a journal for all to read, not just presented to a few hundred people at a meeting or revealed in an interview.

Instead, Mathews' story was a simple and rather effective way for the FDA to quickly throw cold water over the whole issue without publishing. There likely was concern about Susan Brink's article and the "spin-offs" it spawned; now they wanted to publicly distance themselves from us as much as possible. Yet, a news report, rather than a scientific paper, might indicate that there was still a worry that Grieshaber at al. could be wrong in their negative findings. Why not wait for further lab or epidemiology studies to emerge before actually publishing the FDA studies in a journal?[89] Nothing would be worse than to end up with egg on their face if the federal lab was wrong about such an important matter.

Was that the end of the story? Just an unfortunate series of aberrant laboratory results and clinical misinterpretations that "created a stir where a stir should not have been created"?

No. Despite the FDA position, serious questions remained. The interest of epidemiologists and toxicologists was not dampened. But when real evidence for tumor stimulation in humans finally emerged five years later, it arrived not in epidemiology studies but, as will be told, in the "failed" MA.19 clinical trial of DPPE and doxorubicin!

---

89   The FDA results were not published in a peer-reviewed journal until almost nine years later (2003), and after Charles Grieshaber and Ralph Parchment had left the FDA for the private sector and academia, respectively.

CHAPTER FORTY-THREE:

Empty Plates And Cracked Beakers

In March, 1995, I received a letter from Dr. Young at *JCO*. Apparently, two additional "experts in the field" did not share Dr. Einhorn's serious concerns and our prostate cancer study was accepted with only minor revision. "Gre-e-e-yat," Ernie exclaimed when informed of the decision. I couldn't have said it better myself.

Now recovered from my shock over the events of December, I decided once again to contact Lee Schacter at Bristol-Myers. After thanking him for giving me the lead about Sparta, I told him the sad details of our recently-failed business deal. He felt badly. "That's always the problem with these small pharmaceutical start-ups," he lamented. "Most just don't have the deep pockets required to develop drugs." Given what had happened, I obviously could not disagree with that viewpoint.

Changing tack, I raised the subject, yet again, of possible Bristol-Myers interest in DPPE. "Lee, we have just had a paper accepted in *JCO* reporting on a promising study of DPPE and cyclophosphamide in advanced prostate cancer. Based on the results, we have just filed a new use patent. I would be happy to send a preprint your way if you are interested." He definitely was.

A few days later, Lee called back. "Your timing is good," he said. "When we last spoke, our plate was full, so-to-speak. At the moment, that plate is closer to empty. Give me some time to work on this. I think I can definitely stir up interest within the company. New therapies for prostate cancer are definitely on everybody's agenda these days." He ended by promising to get back to me as soon as he had more news. *Hmmm*. Maybe my "high flyer" strategy, developed after our previous encounter, was about to pay off. Maybe this would be *the* one. Maybe, maybe, maybe….maybe doesn't count. I did not want to get my hopes up. Three months later Lee wrote to say he was still working to get DPPE "on the agenda". It seemed that prehistoric glaciers melted faster than the time it took for decisions to be made at Bristol-Myers.

While Lee toiled away on my behalf, so did I. Since it appeared to everyone that good things were happening, pressure mounted to treat more and more patients with prostate and breast cancer. But with each new patient, the work piled up for Susie and me. In addition to the extra time spent in the clinic, there were the hours spent making ever more DPPE. By default, I was the world's supplier for a single client…me! With that dubious distinction came the stark realization that I had an obligation to my patients to make sure we didn't run out of the drug.

One night as I worked alone to make yet another hundred grams of the precious white powder, some alcohol used in the procedure slopped over the side of a hot beaker sitting atop a Bunsen burner and burst into flames. As the apparatus was contained in the fume hood, there did not appear to be any immediate danger to the lab. I figured that, within a minute or two, the fire would simply die out as the wayward alcohol burned itself up. Unfortunately, that script changed within seconds when the bottom of the beaker suddenly cracked open from the heat and its flammable contents leaked out to feed the flames. The inside of the hood rapidly became an inferno. This was definitely a bad hair moment.

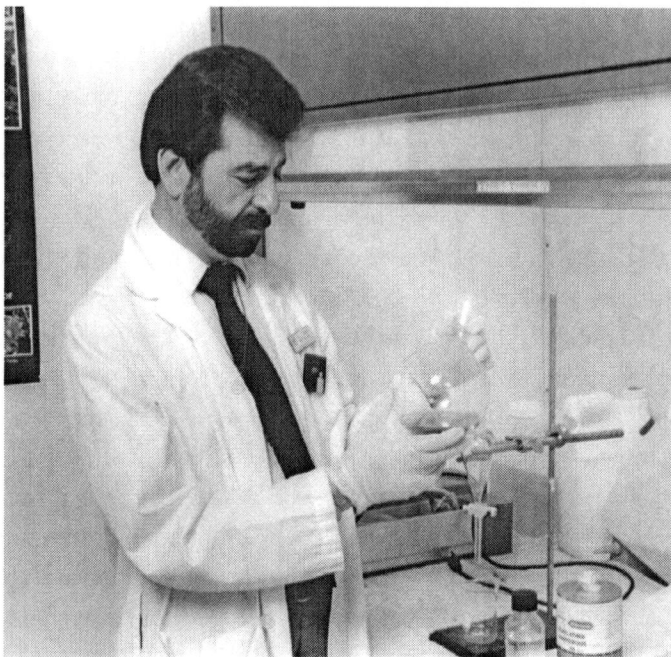

Making DPPE in my laboratory (CancerCare Manitoba Archive)

Running through the lab, I frantically scanned the walls for a chemical fire extinguisher. None was to be seen. *Incredible.* How could there not be a fire extinguisher nearby? Apparently there wasn't. I ran out into the hallway. A few steps down the hall, behind a rectangular glass window on which was stenciled the word "FIRE", was a wall receptacle containing a fire hose. I pondered my next move. *"You don't pour water on a liquid chemical fire!"* my high school chemistry teacher yelled deep within the recesses of my brain. *Absolutely right, sir.* So where was the bleeping fire extinguisher?

I ran back into the room. Although still contained, the flames were now roaring up the wall at the back of the hood. It would not stay that way for long. Time had run out. There was only one thing left to do. I pulled the fire alarm. Bells clanged throughout the building. The fire department would be on the way. But would they get there soon enough? Suddenly, a colleague from another lab ran in, trailing that fire hose. Water was dribbling out the end, awaiting only a simple twist of the nozzle to roar forth, full force. "Don't do it!!" I commanded as I ran back to the wall receptacle in the hallway to turn off the tap. I could hear distant sirens. *Oh, man. Get here already!!*

Suddenly, I stopped in my tracks. There, at the back of the receptacle, behind the now-empty hose reel, was a large red fire extinguisher. A sticker proclaimed that it was to be used for chemical fires. I quickly yanked it out of the wall and ran back to the blazing fume hood. Pulling the safety pin, I pointed the wide black nozzle at the fire and squeezed the handle for all it was worth. A thick yellow chemical cloud immediately shot out with a loud who-o-o-sh. The flames were smothered within seconds.

Literally at that moment, three firemen, axes in hand, came bolting through the lab door. One carried a large hand-held chemical extinguisher. It was no longer needed. All that remained in the hood was a smoking, blackened gooey mess that was once destined to be DPPE. This batch would not make it into the clinic! The yellow chemical powder that had quenched the flames thickly coated everything.

"Hello, gentlemen," I said sheepishly as we all stood looking at the charred residue and blackened walls inside the hood. An over-weight fire captain, breathless from running up the stairs, walkie-talkie crackling, suddenly appeared on the scene. My explanation was requested and given. I told him that a disaster had been averted only at the last moment when the fire extinguisher had finally been located. Thank goodness for my somewhat misguided colleague who unreeled the fire hose, exposing the extinguisher's camouflaged location at the back of the wall receptacle. The cap-tain's eyes rolled as I continued to explain how my cancer drug had gone up in smoke. He wrote down this sad information in his soiled, dog-eared notepad.

By order of the Winnipeg Fire Department, within days all laboratories had new red chemical fire extinguishers bolted to the wall. If nothing else worked out for me, at least I had made one visible contribution to the place.

CHAPTER FORTY-FOUR:

Mr. Goldberg

Mr. Goldberg was an assessor in the U.S. Patent Office. I did not know his first name. Maybe it was just "Mister." All I did know was that his signature kept appearing on rejection forms sent to Michael Stewart. Mr. Goldberg was in charge of the file for our "Method of Cancer Treatment" patent application. For almost two years, he had raised objection after objection to our claims. A mountain of paper outlined the "actions" taken by him...in our case, disallowing this, that or whatever.

When objections are raised by an assessor, applicants are always given a period of time, usually sixty days, to respond. For each response to be considered, a fee must be paid. With whatever patent office he was dealing, Michael would most often handle a response to an objection himself. He would modify wording or "trade off" one minor objectionable claim to gain acceptance of another that was strategically more important to our case. More often than not, this did the trick. On other occasions, if techni- cal input on a scientific point of inquiry was needed, he would ask me to advise him on how to respond. Whatever the approach required, Michael was almost always successful in finding a compromise that resulted in an assessor reversing a rejection....that is, every assessor but Mr. Goldberg.

It should be stated that Mr. Goldberg held no personal animosity towards us, at least none that was obvious. Patenting is a very capricious exercise at the best of times. That is because, to obtain maximum protection for a drug like DPPE, patents are usually filed in multiple countries or, in the case of the European Union, blocks of countries. In the patent office of each country or jurisdiction, every application is judged autonomously, without regard to decisions, positive or negative, made in another.

When a new patent is filed, the first step is a search to determine what is called "priority". During this time, an assessor may discover a journal paper or another patent filing published prior to the date of the current patent application. Such a document would then be cited by the assessor as constituting "prior art". If such a citation cannot be rebutted successfully, the patent application is dead in the water. If the search fails to find evidence of prior art, the patent is then examined to determine whether the claims are supported by the facts provided by the inventor. For example, is the claim that X results in Y justified?

The crazy thing about patent filings is that you never know what objections will be raised, and on what basis, by any given assessor. A patent can fly through one country's patent office and be granted with no objections in a few months. The same patent in another country...well...you get the picture.

In this particular case, the "Method of Treatment" patent had already been granted in many countries, including Canada and the E.U. In the case of the U.S. Patent Office, however, we were at an impasse. Michael had done as much as he could and, in March, 1995, felt the time had come to visit Mr. Goldberg for a face-to-face meeting. He wanted me to accompany him to Washington. "It often helps for the inventor to be present at these discussions so that the assessor sees that there is a real person at the other end of all the paperwork," Michael advised. He had been a patent agent for many years and knew every angle. I always listened to him.

I called Janet Scholz to tell her of Michael's plan. She agreed that I should go along and made arrangements for the University to cover my travel costs. It wasn't a "freebie". As with everything else related to the patent costs for DPPE, my trip would be added to the "bill", to be paid back at the end out of monies flowing from, we all hoped, a licensing agreement.

Arriving in Washington, Michael and I stayed at the same hotel so that we could go over the file ahead of time. Michael instructed that, during the meeting, I was to sit quietly and not interject while he and Mr. Goldberg tried to work out some sort of agreement... unless Mr. Goldberg spoke to me or wanted my input. I readily agreed. After all, this was completely foreign territory to me.

At the appointed time, we walked into the USPO building and took the elevator to the floor indicated on the directory in the lobby. His office door open, Mr. Goldberg waved us in from behind his desk. He appeared to be well into his sixties, thinning hair neatly combed back, tie held in place against his white pin-striped shirt by a gold chain, glasses perched on his nose, grandfatherly, really quite benign-appearing. His office was old and small, with filing cabinets lining walls desperately in need of new paint. The furniture was typical civil service issue, dating from the 1940s or 50s...an old battle-scarred wood desk and swivel seat. Two old chairs with cracked leather cushions, their stuffing uneven and flattened from years of use, faced his desk. Hanging slightly askew on the wall behind Mr. Goldberg was a small black-framed certificate attesting to his long and faithful service.

"Please sit down," he instructed, smiling slightly as he motioned for us to use the two chairs. Michael preferred to stand, like a lawyer presenting his case to a judge. He went through the obligatory "thank you for seeing us" routine and then started to briefly outline the issues as he saw them. He was only a few words into this part of his spiel when Mr. Goldberg interjected. "I'm prepared to give you a Markush on your first claim, but I can't grant the others," he said, hands clasped across his belly. *What had he just said?*

"I'll gladly take the Markush, but I can't give up the other claims," Michael replied. *Markush?? What were these guys talking about?*

As the two old hands then sparred back and forth in technicalise, I just sat there, a stupid smile frozen on my face, my head and eyes turning from one to the other as their lips moved. *Don't interject? I couldn't if I had wanted to.* What was happening to my brain function? They were speaking in tongues. Even a translator from the United Nations would have been useless here. It continued on like this for another few minutes.

Suddenly, Mr. Goldberg leaned forward, clasped his hands in front of him on the desk and spoke to me in English. "What Mr. Stewart and I are arguing about is this. I am willing to give you the other claims in the patent only if you can prove to me that DPPE has to be given *ahead of time* to protect the bone marrow from a chemo drug," he stated matter-of-factly. I suddenly realized that this grandfatherly assessor was as sharp as a tack, having picked up a fine point missed in every other country where the patent had been granted.

The issue arose from the wording in the "Method of Treatment" patent, stating that "an antagonist of intracellular histamine binding (in this case, DPPE) is *first* administered...." The experiments that we had published in our *JNCI* paper did not determine *whether* DPPE must be given first to protect the bone marrow, only that *when* given first, it did. If DPPE could also protect the bone marrow when given *after* the chemotherapy drug, the claim in our patent was invalid on a wording technicality.

Not to be cornered by this wise old goat, I assured Mr. Goldberg that I would speak to Rob Warrington. The experiment could be repeated, comparing the survival of bone marrow cells when DPPE was given before or after the mice had received the chemotherapy drug. He nodded in approval, assuring me that if the protection by DPPE could be demonstrated before, but not after, administration of a chemotherapy drug of our choice, the patent would be granted. We all shook hands and the meeting was over.

"What on earth is a Markush?" I asked Michael as we went down the elevator. My head was still spinning from the encounter. Laughing, he explained that Markush was actually the last name of an inventor. His first name was Eugene. In the 1920s, he had won a landmark case in the United States Supreme Court against the USPO. Prior to that time, so-called "variations on a theme" could not be claimed when patenting a chemical. Markush won the right to do so. Ever since, his name has been immortalized in the phrase, "Markush groups (or structures)". *Patent Law for the Nonlawyer* (*Second Edition, 1991*) explains it this way: "...it is sometimes important to claim, as alternatives, a group of constituents... referred to as a 'Markush Group' that are considered equivalent for the purposes of the invention."

In plain English, based on the Markush case, Mr. Goldberg was willing to allow Michael's claim of several chemical variations of the structure of DPPE in our patent. The "Markush" application would then have the effect of preventing someone else from trying to patent a DPPE-like drug simply by tweaking the molecule. However, unless I could prove that DPPE only worked if given prior to a chemotherapy drug, granting the Markush would be of no use to us.

This episode had not one, but two good endings. First, Rob Warrington was only too happy to carry out the required experiments. A few weeks later, he sent me the results. They could not have been more definitive. DPPE was effective only when given before chemotherapy. True to his word, Mr. Goldberg granted the "Method of Treatment" patent, complete with "Markush" claims.

Second, I got to thank Senator Edward M. Kennedy in person for a kind favor he had done for me ten years earlier. The encounter with the senator occurred while I was waiting at Washington National (now Ronald Reagan) airport for my flight back to Winnipeg on Friday afternoon. The local weather office had issued a winter snow storm warning. As much as three inches of the white stuff threatened chaos in the nation's capitol. I was amused by the panic this announcement was causing. In Manitoba, three inches would be considered merely a "dusting". In any event, the airport became crowded with various government officials trying to flee the city for the weekend before the snow shut down the runways.

As I stood in the main lobby of the terminal, I suddenly became aware of a familiar person standing right next to me. It was Ted Kennedy, no doubt about it. He seemed to be alone. As we smiled and nodded at one another, I saw my opportunity to tell him something. Sticking out my hand to shake his, I introduced myself. "Senator, I wonder whether you might remember what I am about to tell you," I said. He made no attempt to avoid this intrusion on his privacy. On the contrary, he asked me to go on, his eyes firmly fixed on mine.

Ten years earlier, I had treated a young man for bone cancer in his leg. He had gone through heavy-duty chemotherapy and then had the leg amputated. While surgeons now do limb-sparing procedures where the cancerous bone is removed and replaced by a titanium prosthesis, amputation was the rule in those days. Senator Kennedy knew this all too well. His own son, Edward Jr., had gone through the same ordeal about eighteen months before my patient. He had made headlines around the world when a picture of him skiing on one leg was run in every newspaper.

Unfortunately, my young patient was not so lucky. A few short months after his amputation, the cancer came back with a vengeance and spread to both lungs. Surgery to remove the metastases was not possible. There was nothing we could do except to try to buy time with further chemotherapy. He was inconsolable. His parents were devastated. For once, words failed me. Remembering that picture of Edward Jr., I wrote a letter to the senator, telling him about my patient and asking whether he might send a note, care of me, that I could give to the young man.

Ten days later, an envelope bearing the official seal of the United States Senate arrived in my mail box. It was from the office of Senator Edward M. Kennedy. Wow! I took it right up to the hospital ward. "There seems to be a special letter here for you," I said. As the young man opened it and read the personal message of hope, tears welled up in his eyes. That letter remained with him at his side until he died a short time later. I had always been grateful for the senator's act of kindness and now had been able to thank him in person myself. The circle had been closed.

"Doctor, tell me. How are we *really* doing in the war against cancer?" Senator Kennedy asked after I had finished my story. "One step forward, a half-step back...but I remain hopeful," I replied. He nodded as we shook hands again and then left for our respective gates. It was a very special moment, compliments of Mr. Goldberg.

CHAPTER   FORTY-FIVE:

Funding Woes

As I continued to wait for Lee to fill Bristol-Myers' plate with DPPE, I had to contend with unhappy news from NCIC. My major grant, researching histamine, had not been renewed in the spring, 1995 competition. During our studies on the antihistamines over the previous two years, Frank and I thought that we had amassed enough compelling data linking the AEBS and histamine with P450 enzymes to satisfy the harshest critic. Moreover, we had recently discovered that, just like DPPE and the antihistamines and antidepressants, the female hormones, estrogen and proges- terone, and the male hormone, testosterone, also competed for histamine binding. In fact, adding any of these substances to the liver microsomes actually knocked radiolabeled histamine right off the iron molecule to which it attached on the P450 enzymes... a *YinYang* effect. Why should this be? Perhaps naturally-occurring intracellular histamine was keeping the enzymes "quiet", in the steady state; when it was displaced, the electrical charge on the iron would change, possibly activating the enzyme to metabolize whatever substance had caused the histamine to leave its perch.

We thought that the observation was potentially important, and proposed in the grant application that we investigate this intriguing phenomenon in depth.

Unfortunately, nobody on the grants panel seemed to share our enthusiasm. Maybe they just didn't get it. "Ah, yes," they said, "you have made these interesting observations, but what do they mean? You have previously shown that newly-made histamine in platelets causes them to clump, but in the work you have recently published, you have shown only correlations, not the *direct proof* that intracellular histamine is causing cells to divide. Moreover, we do not think that the experiments you now propose will nail down the answer. Therefore, we can not enthusiastically rate your grant." There would be no NCIC money for Brandes and LaBella on this go-around. Once again, we had fallen off the funding bandwagon.

Equally disconcerting, despite the FDA position that tumor stimulation by drugs was a "non-effect", we had prepared a second NCIC grant application to further our studies of this issue. It was a very ambitious project. Frank and I filled the pages with our proposal for new experiments, including an investigation of a potentially important observation, recently published by investigators in Palo Alto, that amitriptyline and fluoxetine acted as tumor promoters by preventing cell death ("apoptosis"). Since, in the natural course of events, some proportion of cancer cells in a tumor constantly die off, any effect of these drugs to prevent apoptosis might be linked to stimulation of tumor growth.

Sadly, this one lost on a split decision, resulting in a rating below the cutoff. Two referees liked it and recommended approval. However the third referee wrote that funding for this type of project should be sought from pharmaceutical companies, not a federal granting agency. We wondered what kind of pharmaceuticals he was on to come up with that one.

Luckily, my other NCIC grant, researching how DPPE makes chemotherapy more effective, was approved for another two years. Nonetheless, I was again in a cash-crunch despite receiving a one-year award of thirty-five thousand dollars from the Thorlakson

Foundation.[90] As loss of the NCIC funding still left a shortfall of seventy-five thousand dollars a year, there was no alternative but to make cuts to my staff. Cheryl had recently left after deciding to go into business with her brother, but I still had one assistant too many on the books. I reluctantly called Tong into my office and gave him the bad news that I could no longer afford to pay his salary. He listened quietly as I explained the situation. He had not seen this coming and was both shocked and upset. Who wouldn't be? I just hated that moment. His reward for doing everything that I had asked of him was to lose his job. It wasn't fair, but with "soft" grant money to pay my assistants, that was the stark reality.

A second stark reality was that, as Michel Dy had also learned, attracting money for this type of histamine research was not easy. What we were investigating had never been considered a mainstream endeavor by the *mavens* who doled out the dollars for cancer research. At most, we were just on the cusp. By continuing to pursue Kahlson's intracellular histamine hypothesis, we were taking a big gamble. A letter that Richard Schayer had written me in the spring of 1993 seemed to prove the point. Wilfried Lorenz had just sent him a copy of our *Biochemical Pharmacology* review paper, "*Histamine as an intracellular messenger*", and he was excited.

His letter read in part, "...I am delighted that you and your colleagues have such good support for the existence of the H_{IC} receptors. I have firmly believed this for more than thirty years but had no way to prove it....*Kahlson's theory was never really accepted.* In his rapid growth studies, an expansion of the microcirculation

---

90   Established by Dr. Paul Thorlakson, a pioneering Winnipeg surgeon who founded the University's Department of Surgery, it was administered, in part, by his sons, both cancer surgeons. One of them, Ken, had shown me great kindness over the years and was only too happy to do what he could to support my work. Ironically, in another of life's random events, one of his own children would later become my patient and receive DPPE.

could be an underlying factor."[91] So there it was. "They" didn't believe Kahlson then, and "they" were highly skeptical of us now.

I met with Frank to plan strategy. Any tensions caused by his refusal to be in that photograph now behind us, we remained the two amigos. If Frank believed a project had scientific merit, he, like I, would stick with it no matter what reviewers had to say. "It's always easy to criticize under the cloak of anonymity," he would observe when, in his opinion, unnamed reviewers widely missed the mark. Rejection had been an all-too-frequent occurrence in his own long and distinguished career, let alone in mine.

Unfortunately, there was virtually never a comeback when a grant was turned down. All one could do was scramble for local sources of funding, wait for the next major competition six months down the road and, when writing up the new proposal, try to anticipate criticisms and somehow avoid them. No matter how much money had been awarded in the past, at grant time there could be no room for complacency in the mind of any researcher. One perceived stumble and the funding agencies that giveth would brutally taketh away.

Despite the relentless criticisms of the grants panels, and knowing that we remained on the critical list for future funding, we made our decision. Whether or not others were excited by our findings, we would continue to soldier on, focusing our experiments on the interaction of drugs and hormones with histamine on P450 enzymes. Unfortunately, further experiments on tumor

---

91   Dr. Schayer believed that, rather than making cells divide, Kahlson's newly-formed histamine actually controlled the tiny blood vessels that form when needed to supply rapidly growing cells and tissues with oxygen and other nourishment. He was way ahead of his time, his theory predating that of Dr. Judah Folkman, whose research (as I will discuss in a later chapter) has championed the importance of tumor angiogenesis (blood vessel formation) in cancer growth. Dick Schayer's hypothesis linking intracellular histamine with the microcirculation took a leap forward when my Swedish colleague, Klas Norrby, made a remarkable discovery that DPPE works with histamine to increase blood vessel growth in mice. That may, in part, explain the ability of DPPE to stimulate tumors.

stimulation would have to be put aside, a victim of this reversal of fortune. I would carry Patty on my grant and Frank would continue to employ Gary and Doug on his. The roller coaster ride that characterized our research continued.

CHAPTER FORTY-SIX:

"A Gift To The World"

Nineteen ninety-six turned out to be "my year". I do not recall that there had been anything to indicate this fact in the fortune that fell out of my "cracker" at the Russell's annual December dinner. So much for premonitions and fortune tellers. And since poor Lee Schacter was still going around in circles with his bosses six months after he had undertaken to interest Bristol-Myers Squibb, I now held out little hope that anything would materialize on that front. But then, early in the new year, the results of two previous phone calls changed the course of events for the better.

The first had been to Arnold Portigal in late September, 1995. Arnold had recently stepped down as board chairman of the Cancer Foundation and relocated to Phoenix where, some years earlier, he had established a branch of his investment company. Now in his sixties, he had decided to close down his Winnipeg office rather than to split his time between the two cities. Talk about weather extremes! What was more unpleasant...freezing Manitoba winters or sizzling Arizona summers? It was a draw, he would laughingly tell me.

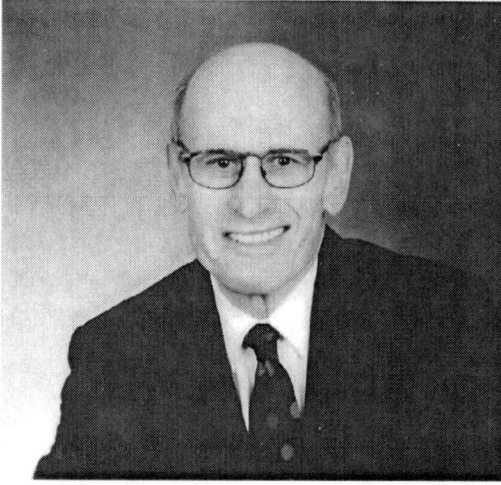

Arnold Portigal (Photo courtesy of Arnold Portigal)

Despite the distance, we kept in close touch. I continued to appreciate all that he had tried to do in furthering DPPE and often called just to talk or to report on new developments. On the September day that I called him, the subject of Lee Schacter and the reticence of his company to make a decision came up. "Arnold, would you be willing to stick your chin out one more time?" I asked on the spur of the moment. After seeing him in action with Bill Sullivan, I knew that if anyone could succeed with Bristol-Myers, it would be Arnold Portigal. "Maybe you are just the one to move things forward with them," I added for good measure.

I needn't have pressed him. He often traveled to the east coast. If the opportunity presented itself, he might be able to meet personally with Lee Schacter and his colleagues at their office in Princeton, New Jersey. One potential problem with my request was that Arnold was no longer officially connected with the Cancer Foundation. True to form, that mere fact didn't bother him at all. He was willing to vet my request with Brent Schacter and his successor as board chairman. If they agreed, he would see what he could do.

Soon after, Arnold called to say that the two had no objections. I was to send him an executive summary outlining my thoughts on the potential of DPPE in cancer therapy. Once he had read it, he would contact Lee Schacter. Arnold may have been a layman but, if well briefed, he had no compunction about meeting with the drug company executives to advocate the merits of DPPE on our behalf. The term "shrinking violet" was not in his vocabulary!

The second call had been made a month later to Dr. David Beatty, successor to Peter Scholefield who had retired as executive director of the NCIC. Over the previous three years, I had tried unsuccessfully to garner the interest of his organization's Clinical Trials Group (abbreviated NCIC-CTG) to test DPPE in their phase two investigational new drug (IND) program. The problem was that it was hard for me to compete with a host of major pharmaceutical companies with promising drugs in their pipeline and lots of money to pay for testing. They continually vied with one another for the group's new studies. From the drug companies' perspective, a clinical trial carried out by a well-regarded organization such as the NCIC-CTG provided an excellent opportunity to generate high-quality data that, if positive, could help lead to regulatory approval for their products.

David and I knew one another quite well, although we had not been in touch for some time. Years earlier, he headed up surgical oncology at our institution and, with his wife Barbara, an immunologist, had been involved in a research project with Frixos Paraskevas at the Institute of Cell Biology. Now it was time to enlist his help. Specifically, I wanted him to intercede with CTG director, Joe Pater, and the head of the IND program, Elizabeth Eisenhauer. "It just doesn't make sense that the premier Canadian clinical cancer trials organization wouldn't be willing to test a 'made-in-Canada' drug," I told my colleague. He listened intently as I vented my frustration at continually having to go it alone. When I had finished, David promised me that he would take up the matter with the others.

Elizabeth called me a short time later. From our few previous contacts I both liked and admired her. In addition to her skills in carrying out clinical trials, she had great people skills, always diplomatic and honest in her dealings. Of course, it didn't hurt that she was also very pretty and that her spiffy attire gave her that "just stepped out of Vogue" look. I wasn't alone in noticing that. Many a male colleague agreed with my assessment. Once, a couple of years earlier, she suggested that I present a lecture about my work at one of the semi-annual NCIC meetings. I was pleased and willing, but nothing had come of it because apparently she couldn't get to first base with the program planners.

Now, in reviewing the latest developments with Elizabeth, I explained that, in all my years as an oncologist, I had not seen the kind of rapid, and often complete, responses that I was observing in the latest breast cancer trial combining my drug with doxorubicin. Having treated just over twenty patients in the last eighteen months, I had documented seven complete remissions and had even taken several of these women off treatment to observe them. More recent subjects were still undergoing treatment, but the signs pointed to significant tumor shrinkage in at least nine of them. Overall, it appeared to me that approximately seven out of every ten patients were responding to the DPPE/doxorubicin regimen.

Elizabeth was definitely intrigued with this information because the CTG had previously carried out a phase three trial comparing doxorubicin alone to the combination of doxorubicin and another chemotherapy drug, called vinorelbine, in a similar group of women with breast cancer that had metastasized. Only three out of every ten women in that study had responded to the doxorubicin, no matter whether it was given alone or combined with vinorelbine. It appeared that, in a comparable group, I was seeing over double that response rate by combining DPPE with doxorubicin.

Elizabeth had an idea. She wanted Winnipeg oncologist Dr. Kong Khoo, a member of her IND committee, to review the charts and X-rays on these patients. If he confirmed my findings, she would be willing to advocate that DPPE and doxorubicin be tested by the NCIC in a phase two "confirmatory" study. I thought that Kong, a very bright and enthusiastic member of our department, was an excellent choice and immediately agreed to her suggestion.

"By the way, who is manufacturing DPPE for your studies?" she asked.

"I am," I replied nonchalantly. I think she was taken aback. "Don't worry," I quickly added, "it's easy to make and comes out as a pure powder. It's been approved for use in humans by Agnes Klein. I can easily supply it if you decide to conduct a trial."

Two weeks later, Kong sat in front of an X-ray view box in the clinic. I had given him eight representative charts and placed a stack of X-rays on the desk at his side. Two hours later, his verdict was in. In a letter to Elizabeth on November 21, 1995, he stated, *"Lorne has something important here but the proper study to assess the many features of DPPE in metastatic breast cancer has to be done."* I couldn't have agreed more. A flicker of optimism crept in. Maybe at last we were going to make headway with the NCIC. I called David Beatty to tell him of Kong's positive response and to thank him for keeping his promise. He was pleased to have helped me out, and wished me luck.

As this was happening, Arnold contacted Lee Schacter. By that time, Lee was probably delighted to have some outside help. His ministrations so far had been frustrating. The most he could show for his efforts was a chronic headache. Lee put Arnold in touch with Roslyn Feder, the new head of worldwide licensing. She seemed to travel constantly. After a few weeks of playing telephone tag, they finally spoke. The following day she sent him a fax suggesting her interest in starting "an *ongoing* dialog". No wonder Lee had a headache!

"Now the fun is beginning!" Arnold wrote me.

But the fun soon turned into frustration. It seemed that they were playing "revolving door" at Bristol-Myers as executives came and went over the next few months. Among them was Roslyn Feder. Enter Alice Leung, the new oncology licensing director.

Soon Alice and Arnold were making progress. After several more months of faxes and phone calls, a face-to-face meeting was finally set up in Princeton to coincide with a business trip that Arnold was making to New York in April. In addition to Lee and Alice, Oncology VP, Renzo Canetta, would attend.

To this day, I am not exactly sure what was said that tipped the scales with Bristol-Myers. I only know that shortly after the meeting I received two calls. The first was from Arnold, reporting that things had "gone well" from his perspective and that Bristol-Myers was "definitely interested" in DPPE. The second was from Lee, to say that prior to Arnold coming on the scene, DPPE was "not on the table". Now, as a result of the meeting with Arnold it was "firmly on the table". There was no doubt about it. Lee believed that Arnold had pulled off a coup. I wasn't surprised. They were dealing with the master.

Lee indicated that the company was especially interested in the prostate cancer data. Due diligence, including a patent review would commence immediately. If no problems were identified, Alice Leung and her team would carry the ball and make a project presentation to senior management. If that hurdle was success-fully passed, all stops would be pulled out to sign a licensing agreement. It would take some time, but the train had finally left the station.

I allowed a second flicker of optimism to creep in. However, based on what Lee had said, there was now a worry in my mind that the breast cancer data might be pushed aside. Drug company decisions are driven by many factors, not the least of which is marketing strategy. There were a lot of breast cancer therapies competing in the marketplace, whereas the field was wide open for new prostate cancer treatments. I firmly believed that DPPE had the potential to make a difference in many types of cancer… maybe in most cancers. Rather than being disease-specific, it was more generic in its action, a so-called "add-on" drug, intended to make existing therapies more effective. I absolutely had to get that point across to the decision-makers at Bristol-Myers.

Rather than Lee, I decided to press the case with Alice Leung. Arnold was very impressed by her and thought she was a sharp cookie. Sharing my concerns with a woman also made the most sense, as she was likely to be highly sensitive to the "other-than-prostate-cancer" indications. It took almost two weeks to make contact because, like almost every other executive in the company, Alice's job required that she travel around the world.

"Alice, I am calling because I am very concerned that Bristol-Myers not have tunnel vision about DPPE. It has potential far beyond prostate cancer," I told her, making clear my belief that it held great promise in breast cancer. I also apprised her of a recent study by a group of researchers in Japan who had carried out experiments showing that DPPE made cis-platinum, a chemo-therapy drug marketed by Bristol-Myers, more effective against human ovarian cancer tumors transplanted into nude mice.[92]

Alice promised me that she would keep this information firmly in mind. I spoke to her again three months later, just before she was to put the project to senior management. She told me that her group had put a lot of effort into preparing their presentation. It would include the other potential applications I had discussed with her. She allowed that she was quite nervous. In a huge pharmaceutical operation like Bristol-Myers, new-candidate drugs compete for licensing approval not only within a division such as Oncology, but also *against* other divisions, such as Cardiovascular, Neurology or Endocrinology. This meant that DPPE could be turned down in favor of promising drugs that lower cholesterol, fight obesity, treat high blood pressure or improve Alzheimer's disease, all worthy in their own right. I wished her luck and kept my fingers crossed.

---

92   Nude mice are so-named because they are hairless. More important, these genetically-inbred mice lack a functional immune system. As a result, human tumors can be transplanted into them without being rejected as foreign tissue. In this way, the response of human cancers to various treatments can be assessed in the mice.

A week later my prayers were answered. Alice rang to tell me that the presentation had been well received. Senior management had bought the story. The train had not only left the station but was now heading towards its destination…a licensing agreement! Once again the lawyers, including mine, would be busy. I excitedly informed the University and Cancer Foundation of this important development. I also informed Elizabeth. By now, her IND committee had endorsed the plan to test DPPE and doxorubicin in patients with metastatic breast cancer. A draft of the treatment protocol, involving Winnipeg and three other Canadian centres, was being developed.

"It looks as though Bristol-Myers may acquire the rights to DPPE," I told her. Elizabeth did not see this as a problem for NCIC unless the drug company was against the proposed study. Given Alice's assurances, I could not imagine that it would object, but called Lee Schacter to be sure. To my relief, he viewed the involvement of NCIC as positive and believed his company would as well. I passed along his comments to Elizabeth. Now there were two trains, Bristol-Myers and the NCIC, traveling in the same direction on parallel tracks. I could only pray that, this time, nothing would happen to cause a derailment.

The summer was spent fine-tuning the agreement, but two aspects of the deal got my goat. First, the "up-front" money offered by Bristol-Myers was a paltry one hundred and fifty thousand dollars, not even enough to repay all the cost of the many patents. I personally would not share in that initial money because I had signed a prior agreement that the University and Cancer Foundation would first have to recoup the money they had spent along the way. I understood. It was only fair. Subsequent "milestone" payments would become progressively larger and, with the patent debt repaid, I would share them equally with the two institutions. The first such milestone payment would be triggered if the outcome of the soon-to-start NCIC confirmatory phase two breast cancer trial, now known as "IND.97", was judged to be positive. If the drug then passed several other clinical trial milestones in breast and prostate cancer and was ultimately approved by the FDA, royalties would flow. *We should only be so lucky.*

Second, although they were willing to pay me as a consultant, Bristol-Myers would not up the ante to fund my laboratory research. Try as he might with Alice Leung, even Arnold could not squeeze that concession out of them. "They are hard-nosed business people who regard this as an unproven drug. Their aim is to pay the least amount of money for the maximum gain. They know that we need them more than they need us. If DPPE proves successful in the short term, I believe their thinking will change about funding you," he told me.

I accepted the wisdom of his comments, but was insulted nonetheless. Why shouldn't I be? My research had made possible the drug they were licensing. I discussed my frustration with Brent Schacter and Terry Hogan. Without some sort of infusion of funds, the current research money would run out in less than a year. Given our recent track record, I was not optimistic that Frank and I would be successful in the next grants competition.

After huddling with their respective boards, Terry and Brent agreed that I would be given seventy-five thousand dollars from their share of the licensing money. It would be designated as a research grant so that the money would not have to be repaid. Moreover, we could apply for matching funds from the University/ Industry program that the Manitoba Health Research Council had in place for just such situation. It was a magnanimous move on their part and went some distance in mollifying me.

Then, just when I had come to terms with the hard bargain driven by Bristol-Myers, Lee Schacter broke the sad news to Arnold Portigal that, after many years with the company, he had come to the end of his rope and would return to academia before the licensing agreement became a reality. Arnold and I both believed his frustration over getting Bristol-Myers to commit to DPPE was the straw that broke the camel's back. From Lee's perspective, licensing DPPE was a no-brainer and should have been taken up quickly. He just couldn't stand the stultifying corporate bureaucracy that allowed months and years to go by without making business decisions. I thanked Lee profusely for all his help but wished he could have stayed on to head up the DPPE project. He told me that his replacement would be Dr. William Slichenmyer, a fellow oncologist with the company. I did not know him.

Although the actual document was officially signed in late August, it was decided for public relations reasons to have a ceremonial signing at the Cancer Foundation on September 5. A joint announcement appeared that day on the wire services:

"DPPE a Promising Therapy for Prostate and Breast Cancers"

PRINCETON, N.J., MONTREAL, and WINNIPEG, Manitoba, Sept. 5 /PRNewswire/ —

"Bristol-Myers Squibb Company (NYSE: BMY), the Manitoba Cancer Treatment and Research Foundation (MCTRF), and the University of Manitoba, Canada, announced today a license agreement under which Bristol-Myers Squibb will develop and market DPPE, a novel treatment for cancer. In preclinical tests and in clinical trials conducted at MCTRF in patients with prostate and breast cancer, DPPE appears to enhance the cytotoxic effects of chemotherapy with no additive unwanted side effects.

"Under the terms of the agreement, Bristol-Myers Squibb, the world leader in cancer chemotherapy, will assume responsibility for worldwide development and marketing of DPPE, which has demonstrated activity in a Phase II trial as combination therapy in patients with hormonally-resistant prostate cancer. In addition, the National Cancer Institute of Canada is undertaking a Phase II trial with DPPE in combination with doxorubicin in the treatment of patients with metastatic breast cancer. Bristol-Myers Squibb will provide upfront and milestone payments to MCTRF and the University of Manitoba, as well as royalty payments after marketing. Details of the financial terms were not disclosed....

"'Despite significant advances in the war against cancer,' said Sol Rajfer, M.D., senior vice president, Worldwide Clinical Research and Development, Bristol-Myers Squibb, 'treatment options remain limited for all too many patients with cancer. DPPE is an exciting therapy which, in combination with other chemotherapy drugs, may help fill a largely unmet medical need for patients with hormone-refractory prostate cancer, metastatic breast cancer, and other cancers. In addition, we expect that DPPE will complement Bristol-Myers Squibb's broad oncology product line. We are delighted to have the opportunity to collaborate with MCTRF and the University of Manitoba and we look forward to a mutually beneficial collaboration'....."

The signing ceremony was expertly co-ordinated by Julia DeFehr, the Cancer Foundation's head of media and public relations. It was held....guess where?...in the boardroom (the famous table had been moved off to the side to hold the food and refreshments). Various dignitaries were present: representing the Cancer Foundation were Brent Schacter, board chairman Rick Hester, and "my man", Arnold Portigal, who had flown in from Phoenix; Janet Scholz, Marion Vaisey-Genser and President Emöke Szathmáry represented the University; front and center for the provincial government were Premier Gary Filmon, accompanied by his wife, Janice, and Minister of Health, Jim McCrea; the Bristol-Myers

Squibb contingent consisted of Alice Leung; VP of International Development, Dr. Michael B. Stewart (no relation to our patent agent); and Canadian VP of Scientific Affairs, Dr. Sophia Fourie from Montréal.

From my perspective, the most important attendees were in the audience. First and foremost were Jill, Jason, and Carolyn. In addition, my mom and dad had flown in from Windsor, Ontario. It's one thing for them to have a son, the doctor. But this? There were no words possible, only tears of pride and joy. I was just happy that they were still in good health and could be present to enjoy the moment. Mom's breast cancer had remained in remission on tamoxifen and she felt and looked wonderful. Dad, a former haberdasher, was dapper as ever in his dark business suit. At eighty-two, he was in excellent shape and still appeared ten years younger than his age. Susie Bracken saw the three of us walking down the hall to the boardroom and, camera at the ready, snapped a sensational picture that, to this day, sits front and center in a frame on my desk.

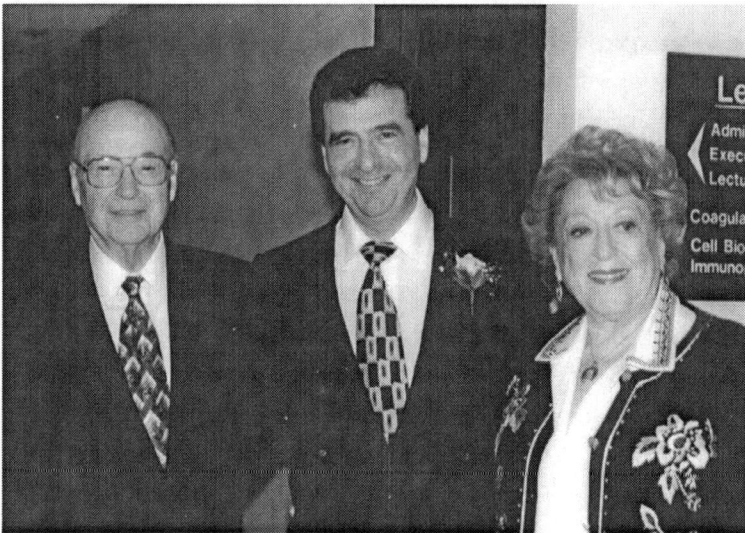

With mom and dad before the signing ceremony (Photo courtesy of Susan Bracken)

Among many invited close friends and colleagues was Gerry Arron, who beamed at the accolades coming my way. Lyonel, standing next to Arnold Greenberg, looked on proudly from the back of the room. And of course there was Susie. None of this would have been possible without her nor, for that matter, all the other dedicated people who worked so hard on my behalf: long-time clerk Michelle Powder, Linda Friesen, and Nancy Johnson.

Also in the boardroom that morning were three specially-invited guests: Clarice Silver, whose husband Paul had gained a year and a half of good-quality life on DPPE before succumbing to his disease, and Dr. and Mrs. Ken Thorlakson, whose daughter Carla, a brilliant career diplomat, also appeared to have her young life prolonged by the drug. The gratitude they showed by their presence that day gave me a feeling that no money on earth could buy. Sadly, Katie Brown, Arnold's widow, was still trying to cope with his death. She sent her regrets and best wishes.

Following the signing ceremony, *Winnipeg Free Press* reporter, Catherine Mitchell, briefly interviewed me and then left to file her story. Later that afternoon, after I returned from a posh celebratory lunch at the Westin Hotel arranged by Julia and Arnold, Catherine called me at my office. "How old is your suit?" she asked. After I got over her chutzpah, I estimated that it was eight years old.

"I must tell you that it happens to be a very good suit, made in Italy," I hastily proclaimed to hide my embarrassment. *Sigh.* I had dealt with the press long enough to know that the age of my suit somehow would be vital to her story.

Under the next day's page-five story headline, "*New cancer drug a 'gift to the world'* ", she wrote, "Sporting an eight year-old suit and a white rose in his lapel, Brandes watched as representatives of Bristol-Myers Squibb, U of M and the [Cancer] Foundation signed over development and marketing control to Bristol-Myers Squibb. 'This is Manitoba's gift to the world today,' said Premier Gary Filmon, whose friend and mentor, the late Arnold Brown was among the first to use DPPE to fight his cancer."

Despite Gary's heart-felt, optimistic words, I knew that only time would tell whether that "gift" would become a reality. The road ahead remained long and uncertain.

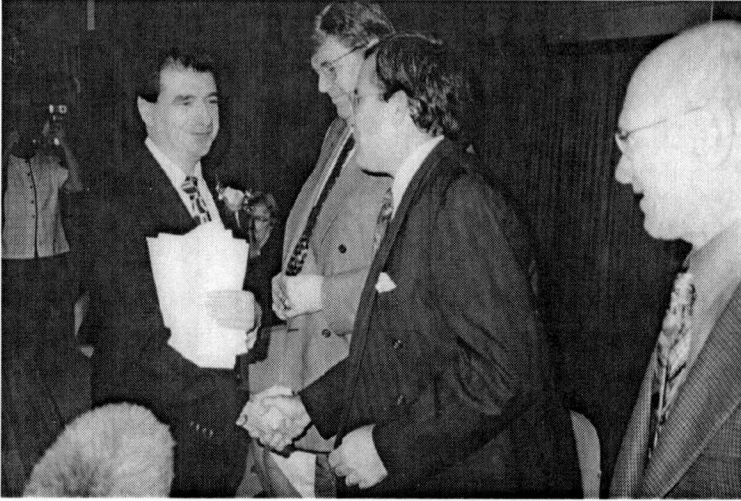

Premier Gary Filmon congratulates me. Arnold Portigal is at far right. (Photo courtesy of Susan Bracken)

Winnipeg Free Press, Friday, September 6, 1996   A5

Local

New cancer drug a 'gift to world'

Local doctor sells patent rights to pharmaceutical giant

By Catherine Mitchell
Staff Reporter

IT TOOK Dr. Lorne Brandes and a team of nurses 12 years to prepare for the stroke of a pen that yesterday handed over their cancer drug's future to a major pharmaceutical company.

Described as a momentous occasion for Manitoba as well as for medical science, Brandes sold the patent rights of the drug known as DPPE to Bristol-Myers Squibb.

Officials say if all goes well, DPPE should be on the market in a few years.

For the rights, the drug company will make upfront payments to the University of Manitoba and to the Manitoba Cancer Treatment and Research Foundation. "Milestone" payments — such as after periodic successes from clinical trials and again when the drug is licensed for use — and royalties once it is on the market, will flow to both public bodies.

No one, however, was revealing how much DPPE's development will be worth to the university, the foundation nor Bristol-Myers Squibb.

"What we're doing here is taking a giant step forward," said Brandes, a professor of medicine at the university and an oncologist at the foundation.

Sporting an eight-year-old suit and a white-rose on his lapel, Brandes watched as representatives of Bristol-Myers Squibb, U of M and the foundation signed over development and marketing control to Bristol-Myers Squibb.

"This is Manitoba's gift to the world today," said Premier Gary Filmon, whose friend and mentor, the late Arnold Brown, was among the first to use DPPE to fight his cancer.

In 1992, the provincial government gave $500,000 in special funding to usher DPPE through experimental clinic tests. The money was said to salvage the research, at risk from funding cuts, and the drug was credited with extending Brown's life by 18 months.

Sitting in the audience of the foundation's small boardroom, Clarice Silver watched the signing with joy and sorrow.

Nine weeks ago, her husband Paul, 62, succumbed to leukemia diagnosed about 18 months earlier.

He was given three to six months to live but after three months of conventional treatment, it was clearly not working, his wife said yesterday.

Failing quickly, Paul Silver went to

> *'What we're doing here is taking a giant step forward.'*

Brandes and joined the group of 170 patients using the experimental drug.

"It made a significant difference to his quality of life, extending his life a year and a half," said Clarice Silver.

Paul worked at his distribution company to the end, and in March, they visited their new granddaughter in Toronto.

While smiling from the shower of accolades thrown his way at the news conference, Brandes was careful to thank the people like Paul Silver who made the drug's development possible.

He singled out oncology nurse Susan

Bracken, who developed the treatment protocol for the patients, and Dr. Marion Vaisey-Genser, who, as the university's vice-president of research, took a leap of faith in 1984 and started the quest to patent the drug.

Dr. Arnold Portigal, the foundation's past-chairman, was the chief negotiator in securing the agreement with the drug company, he said.

Brandes said the signing yesterday marks a rare event in medical research.

It is unusual for a drug to be taken off a professor's lab bench and into hospital use for experimental use before a drug company gets involved, he said.

He could recall only one other occasion in recent medical history in which an individual — a University of Michigan professor in the 1960s — developed a drug through to advanced clinical stages. "Drugs are normally discovered in pharmaceutical labs, or people run out of steam, or they run out of money before they attract the interest of (private) labs."

DPPE, heralded as a cancer success story destined to put Manitoba on the map, is an antihistamine that appears to make cancer cells more susceptible to chemotherapy.

Used alone, DPPE will hasten the production of diseased cells. But in conjunction with chemotherapy delivered an hour later, it helps knock out diseased cells.

DPPE appears to fight prostate cancer that no longer responds to hormones or radiotherapy, and has been found to be effective, in combination with other drugs, with colon cancer, lymphoma and other cancers.

It has entered new trials on breast cancer patients, just under way in Winnipeg, Thunder Bay, Hamilton and London.

Story in the Winnipeg Free Press, September 6, 1996

CHAPTER FORTY-SEVEN:

The Cat's Meow

The following morning, Julia DeFehr received a message from her contact in the public relations department at Bristol-Myers. Apparently the company had received a private request for DPPE that they would like to discuss with me. If I would be so kind as to call the public relations office, I would be given further details. That was intriguing. I phoned the number Julia had given me.

"Oh, Dr. Brandes, it is so nice to speak to you personally, at last. Thank you for getting back to me," bubbled the lady at Bristol-Myers.

"My pleasure. What can I do for you?" I replied, feeling quasi-important.

"We have had a somewhat unusual request," she said. I listened with increasing amazement as she spelled out the details. A senior executive in the news department at one of the major U.S. television networks had a cat who suffered from non-Hodgkin's lymphoma. He wanted to obtain DPPE to treat the poor animal. I quickly conjured up a vision of a lonely, aging bachelor in a smoking jacket sitting on a Victorian sofa in his Manhattan

apartment, sipping from a martini glass in one hand while stroking the sickly cat, perched on his lap, with the other.

How had he learned about the drug? Apparently from the
company's press release on the financial newswires announcing
the licensing agreement. "You now own the rights to DPPE," I
explained to the woman. "I would assume that any decision on
such requests would be made by Bristol-Myers."

"Yes (throat-clearing noise). Apparently it *was* discussed by
senior management. They have suggested that you would be the
best person to handle this," she explained, trying to suppress
a giggle.

I did not think it was quite as humorous as she did. I also
understood the not-so-subtle message. The company wanted
nothing to do with this crackpot and punted him to me. If I said
"No" to the man, Dr. Brandes was the bad guy, not beneficent
Bristol-Myers Squibb. Given his apparently influential position, the last thing they wanted was a possible "human interest"
story on the network's evening news about a poor sick cat that a
major pharmaceutical company with a potential "curative drug"
would not help. What a way to start off a business relationship. I
thanked her and filed the request for future consideration …far
into the future.

Unfortunately for me, the future arrived quickly, with an e-mail
that afternoon. The message, from the news executive's assistant,
repeated the urgent request for DPPE. With that, I realized I was
no longer in a position to ignore the issue. Bristol-Myers had
obviously supplied his office with my e-mail address. Hitting the
"reply to sender" button, I immediately typed out my message
telling the man that DPPE was still an investigational drug and
that, until it was manufactured by Bristol-Myers, I had the only
supply. Unfortunately, all of my DPPE was committed to treat
human patients in clinical trials. I was sorry not to be able to help
his cat. I trusted that he understood.

He did not. The next morning a fresh e-mail arrived, outlining
in detail the cat's medical history. It had been diagnosed with the

lymphoma three years earlier and treated with surgery followed by radiation therapy. A year later the cat had relapsed and was then treated with various types of potent chemotherapy drugs. Despite all that treatment, the lymphoma had recurred yet again. DPPE was the cat's last hope. The executive looked forward to hearing back from me as soon as possible so that the cat could receive my drug.

As a former pet owner myself, I have great sympathy for sick animals and the angst that an ailing pet causes its human master. Many animals develop cancerous tumors and there are specialized clinics to treat them. That is all well and good under appropriate circumstances. Nonetheless, I believed that, given the history of multiple relapses of the lymphoma, this particular pet owner had now crossed the line from trying to help his cat, to potential animal abuse. If the man was not acting out of personal selfishness, at least he was in total denial about what would be best for his cat. *No way, José.* I did not reply.

The following day, a veterinarian left a voice-mail on my phone. She was sorry to have missed me and asked that I call her back to discuss a DPPE dosing protocol for the cat. "Forget it," I mumbled to the phone and went back downstairs to my clinic. One day later…two days later….no more e-mails or phone calls. I was starting to feel safe. My lack of response had finally done the trick. How wrong I was. The telephone rang.

"Hello?"

"Dr. Brandes?"

"Yes."

It was the veterinarian!

"I am a pharmacologist at the College of Veterinary Medicine and have been contacted by Mr. Smith (not his real name) to determine the proper dose of DPPE to be administered along with chemotherapy to his cat. If you could please provide me with information on its half-life in the bloodstream in humans, I will then work it into my calculation for the cat."

"I am sorry but I am unable to help you out," I replied.

"Look, I am being paid by Mr. Smith to provide this information, but I can't if I don't know the half-life."

"I cannot supply any DPPE for the cat," I told her.

"Are you saying that you will not co-operate?" she asked incredulously, her voice rising as she sensed, to her horror, that a significant retainer was about to go down the drain.

"That is correct," I answered blandly.

When she persisted in her invective, I simply said goodbye. Her nattering continued until the phone finally came to rest on its cradle, cutting the connection.

The next morning, an e-mail from the executive's assistant severely admonished me for being uncaring in my indifference to the poor cat. My initial reaction was, "Enough is enough!" I would not respond. However, after further consideration, I decided that the deck needed clearing once and for all: "Tell your boss that my time is taken up caring for sick humans. He should recognize the difference between continuing his quest to treat the cat and causing it to suffer. There comes a time when the most humane act is to put a sick animal down. Now is that time. The cat is beyond help. Put it out of its misery and get a new one."

As there were no more e-mails in either direction, I have no idea whether he took my advice. I hope so. As they use to say on that 1960s TV show, "There are eight million stories in the Naked City. This was one of them!"

CHAPTER FORTY-EIGHT:
Bill, Jeff And The Audit

My first contact with Bill Slichenmyer did not bode well for a happy future. I had expected to hear from him by late August. When he did not call me after the signing ceremony, I phoned his office. His response to my call was very tip-toe and generally quite distant. There was none of the repartee and enthusiasm that I had associated with Lee Schacter. Somewhat dismayed by the icy reception, I decided to go on the offensive. "Bill, I have worked very hard to get to this point and need someone to share my passion about DPPE. I hope you will be that person. Otherwise, as far as I'm concerned, we're in trouble." He definitely hadn't expected that.

"I have just taken over the file on DPPE from Lee and need to review it," he replied.

"That's fine. Maybe you can call me once you have," I countered.

Two days later, Bill sent me a fax, his tone much more conciliatory and warm, a totally different response than the one I had encountered over the phone. Perhaps his boss, Renzo Canetta, told him to stroke me. His letter congratulated me on all the work

I had done on DPPE. "It must give you great satisfaction to see your many years of effort achieve such recognition," he wrote. He then assured me of the company's commitment to develop the drug and ended by suggesting that I visit and present a major review of my work to his whole group. "Looking forward to getting our studies with DPPE underway at long last and having an opportunity to meet you in person soon," he ended. That was better. Of course I would be happy to go.

Two weeks later I arrived at Newark airport and was met by a company limo driver who chauffeured me the hour's drive to Bristol-Myers' impressive Wallingford, Connecticut facility. On my arrival, Bill and Renzo came to the reception desk and warmly introduced themselves. In contrast to the bearded studiousness and informal, open-collared paunch of the shorter Renzo, Bill was tall, slim, bespectacled and clean-cut in an earnest, shirt and tie, rah-rah midwest college cheerleader sort of way. Any remaining tension now evaporated. "Do you have all your stuff?" Bill asked as he led me into the large auditorium where I was to give my talk. I assured him I did. As we entered the door I found a crowd awaiting my talk. *Wow.* There must have been at least two hundred people in the seats, all with…..you know what…in hand.

Since Bill had given me carte blanche to cover the landscape, I compressed twelve years of work into two hours. If I must say so myself, it was a tour de force. I was on a tear. I kept looking at the audience for signs of restlessness. There was none. They were with me. Loud cheers and laughter erupted when I reviewed the history of DPPE, pointing out that we had just licensed back to Bristol-Myers the very compound they had invented, patented and left on the shelf over thirty years earlier. I ended the talk by showing X-rays and CT scans of several patients on my studies who had experienced dramatic responses.

Afterwards, many of those assigned to the project came up to introduce themselves to me. To a person, they told me how excited they were by the "DPPE story" and how pleased they were to be involved in its development. We all then went to an expensive

Wallingford restaurant. Over a scotch, Renzo recounted to me his role in shepherding the clinical development of carboplatin, an important Bristol-Myers anticancer drug.[93] Now he would be leading the development of DPPE. At dinner, red wine flowed and toasts to success were made. The company meant business! I was no longer alone. It was a high point on the long road traveled.

Shortly after returning to Winnipeg, I received an e-mail from Jeff Usakewicz, the clinical research manager who worked under Bill. From the moment we were introduced in Wallingford, I knew that, in Jeff, I had a real friend at Bristol-Myers. We had sympatico. Even more, we had a lot of laughs. He was a great guy. Now, he was contacting me to arrange for a review of the charts of all the patients I had treated with DPPE.

Could he bring a group of auditors to Winnipeg as soon as possible? What about the middle of December? I would have to speak to Gordon Grahame but I did not think he, or his ethics committee, would object as long as patient confidentiality was protected. "Jeff, I get the impression that someone at Bristol-Myers suddenly asked a hard question: 'Has anyone actually seen Dr. Brandes' clinical data?'"

"You've got that right," Jeff laughed.

It turned out that "the someone" was company VP, Dr. Sol Rajfer who, in the newswire story released at the time of the signing ceremony just three months earlier, was quoted as saying, "DPPE is an exciting therapy..." Exciting or not, perhaps as a result of Arnold Portigal's great persuasiveness, a crucial part of the due diligence appeared to have been overlooked prior to licensing! I assumed that Dr. Rajfer was now very nervous. Maybe *he* was, but I wasn't. Knowing that Kong Khoo had already verified my observations in a small number of patients, I welcomed a wider

---

93 Carboplatin was not discovered in-house. It was synthesized by Chester Beatty Institute research chemist, Dr. Ken Harrap, whom I knew from my days at the Royal Marsden in 1970-71. The drug was then licensed to Bristol-Myers Squibb where it underwent clinical development led by Renzo.

audit, especially if it meant that Jeff and I would get to spend some time together.

Jeff and his crew of ten arrived on December 16. Bill also came along to spend a day in the clinic with me. Unfortunately, an early severe blast of winter straight out of the Arctic preceded them by two weeks! The temperature had plummeted to thirty below zero and two feet of snow covered the ground. Even by brisk Manitoba standards, it was a total shocker….February weather in December. One of the auditors, a gal from Corpus Christie, Texas, had only a thin rain coat. No one had boots. A quick trip to the store was arranged so that everyone could stock up on warm clothes. Were they upset? Not on your life. They thought it was a hoot….one of life's greatest experiences. *Hmm.* I hoped they would still think so weeks down the road. According to the weather office, this record-breaking cold showed no signs of moderating. Winter, 1996, was here to stay until the snow wore out four or five months down the road.

Showing Bill and Jeff around the clinic, I introduced them to Susie, who demonstrated the administration of DPPE to a patient. After she finished, I had Bill examine two people who were on my studies, one with prostate cancer and one with breast cancer. He appeared a bit nervous as Jeff and I looked on, but didn't do badly for someone who had been out of clinical practice for a few years. Later that afternoon Bill was back on a plane to Newark, satisfied by what he had seen. Our relationship was on firm footing.

That night I had Jeff over to our house to meet Jill and Carolyn over dinner. He was an appreciative guest, cleaning the food off his plate with gusto. After-dinner talk was sprinkled with laughter, especially when Jeff asked Carolyn about The Palomino Club, a cross-town joint with a checkered past, now popular for nightly line dancing. It turns out that our Jeff and his wife enjoyed that particular form of culture. He would check the place out when he had a free evening.

Early the next morning, I was introduced to the entire group as we sat around a large square table in a quiet corner of the medical records department in the Health Sciences Centre. Large pushcarts filled with charts lined the walls. Many more carts were in waiting. Jeff had brought along boxes of case report forms on which clinical and laboratory data from every patient would be recorded. He explained that the primary aim of the audit was to document toxicities, thereby determining the safety of the DPPE/chemotherapy treatments. Secondarily, the review would assess the tumor responses that I had claimed. The results would all be tabulated in an "Investigator Brochure" that the company would issue to regulators and physicians involved in planned clinical trials of DPPE.

I briefly reviewed how our clinic and hospital charts were organized so that the auditors would know where to look for nursing and physician notes, orders, and laboratory work, including pathology and X-ray reports. One great advantage was that all of our cancer clinic notes were typed. That information was met with smiles and a sigh of relief. Apparently, pages and pages of illegible hand-written scrawl were not unknown to this group. We, and they, were indeed fortunate that our centre maintained a well-staffed steno pool. As a bonus, Susie supplied Jeff with her meticulously-kept folders containing her own highly-legible notes and tables for each patient.

Despite the affability all around, I could tell that there was a certain degree of natural tension at the outset. That was understandable given that the group did not know what was going to emerge from their review. It was one thing to have good charts; it was another to determine whether the charts had "the goods". They needed some time to come to their own conclusion about whether my data were solid. "Just page me if there are questions or concerns," I assured them. They smiled and nodded as I left them to their long task.

When I returned late that afternoon, every eye was buried deep in a chart, looking for data to be extracted and entered on the forms. "Any questions so far?" I asked.

"Hey, Doctor Brandes. We're getting real hungry. Can you suggest a good restaurant for tonight?" asked Gary Sniffen, one of the two lead auditors.

"The Liberty Grill is just across the street from the Westin where you're staying. The food is usually very good. They even fly the Stars and Stripes on the wall to make you feel at home. Give it a try," I suggested. The group smiled in unison and thanked me. As they all prepared to leave after a tiring first day, Jeff looked pleased with what had turned up so far.

I met again with the group the following morning. My restaurant recommendation had been a hit. Perhaps for that, or other reasons, their tension was starting to dissipate. When we finished going over a few questions that had arisen from the chart review the day before, I handed Gary a list of other potentially good eateries. "Tonight I would recommend dinner at Victor's," I said. Everyone assured me they would take my advice. "And be sure to wait for the green light before crossing," I added, vividly recalling my life-saving grab of that other Bristol-Myers visitor, Julius Vida, on Osborne Street all those years ago. The group looked at me, somewhat perplexed, waiting for an explanation. I didn't bother. "Just trust me on that one," was all I said.

"How are things going?" I inquired of Jeff after the others had left on Wednesday.

"Quite well. Your notes are very detailed and the charting is excellent," he replied.

"Did you expect otherwise?" I asked.

"Having done audits for many years, I can only tell you that I have seen it every which way. Some of the worst record-keeping comes out of major hospitals, often involving consultants with big reputations. Your charts are miles ahead of most." *Gee whiz.*

"Would you and your good wife like to join us for dinner tonight?" Gary asked me late in the day on Friday of the first week. I smiled and nodded in the affirmative, knowing the real meaning behind the invitation. It was now clear that the group was happy with their findings. The "goods" were being delivered. It was time for all of us to relax.

Jeff and Gary were salivating at the thought of eating at a restaurant I had told them about in St. Boniface, the French section of Winnipeg. I called for reservations. That night, as the cold wind whipped up even more snow, we could be seen through the large frosted window at Le Beaujolais, laughing over wine and partaking of the mouth-watering gourmet entrées, compliments of "Billy Bristol", Jeff's euphemism for Bristol-Myers.[94]

The two hundred-patient audit finally ended in the spring, with a few breaks in between. To celebrate, I took Jeff to dinner and a men's fashion show that Harry Rosen, a Canadian icon of mens' apparel, was staging at a local downtown restaurant. Harry and I had been acquainted for some time; I shopped regularly at his store and he had known my late uncle, likewise named Harry, who was also in the *shmatta*[95] business in Toronto. After the show had finished, the three of us made small talk over a beer. Later that evening, as Jeff and I sipped a scotch in the plush Palm Room at the Fort Garry Hotel, I popped the question. "Licensing agreement or not, if that review had come up short, Sol Rajfer would have pulled the plug, wouldn't he?"

"No doubt about it," Jeff agreed.

"Well, I guess that's one thing we won't have to worry about now," I replied.

Smiling, we clinked our glasses.

---

94 The company was originally founded in 1887 by William Bristol and John Myers, who paid five thousand dollars for a failing company called the Clinton Pharmaceutical Company, located in Clinton, New York. It merged with Squibb Pharmaceuticals in 1989 to become Bristol-Myers Squibb.

95 "Shmatta" is a Yiddish word meaning "rag". It's a euphemism for the garment industry.

CHAPTER FORTY-NINE:

Taxed By Taxol

Shortly after his visit in December, Bill called me. "Our group has been working on a brand new breast cancer protocol to test DPPE. I want to send it to you for your comments and advice."

"I'll be happy to read it," I replied.

As it soon turned out, I was not at all happy with what I read. Bill and his colleagues wanted to combine DPPE with Bristol-Myers' leading oncology drug, Taxol (paclitaxel) in patients with late-stage breast cancer. The proposal instantly got under my skin.

To begin with, the design of this new study was such that, to be eligible, patients had to be heavily pretreated with other chemotherapy drugs such as doxorubicin. In other words, this was another of those "last-ditch" trials, a significant step backward from what we were trying to accomplish with Elizabeth and the NCIC. I had already been that route with my first studies in Winnipeg. DPPE would be predicted to have its greatest impact in patients with early stages of cancer who had received little in the way of prior chemotherapy, not late in the game where third-or fourth-line treatment of any kind usually pays small dividends, if any. Why bog down my drug in a study like this? I believed that the answer to that question rested squarely with executives at the business end, in the marketing department, who appeared to be far more concerned about the well-being of Taxol than of the still-unproven DPPE.

It was no secret that Bristol-Myers had not successfully developed an "in-house" chemotherapy drug in a very long time. The company had acquired its blockbuster, Taxol, from the National Cancer Institute, a branch of the National Institutes of Health (NIH). The prototype of a family of important cancer-fighters called taxanes, Taxol was initially isolated from the bark of the yew tree. Its antitumor properties were discovered in a government lab in Bethesda several years earlier and the drug was then put into clinical trials at a cumulative cost to taxpayers of approximately seven hundred million dollars.

There had been much bad publicity over the "sweet" business deal struck late in the game between Bristol-Myers and the NIH to commercialize Taxol. Many people, including Senator Ron Wyden of Oregon, a vocal member of the Senate Subcommittee on Science, Technology and Space, believed that the company had severely short-changed the NIH, and thus the U.S. taxpayers, reaping billions of dollars in profit while paying the government agency a paltry thirty-five million dollars up front, followed by a meager one-half percent royalty on sales.[96]

Bristol-Myers countered the criticism with its own arguments. Since the NIH did not have a composition patent on Taxol, it had been a risky venture for the company. Moreover, the NCI had benefited greatly from a vastly increased supply of Taxol, manufactured by Bristol-Myers, for use in many additional clinical trials. An official Government Accounting Office (GAO) report examining both sides of the issue concluded that the public had benefited by the rapid development of Taxol once Bristol-Myers

---

96   Royalties are typically four to five percent of gross sales. Our royalty agreement for DPPE was four percent. Then again, our up front payment was a mere 0.2 percent of the thirty-five million paid to the NIH.

came into the picture, but that the government had not negotiated a good bargain with the drug company.

That aside, a five year exclusivity right to Taxol negotiated under the deal was set to expire in 1999. Some additional protection had been obtained by the successful filing of a new use patent for Taxol that cut many hours off the time originally believed to be needed to safely administer the drug to patients.[97] Nonetheless, generic versions of the drug were certain to appear as soon as the five years were up, severely cutting into company profits. Perhaps the generation of new data in late breast cancer, combining Taxol with DPPE, would result in yet another new use patent to help keep the wolves at bay.

I decided to tackle the whole Taxol issue head on and e-mailed Bill, outlining my firm opposition to the planned study. At the end of a blistering critique, I wrote, "...I believe that, although DPPE is an add-on drug, we should all regard it as a drug in its own right, a drug added to the best regimens, whatever they may be, in an attempt to make them even more effective for a particular form of cancer....I know that Taxol is a very important drug to Bristol-Myers (and, indeed, I think it deserves to be). However, it has not escaped my notice that the direction being taken in the proposed study could be interpreted more as what DPPE might do for Taxol, rather than what DPPE and Taxol might do for each other."

I am sure Bill was completely floored by the vociferousness of my response. The following day, he e-mailed me. "Thanks for being candid...all your points are perfectly valid," he began. Then, to assure me that the DPPE/Taxol study was but a minor component of the overall picture, he summarized an ambitious and comprehensive plan for the development of DPPE that he was putting

---

97   Bristol-Myers had obtained the new Taxol use patent as a result of a collaboration with Elizabeth Eisenhauer and her colleagues at NCIC-CTG. When the patent was awarded, Elizabeth received a large royalty which she magnanimously donated to her alma mater, Queens University, to establish a Breast Cancer Chair in memory of her late mother who had died of the disease.

forward to the company. As I read his long summary of "things to do", I was very impressed by the scope of his ideas. But in the end, Bill admitted to what I had suspected all along. "The reason that the Taxol/DPPE study is the first one getting launched is related to internal politics. The best way for the entire plan to get approved is for marketing to like DPPE. The best way to get that done is to start with a study that marketing likes; hence, Taxol/DPPE. This may be distasteful but it is the political reality that I face here," he wrote.

My suspicions now confirmed in black and white, I replied as follows: "The big picture you present is very reassuring....I feel much better now about where we are going with this. However, I would like to point out to marketing that life does not begin and end with Taxol. The success of DPPE in the many initiatives you have outlined will carry many other drugs along with it, including Taxol. In addition (and I know that you and Renzo share this view) the main goal should be to save lives early in the disease. I don't think that people in marketing give a lot of thought to this issue, as they only see the dollar signs to be made from cancer on a balance sheet, rather than cancer in real people in the real world of the clinic. I hope I am not being too cynical in expressing this view."

A short time after this exchange of e-mails, the DPPE/Taxol proposal was quietly shelved. Whether my candid comments played any role in this policy reversal is unclear. The result of the "Taxol" episode was to put me on my guard. I now suspected that people above Bill, and maybe even above Renzo, those with real authority in the company, were not particularly enamored of DPPE. Perhaps this was because it was an "outsider", developed by some obscure guy in a lab in Canada and foisted upon them by a fast-talking entrepreneur. Moreover, our research findings notwithstanding, they simply had no sense of how the drug might work, let alone *whether* it would work. Ultimately, DPPE represented just another budget line on their books. One hiccough and it would be jettisoned in a flash.

The stark reality was (and is) that, despite vociferous protestations to the contrary, pharmaceutical development is almost always driven, first and foremost, by market pressures and pure profit motives....the prototype clash between money and morality, between doing what is right for the shareholders and what is right for the public. Without very strong advocates to keep the development of drugs like mine squarely on course, patient welfare could easily suffer. When it came to prevailing over such forces, was my "team" at Bristol-Myers strong enough to advocate for DPPE? Now, just a few months into the relationship, I was not at all sure.

CHAPTER FIFTY:
Behind The Sofa

By May, 1996, three months before the licensing agreement was finally inked, the phase two NCIC confirmatory trial, called "IND.97", was up and running in women whose breast cancer had metastasized. After signing on the dotted line, Bristol-Myers agreed to help cover the costs of the study. Although the company planned to manufacture the drug, it would take a year or longer before the final product received regulatory approval for use in humans. Since everyone wanted to move forward without delay, it was agreed that my DPPE powder, having already been approved by Agnes and her colleagues in Ottawa, would be used for the study.

The Clinical Trials Group, led by Elizabeth and Kong, collected, monitored and analyzed the data. At the time the trial started, Elizabeth told Alexandra (Alex) Paul, a medical reporter at the *Winnipeg Free Press*, "Lorne feels, and I agree with him, that it's time this treatment was tested in more than one centre." Suddenly my client base for DPPE increased by four hundred percent! With all that new powder to make, it was a good thing that the fire extinguisher was now mounted on the wall in close proximity to the fume hood.

The design of the study allowed women to have had prior chemotherapy, but only as an "adjuvant" treatment that was intended to prevent the disease from coming back after the breast surgery, or on one occasion after the disease had recurred and spread. Doxorubicin must not have been a component of that prior chemotherapy. To begin with, fifteen patients who had developed spread of breast cancer that could be detected on examination or by various X-ray tests, would be treated to confirm whether DPPE plus doxorubicin produced a high rate of tumor shrinkage, including at least one case of complete remission. If that goal was achieved, another fifteen women would be treated. The trial would also assess side effects, such as the mild hallucinations that Susie and I had reported.

Within a few short months, two Winnipeg patients had complete remissions, one treated by David Bowman, the other by me. Len Reyno, a Hamilton, Ontario, oncologist participating in the trial, was also very impressed by the rapid and significant tumor shrinkage he was observing in many of his patients. Len had done his cancer training at Roswell Park in Buffalo and was especially interested in testing new agents. Now he was becoming increasingly impressed by DPPE. "It's a pleasure to see my protocol nurse enthusiastically recruiting people for a study," he commented during a phone conversation. I called Elizabeth to report the good news about our two patients. Under the rules, we were "go" for another fifteen.

Then, for some inexplicable reason, the number of new recruits in Winnipeg slowed to a trickle and then ground to a halt. I knew they were out there. They always were. Yet, for some reason, they were not being referred. As much as I hate to say so, I suspected that, for a variety of reasons, some of my colleagues were reluctant to give up eligible patients. Perhaps if the women themselves had a "heads-up", they would raise the issue with their oncologist and more would come our way. I called Bill. "What would you think if

I contact Alexandra Paul at *The Winnipeg Free Press*, tell her about the progress of the study, explain that we have met the requirement to continue on for another fifteen patients and make a pitch for more referrals?" I asked him.

The previous June, Alex had written a front page story, "*Cancer drug put to test*", announcing the NCIC trial of DPPE. The article was accompanied by a longer piece on an inside page, "*Hard work pays off*", that chronicled my travails in developing the drug. The background story featured interviews with Georgie Hogg, Arnold Portigal and Premier Gary Filmon. As well, Alex highlighted the cases of Frances Gunning and Rita Drawbridge, two women with metastatic breast cancer treated with DPPE and doxorubicin; each had gone into remission and were being followed off treatment. It was a well-researched and wonderfully-written story that made everyone who read it feel good. The whole community was very excited and proud. The positive feedback persisted for months.

Now, a brief update on the trial by Alex in her newspaper might stimulate the new referrals we needed to finish the study. After some discussion, Bill agreed with the idea and gave me the go-ahead. That afternoon I reached Alex at the news desk, filled her in on developments since her last story and explained the motive behind my call. She appeared to understand and wanted to help. She would definitely file a story for the next day's paper.

The following morning, I went downstairs and retrieved the newspaper from the front porch. My mouth dropped as I saw the banner front page headline, "*Cancer drug passes the test*". Under the headline was written, "*Local researcher startled by early promising results*". It got worse. The story carried over to the second page, under the heading,

"*DPPE hailed as cancer success story*". Startled?? Try nauseated. I truly thought I would vomit. I shook my head with disbelief as I read the overblown story that made it sound as though we had rapidly proven that DPPE was all we had hoped it would be. What was going through Alex' and her editor's mind to write a ringer like that? A slow day for news? More likely a simple case of local

pride, perhaps, but no real understanding of what it would ultimately take to bring DPPE to the marketplace.

Cancer drug passes the test

Local researcher startled by early promising results

By Alexandra Paul
Medical Reporter

CANCEROUS BREAST tumours shrank by more than half for nine of 15 women treated with a drug developed in Winnipeg — and a tenth woman's cancer is in complete remission.

The promising results have quickly spawned another nationwide test.

But for Winnipeg's Frances Gunning, who received the drug last year before this latest trial, the medicine is already a miracle. Gunning has been free of breast cancer for almost a year.

"I had a bonus, too," she joked last night. "My hair grew in curly."

Oncologist Dr. Lorne Brandes led the team that created the promising drug DPPE over a decade of painstaking research at the Manitoba Institute of Cell Biology at the Manitoba Cancer Treatment and Research Foundation.

"When the positive results

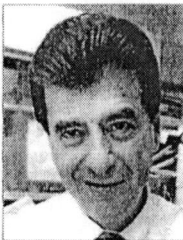

Brandes: 'encouraging'

come this early it's an encouraging sign," Brandes said yesterday.

The National Cancer Institute of Canada conducted the latest trial, involving 15 women in four cities across Canada including Hamilton, Thunder Bay, London, Ont. and Winnipeg.

The women were given treatments of DPPE and the chemotherapy drug Adriamycin every three weeks for six months.

Continued
Please see DPPE /A2

Winnipeg Free Press story that backfired

Of one thing I was sure: this would be a very bad day for me once my colleagues read the paper.[98] As they say, news travels fast; bad news travels faster. I desperately wanted to go back to bed and pull the sheets up as high as they could go. But what would that accomplish? They would simply track me down at home. *Oh, to be able to drop off the face of the earth!*

Barney, the timid family pooch, must have known instinctively what was going through my mind. He glanced sorrowfully my way and then scooted behind the living room sofa, his favorite hiding place. For once, I wanted to join him. I was sure that his doggy sense sniffed trouble with a capital "T". It was one of the very few times in my life that I did not look forward to going to work.

My fears were well-founded. As I entered the corridor leading to the Cancer Foundation, I passed Julia DeFehr's office. From inside the door, she shot me an "if looks could kill" stare. Demoralized by her less-than-warm greeting, I kept walking and trudged up the stairs to the lab. Opening the office door, I saw the voicemail light flashing on my phone. Bill had left a curt message to call him urgently. My computer screen signaled that I had new e-mail. It was a furious missive from Kong Khoo, excoriating me for what I had done. He had faxed a copy of the newspaper article to Elizabeth at NCIC. I assumed that, like her royal namesake at Buckingham Palace, she was not amused. *No wonder Barney ran behind the sofa!*

I reluctantly returned Bill's call. While agreeing that he had given me permission to talk with the newspaper, he had no idea that the story would be played that way. "Welcome to the club, my friend," I replied glumly. Although he would not admit to it, I suspected that Bill had been roundly reprimanded by Renzo for his part in this fiasco. However, it was now clear as a bell that I, rather than he, was in everyone's bad book. I thought that was unfair. After all, I had acted in good faith, both seeking and receiving

---

98 "I am writing to express....chagrin....at the untimely and unseemly publicity accorded an unfinished clinical trial...," an irate Brent Schacter wrote Free Press editor, Nicholas Hirst, on December 13, 1996.

Bill's approval to give the interview. With the benefit of twenty-twenty hindsight, our plan was, at best, ingenuous and had back-fired badly. Nonetheless, Bill could have shown more backbone in supporting me and shouldering his portion of the blame for what had happened. That he did not was very disappointing. I had just learned a hard lesson, the one about success having many fathers and failure being an orphan.

Later that day, Bill and Renzo held a conference call with Elizabeth and her group to discuss the implications and potential repercussions of the story. Shortly after, a long and sternly-worded e-mail arrived from Renzo. He read me the Riot Act, pointing out, in true Jesuit fashion, my mortal transgression in talking with the press. However well-intentioned my motive, Bristol-Myers[99] and NCIC took a very dim view of what I had done. I was officially put on notice. This grievous act was not to be repeated…ever!

I fashioned a reply in the only way I could under the circumstances. I fell on my sword, agreeing that I had been sitting on my brains when I gave the interview. The reporter should not be blamed, no matter how misguided her report. The buck stopped with me. Everyone could rest assured that the lesson had been well-learned and this would not happen again.

Silence then descended. Everyone cooled down. The entire incident appeared to blow over within another twenty-four hours. Then an interesting thing happened. Within two weeks, several requests for a "second opinion" resulted in three new women entering the trial. After seeing the story in the paper, they had asked their oncologist whether they might be candidates for DPPE. This was one case where that hackneyed phrase, "Ask your doctor", so often heard in drug company-sponsored television commercials, paid off!

---

99 Some years later, Julia DeFehr wrote: "Another intriguing nuance of the Four Inch Headline Episode was that, patients aside, the great fear [of Bristol-Myers] was how this would play out on the NYSE. Since it didn't even cause a blip, Bill was off the hook and the incident de-escalated. (I wouldn't go so far as to say it was a tempest in a tea-cup.)"

CHAPTER FIFTY-ONE:

On The Up Escalator

By mid-1997, thirty-two women had been entered on the IND.97 study. Many had already completed their planned six cycles of treatment,[100] while others were still undergoing therapy. At that point, a conference call was held so that Elizabeth and the investigators from the various centres, including Kong and me, could discuss the findings and offer opinions on the clinical potential of DPPE. Listening in from Wallingford were Bill and Jeff. It took but a few minutes for everyone to agree that a high response rate to DPPE and doxorubicin had been observed in this relatively small number of women. Naturally, I was both relieved and delighted with this outcome.

We then turned our attention to a discussion of side effects. As Susie and I had observed previously, a few patients reported visual or auditory hallucinations, generally of a pleasant or humorous nature, with their first treatment. There was some laughter among

---

100 A "cycle" means a treatment, followed by a rest period, usually three weeks. Then the next cycle begins. Only six treatment cycles of DPPE and doxorubicin were permitted because of the increasing potential for heart damage by doxorubicin if given more than six times.

us as a few anecdotes about the hallucinations were traded back and forth. From my point of view that was a good sign, since other doctors considering this treatment could be reassured by those who had experience with the drug that any hallucinations associated with DPPE were no big deal. In fact, given that the patients generally seemed to enjoy them, they might even be considered a benefit. After all, who enjoys receiving chemotherapy?

Of more concern to the group was a perceptible increase in nausea and vomiting in some patients that lasted for several days after treatment, again similar to what Susie and I had found. It appeared to be the price paid for using DPPE at the high dose to increase its punch with chemotherapy drugs such as doxorubicin. Fair enough, but could we find a way around this unpleasant side effect?

Len Reyno put forward a plan to add dexamethasone, a nausea-fighting steroid medication. Along with lorazepam and the powerful antinausea drug, ondansetron (Zofran), the dexamethasone would be given intravenously before the DPPE and doxorubicin, and then both dexamethasone and ondansetron pills would be prescribed for four days afterwards. Everyone thought it was a good idea, worth trying. I also had a suggestion. An injection of the anti-motion sickness drug, scopolamine, also available in the form of a patch worn behind the ear by many passengers on cruise ships, seemed highly effective when all else failed. The others agreed to try it if the dexamethasone did not work.

"Is Bristol-Myers willing to fund us to test this modification in an additional ten women?" Elizabeth asked.

"I am sure that will be no problem," Bill replied confidently.

The conference call having ended, Bill, Jeff and I held a "post-mortem".

"I thought overall it was very positive," Bill said, referring to the tenor of the discussion. Jeff agreed. "The fact that everyone wanted to work together to decrease nausea and vomiting is a very good sign. If they didn't believe they were seeing a positive benefit of DPPE to increase remissions, they wouldn't waste their time trying to minimize the side effects," he explained. The correctness of this insight was immediately obvious to me.

Three months later, the spring meeting of the NCIC Clinical Trials Group took place in Montréal, one of the most charming and cosmopolitan cities on the continent. Everyone looked forward to the meeting being held there because, in addition to the razzmatazz of Canada's largest French-speaking city, the cuisine was, as they say, magnifique. Pharmaceutical company-sponsored dinners were held at various restaurants around town as a gesture of thanks to investigators for participating in tests of their oncology drugs. An invitation to dine, compliments of such and such a company, was seldom turned down after a long day of meetings.

Bill, Jeff and other Bristol-Myers people were there, as were all the Canadian investigators involved with the DPPE study. The meeting spanned several days to allow discussion of the many different cancer trials that were either planned or in progress. The IND.97 study report was scheduled to be presented with the other phase two studies on the morning of the second day. I assumed that it would be a dry affair, a summary of the trial's progress in the first thirty-two patients and the modified treatment plan to control nausea and vomiting in an additional ten. Several in the latter group were already receiving the additional medications suggested by Len and seemed to be doing better. I sat restlessly in my chair for over an hour as reports on trial after trial were presented.

Then something totally unexpected happened. After a short introduction describing the IND.97 trial, Elizabeth announced that, although the study had not yet finished, an analysis by the group's statisticians showed a response rate in excess of fifty percent. The results were unlikely to be changed by the ten additional patients, some of whom also had significant shrinkage of their tumors. The Clinical Trials Group felt that my findings had been confirmed in this small study. Even as the trial was wrapping up, Dr. Kathy Pritchard, chair of breast cancer trials, and her group of NCIC investigators, would begin the process of designing a formal phase three trial comparing DPPE and doxorubicin to doxorubicin alone as first- or second-line treatment in women with metastatic breast cancer. *Ohmygosh!!*

I was truly stunned by this announcement. With the phase two trial still in progress, I had not remotely expected such an early decision. For the first moment I just sat quietly, eyes closed, sucking it all in, listening to the murmurs rising in the room. "G-e-e-e-z, that's amazing," muttered someone a few rows back. Bill and Jeff were clearly delighted with the news.

"Good show!" Jeff exclaimed, as both he and Bill pumped my hand.

"I can't believe it," I replied, a great wave of relief washing over me.

Looking back over the room, I suddenly spotted Agnes Klein. She usually attended NCIC meetings and this one was no exception. I immediately sauntered over and gave her a big hug. "You know this would not have been possible without your help," I reaffirmed. She returned the hug, telling me how pleased she was. "But just remember," she whispered, "there's a rule of thumb that drugs usually perform better in phase two than in phase three."

Although her words were like a splash of cold water, I understood her point. The "single-arm" phase two study of DPPE and doxorubicin that had just been declared successful did not have a control group. The phase three trial would be a much more stringent test because it would randomly assign patients to receive doxorubicin alone, or DPPE plus doxorubicin. This procedure minimizes any chance differences between the two patient populations, such as age and performance status, that could affect the outcome. It also corrects for any unconscious bias in entering patients on a study, for example, those who might be more likely than average to benefit from a test treatment. In giving me this "reality check", Agnes was trying to be protective. She wanted DPPE to succeed, but was trying to keep me from getting my hopes too high.

At that moment, Bill suggested that he and I go to lunch where we could talk privately. There was an informal restaurant off the hotel lobby where a sandwich and coffee could be ordered. After we sat down in the booth facing one another, Bill told me how pleased he was that the IND.97 trial had been an early success. He then stunned me with the news that he was leaving Bristol-Myers to join a small biotech company near Boston. He became quite emotional as he told me of this decision, his eyes glistening as he talked. Typically, Bill gave few details. "It wasn't that newspaper interview, was it?" I asked. He just smiled, shaking his head. He had enjoyed our association and told me so.

Any attempt at humor quickly subsided as I became quite downhearted. After rejoicing over the unexpected and happy news announced that morning from the podium, I now had been hit with a sudden, not-so-happy bombshell. Whatever our initial differences, I had come to respect and admire Bill. He was a very political animal, a needed attribute to succeed in large corporations. He was also a person with strong convictions who had gone to bat for DPPE. I suspected that, in the process, he had developed irreconcilable differences with his company[101] and maybe even with Renzo Canetta. The thought of him departing within the month left an empty feeling in the pit of my stomach. I would now have to deal with someone entirely new. His name was David Lebwohl. "What's he like?" I asked.

"He's okay," was Bill's terse reply. *That was an effusive endorsement!*

Sensing my discomfort, Bill then uttered this gem: "Lorne, remember this. Whether I stay or go is of no consequence to

---

101 According to Jeff Usakewicz, a serious blowup had occurred between Bill and the company's regulatory VP, Tony Santapaulo, over moving DPPE forward. Bill was enthusiastic about its prospects and wanted to fast-track development of DPPE with the FDA, but Santapaulo took a more "wait-and-see" approach. As there were no flies on the wall to hear what was said, the details are sketchy at best. However, Jeff believed that the sharp disagreement probably resulted in Bill's decision to leave Bristol-Myers.

DPPE. Think of drug development as being on an escalator that is going up. As long as the drug meets or exceeds company expectations, it continues to go up the escalator. When it reaches the top, it has succeeded and will be marketed. If it fails along the way, it falls off the escalator. It's as simple as that." That metaphor stuck.

C H A P T E R   F I F T Y - T W O :

Playing The Hand You Are Dealt

Ah, the sweet smell of success. The first order of business on my return was to call Brent Schacter, Janet Scholz and, as a grateful courtesy, Arnold Portigal, to report the good news about DPPE and the bad news about Bill Slichenmyer. My colleagues at the University and Cancer Foundation shared my concern over Bill's departure but were pleased to learn that we were owed a milestone payment of two hundred and fifty thousand dollars. I was pleased, too. Any remaining development costs would now be recovered in full, with money left over to split among us. From now on, Bristol-Myers would foot the bills. Everyone was gratified that, at worst, the investment in DPPE had not only paid for itself, but generated a small profit to boot. At best? The mountain top beckoned.

That out of the way, I needed to sort through four days of mail. Some wiseacre once observed that the day after you die, your inbox is still full. *Oh! Oh!* The minute I saw the envelope from the NCIC, my heart sank. In the fall, I had applied to the research arm of the agency for renewal of my "DPPE" grant, the one major remaining source of federal funding for my lab program. Now, the receipt of the decidedly-thin envelope was a bad sign, indicative of a short "we're sorry" form letter.

My hopes had been buoyed by the involvement of the NCIC's own Clinical Trials Group in testing DPPE. As a result, I thought that the research program investigating how the drug worked would be a shoo-in for a three year renewal. How much more relevant to the NCIC's mission of conquering cancer could a project be? In preparing the application, I had to carefully explain to the grants panel the nitty-gritty of the licensing agreement with Bristol-Myers, lest they conclude that I was now flush with drug company research money and not in need of their help. That was not the case at all, I wrote. As strange as it may seem, the licensing agreement had not come with funding for my laboratory program. I needed money from NCIC.

That embarrassing admission aside, I went on to describe exciting new experiments that Frank and I were carrying out. Tiny fruit flies could be infected with viruses that, in addition to their own genetic material, carried a specific fragment of human DNA that coded for a specific P450 enzyme. Employing this technique, a biotech company was able to supply us with microsomes from the insects that contained a single purified human P450 of our choosing. Using this material, we had just shown quite a strong binding interaction of DPPE and histamine on the CYP3A4 enzyme, the one responsible for metabolizing many chemotherapy drugs and hormones. Other tests showed that DPPE blocked the enzyme.

We were very enthusiastic about the implications of this finding, because the activity of CYP3A4 is closely tied in with that of the P-glycoprotein (P-gp) pump. In chemotherapy-resistant (MDR-positive) cells, the P450 enzyme may be increased, working overtime to break down susceptible drugs while the frenetic P-gp pumps shoots out any remnants that survive the enzyme attack.... quite an ugly affair, as the cancerous tumors happily grow despite the chemotherapy treatments.

Earlier, it had been discovered by other researchers that many drugs which bind to the 3A4 enzyme also bind to the P-gp, in effect, blocking the activity of both; however, Rob Warrington had shown in the test tube that DPPE overcame chemotherapy resistance in MDR-positive cells through some mechanism *unrelated* to the overactive P-gp pumps.

Since DPPE blocked 3A4, was it possible that it worked primarily on that particular P450 enzyme in certain resistant cancer cells, inhibiting them from metabolizing chemotherapy drugs? Were there additional P450 enzymes involved in drug resistance that DPPE blocked? Among other experiments, our new studies would explore these possibilities.

No matter. The work would not be funded by NCIC. The opened envelop confirmed my darkest suspicion. The grant was terminated for any one of a number of arcane reasons. *Picky, picky, picky.* This, then, was my reward for moving DPPE from discovery into human clinical trials. The very research that had led us to this point was now deemed unworthy of continued funding. *Oh, give me a break!!!*

Now we were in trouble....big time. Thankfully, a life preserver was again thrown my way by Peg Sellers and her cadre of sage advisors, but to continue on, to really have a chance, Frank and I needed more money...much more. It was time for Bristol-Myers to fund me. Arnold Portigal had suggested that their pockets would open up once DPPE showed signs of proving itself. Okay. Now was the time to see whether he was right.

I called Renzo Canetta to tell him of my dilemma. "Send me a copy of your grant application and I'll see what I can do," he advised. A couple of weeks later, I received an encouraging letter from Dr. Mariano Barbacid, head of the Oncology Drug Discovery group at the Princeton facility:

"Dear Dr. Brandes:

"We have received copies of your proposal to study the basic mechanism of action of DPPE. Oncology Drug Discovery is fully committed to support the clinical development of DPPE in any way we can......We would like to discuss with you your research plans to determine the most effective ways to support them...."

He then invited me to visit him and his group "at your earliest convenience".

My spirits rose considerably.....until, that is, the apparently understanding and supportive Mariano Barbacid suddenly vaporized. All attempts to reach him were fruitless. *Now what was going on?* I contacted Renzo, who told me that the revolving door had once again revolved. For the moment, the funding issue had to be put on hold. It would take a bit of time for Dr. Barbacid's replacement to be named.

To add to my frustration, I had not heard anything from David Lebwohl, the Roswell Park-trained oncologist who had just taken over the DPPE project. Jeff, who had been very loyal to Bill, now reported to the new man. He was devastated by "Slick's" sudden departure and did not hold Dr. Lebwohl in the same high esteem as he did his former boss. "I guess you have to play the cards you're dealt," he told me. Then, with his usual candor, he confided that, in his opinion, DPPE and I had not been dealt the best hand. It would not be long before I learned what Jeff meant. I got wind that an investigator's meeting had taken place to discuss possible new studies of my drug. Not only had he not asked me to participate, Dr. Lebwohl had not even the good sense to call and introduce himself to me as soon as he succeeded Bill. We needed to talk. I left a message with his secretary for him to call me.

If my first contact with Bill Slichenmyer had been mildly unpleasant, the one with David Lebwohl was an unmitigated disaster. "Why would you hold a clinical meeting about DPPE with other doctors and not invite me?" I asked when he phoned later that morning.

"Well, you know, you're not really regarded in the company as someone who's objective," he replied.

"Not objective? Not objective? Who says I'm not objective?" I shot back, instantly furious.

As the inventor of DPPE, I had an identifiable bias in wanting it to succeed. I was also passionate in my views. Those obvious facts aside, my objectivity had never been called into question before. How could it, when my data had been verified by a large company audit and the results of IND.97? As he tried to justify his remark and thus extricate himself from the mess he had just created, I quickly tired of the blabber and cut him off.

"That's fine. Thank you. Goodbye." I banged down the phone.

I wasn't going to put up with that nonsense and immediately called Renzo to vent my anger. "Do you consider me less than objective?" I demanded.

"Not at all," he replied, promising to quickly get to the bottom of this unpleasant episode.

As I later learned from Jeff, David, pale as a ghost, quickly ran into Renzo's office, only to be confronted by his angry boss who tore a strip off the hapless Dr. Lebwohl. "What did you eat for breakfast this morning that made you say something so stupid?" he is alleged to have asked his red-faced underling. Apparently Renzo's loud voice could be heard far beyond the closed office door.

The next day, a perceptibly nervous David Lebwohl placed a "kiss-and-make-up" call to me. By that time I had calmed down. We all say things that we regret. Maybe it was just one of those times. I accepted his apology.

"We've had an unfortunate start, but I don't hold a grudge. Let's just put this behind us and agree to work together in friendship," I suggested.

"I would like that," he replied earnestly.

"You know David, I fully understand the need for others to move the drug forward at this point, but no one has my knowledge and experience with DPPE. I would think that you and Bristol-Myers would want to capitalize on that fact." He agreed, promising that I would be included in any future meetings, kept informed about all important developments and consulted on a regular basis.

No sooner was that settled than I learned I held another, more dubious, card in my hand.

Renzo called to say that Robert Kramer, who had replaced the hapless Mariano Barbacid as head of the Oncology Discovery Group, would be in touch within a few days. When he was not, I took the initiative and called him. Within thirty seconds of his picking up the phone, I knew that if I were to look up the words "warm and fuzzy" in the dictionary, I would *not* find a picture of Rob Kramer. His abrasiveness left me with the distinct impression that he cared not one whit about me and that I was wasting his valuable time. Our fleeting discussion over, I hung up the phone, exasperated.

Dejected, I again called Renzo to report on my "conversation" with the decidedly unhelpful Dr. Kramer. A few days later, Renzo called to smooth things over. Dr. Kramer and his group would like me to come to Princeton to present a seminar on my research. Renzo and David would be there. Fine, but the wording "present a seminar" did not sound quite as positive as "...discuss with you your research plans to determine the most effective ways to support them," quoted in Dr. Barbacid's letter. I had no choice but to go and find out for myself.

Finally, at the end of June, I arrived in Princeton, a beautiful university town where Bristol-Myers had a very impressive facility. Their large modern building was located on acres and acres of beautifully manicured land that included a marsh complete with swans and ducks. As promised, Renzo and David drove in from Wallingford for my seminar. It was my first face-to-face with David. Formally dressed in a light summer khaki-colored suit, white shirt and tie, he was over six feet tall with short, thinning dark hair. His bespectacled face was kind and he smiled as we shook hands. We were now comfortable with each other.

I was then introduced to the perfunctory Dr. Kramer. "S-o-o-o, you're here to tell us all about your *new* histamine receptor," he said in a tone of voice guaranteed to get under my skin. *What was it with this guy's shtick?* Before I could decide, Dr. Ana Menendez, a lead researcher assessing DPPE in the lab, came to my rescue, introducing herself and several colleagues from the Oncology

Discovery Group. I loved her thick New Jersey accent which, I told her, reminded me of Penny Marshall's character, Laverne, in the *Laverne and Shirley* television sitcom. Luckily, Ana had Penny Marshall's sense of humor and laughed at the comparison.

Over the next hour, I described the results of our recent lab experiments to the assembled researchers. Many of the graduate students and senior investigators, Ana included, interrupted the talk with questions, their level of interest apparently high. In contrast, Rob Kramer sat slumped in his chair, often looking up at the ceiling or into the distance, saying nothing. I decided he was just putting in time, thinking about other, more important things than what I had to say….not a good sign. *Did he know Pedro?*

Afterward, as we grabbed lunch in the cafeteria, Renzo told me that he had been holding talks about DPPE with the FDA. The agency was in the process of "raising the bar" on its requirements for new oncology drugs. Simply shrinking tumors was no longer sufficient to gain approval. There also had to be a significant increase in what is called the "time to progression (TTP)". This term is defined as the interval between starting on treatment and the tumor growing again or spreading to new areas in the body. In other words, in the new phase three trial, no matter how much tumors shrank, the TTP would have to be significantly longer with DPPE and doxorubicin than with doxorubicin alone, or DPPE likely would not be approved.

I was not particularly concerned by the news, believing that the high response rate we saw in IND.97 should easily translate into an improvement in this parameter. That said, I knew that an increase in time to progression usually only translated into an additional two to four months before the patient got into trouble once again. Moreover, it was a "soft" endpoint and usually did not result in a true increase in *survival*. The latter, accompanied by a good quality of life, was what really mattered to patients whose cancer had metastasized.

Unfortunately, up to that time, an improvement in survival in metastatic breast cancer had not resulted from treatment with the most powerful breast cancer drugs, such as doxorubicin and Taxol. Added to that were their toxicities. This could have a decidedly negative impact, even if, over the short term, the drugs increased the time to progression. Based on my mouse experiments, and those ever-thicker charts in many of the patients I had treated, I was hopeful that, with the addition of DPPE, we would achieve that elusive goal of increased survival, above and beyond any increase in time to progression.

Despite that optimism, I was uneasy about some experiments that recently had been carried out by Bill Rose, head of Bristol-Myers' Experimental Therapeutics Division. Bill was assessing the ability of DPPE to increase the killing of cancer cells by several chemotherapy drugs. He had recently faxed me his preliminary results, a hit-and-miss affair, mainly miss. On the positive side, in the test tube, DPPE definitely appeared to increase the killing effects of Taxol in resistant cancer cells that made too many P-gp pumps. However, on the negative side, Bill could not reproducibly show that DPPE improved the response to chemotherapy in mice with tumors.

I had started to sweat the moment I read his report. First it was Chuck Grieshaber and Ralph Parchment with the antidepressants and antihistamines. Now it was Bill Rose with DPPE. "I can't take it," I groused to myself, immediately looking for reassurance in the paper by the Japanese researchers who had shown that, compared to the chemo drug, cis-platinum, alone, DPPE plus cis-platinum significantly improved the survival of the immune-deficient mice transplanted with human ovarian cancer tumors. I could show it in mice. Rob Warrington could show it in mice. This Japanese group could show it in mice. Yet, where it really counted, Bill Rose couldn't show it in mice. *Maybe there was a mouse conspiracy!!*

"Are we in trouble over Bill Rose's experiments?" I asked Renzo after he had finished telling me about his meeting with the FDA. He shook his head. "If DPPE works in humans, as it appears from IND.97, I'm not going to worry about a bunch of mice and neither will the FDA if the new phase three trial is positive," he answered, reassuringly. Rationally, I believed him. Emotionally, I remained very troubled by this development. Too many past memories kept creeping into my mind.

I had one more item on my agenda that day. At my request, Renzo had arranged for me to meet with his boss, Sol Rajfer, whose office was in the executive wing of the Princeton facility. Ushered in by his secretary, I found him quietly working away at his computer.

"Please give me a few minutes to finish this," he requested, glancing over his shoulder at me.

"Of course. Take whatever time you need," I replied, taking a seat beside a small conference table to the right of his large desk. After a short time, he finished and came over to join me at the table. As he sat down, we formally introduced ourselves. Slight of build, bald with rather chiseled fine features, he seemed pleasant but no-nonsense. "I'm pleased to meet you. How can I be of assistance?" he asked.

Dr. Rajfer then listened intently as I discussed my lingering concerns over the "DPPE/Taxol affair". I was very frank as I told him my perception that non-physicians in the company's marketing department appeared to be calling the shots, trying to prop up Taxol with DPPE in dead-end trials, rather than seriously considering the opportunity that DPPE-based chemotherapy presented to patients with earlier stages of cancer. I had hoped for better treatment of my drug by Bristol-Myers.

When he assured me that my fears were unfounded, I told him about my e-mail correspondence with the now-departed Bill Slichenmyer. At that moment, a light suddenly seemed to go on in his head. He started nodding quietly. "Now I understand some of the things that happened around that time," he said.

"Meaning…?" I asked after a pregnant pause of several seconds.

"Meaning…that certain things are now much clearer to me," was all he would say. Our meeting at an end, Dr. Rajfer gave me his card, told me to feel free to call him any time and thanked me for coming to see him.

"What was he talking about? What was now clear?" I kept asking myself as I walked out of his office. I never found out.[102]

---

102 I never spoke with him again. Heaven knows I tried. My e-mails were always returned as "undeliverable" and calls to his office were not returned. So much for sincerity. Rajfer eventually left Bristol-Myers for Aventis. Drug companies must employ people just to keep the revolving door well-greased.

CHAPTER FIFTY-THREE:

Pushing The Envelope

Was anyone surprised when Robert Kramer refused to free up any money from his research budget to fund me? Certainly not I. However, Renzo soon called with a plan. The Oncology Discovery Group would use all their lab resources to sort out the mechanism by which DPPE was *really* working. *Did our findings count for nothing? Apparently.* That notwithstanding, he would give me two hundred thousand dollars out of his clinical research budget, ostensibly to participate in a phase two prostate cancer trial testing DPPE combined with an intravenous chemotherapy drug called mitoxantrone and an oral steroid pill called prednisone. He then made it clear that if I wanted to use some, or all, of that amount for my research, that was entirely my business. In reality, about thirty thousand dollars would pay for the costs of putting fifteen patients on the trial, leaving the rest for the lab. Naturally I would help out with the trial. I thanked him for bailing me out with such a clever strategy.

Although, as promised in the licensing agreement, the company had also started a prostate cancer trial comparing DPPE and cyclophosphamide to cyclophosphamide alone, interest was low among the doctors they were trying to recruit to conduct the study. One reason was the general perception that cyclophosphamide was a weak or ineffective drug in this situation. Not only could they not "sell" the study to their patients, many investigators were themselves against participating, nervous that men who were willing to go on the trial might be randomized to the study arm containing only cyclophosphamide.

A second reason was that, during the time I was carrying out my initial trial of DPPE and cyclophosphamide, the NCIC Clinical Trials Group published a landmark study in *JCO*. Chaired by Dr. Ian Tannock of Toronto's Princess Margaret Hospital, the trial showed that mitoxantrone, a drug not unlike doxorubicin, and prednisone benefited about one-third of patients with advanced prostate cancer who had bone pain. Since the side effects were reasonably low, U.S. and Canadian regulators quickly approved the treatment for patients who no longer responded to blocking testosterone. It soon became the "standard of care". As a result, my protocol, although potentially superior, no longer had much of a chance.

Dr. Derek Raghavan, an oncologist specializing in prostate cancer, and a member of one of Bristol-Myers advisory committees, was very interested in DPPE and convinced the company that combining the drug with mitoxantrone and prednisone would be a better strategy. If a phase two study looked promising, it could then be tested against the "standard of care" in a full phase three trial. It made a lot of sense. Renzo suggested that the new study be carried out in Winnipeg and at the University of Southern California in Los Angeles, where Derek had his clinic. I discussed the proposal with Ernie Ramsey. He thought it was a good idea, and, as usual, was only too happy to send patients my way. If Gordon Grahame and his ethics committee approved the protocol, it would be underway.

That was not the only new development. I was now forging ahead with a new DPPE study of my own in breast cancer. I had been impressed by reports that combining doxorubicin with Taxol produced very high response rates, approaching seventy or eighty percent, in women with newly-diagnosed metastatic breast cancer. The only problem was that, according to some of the studies, the Taxol appeared to substantially increase the risk of serious heart damage caused by doxorubicin, a major drawback.

I was convinced that I could add DPPE to a safer Taxol combination, substituting epirubicin, a first cousin of doxorubicin, that is as strong against breast cancer, but generally less toxic. For example, it takes twice as much epirubicin as doxorubicin to cause heart damage. Strangely, epirubicin had been approved years earlier in every major country except the United states. Despite its better side effect profile, the FDA had ruled against approving the drug, feeling that it did not offer any major advantage to doxorubicin in the treatment of breast cancer.[103] I, and many others, believed that to be a big mistake.

Therefore, during the six months it would take for the NCIC and Bristol-Myers to lay the groundwork for the new phase three trial comparing DPPE and doxorubicin to doxorubicin alone, I was already pushing the envelope with DPPE, epirubicin and Taxol. In addition, I added a twist. While many of the patients would once again have newly-diagnosed spread of their breast cancer, I added a second category: those with newly diagnosed and *un-operated* breast cancer of a very specific, aggressive, type called "inflammatory".

Although thankfully rare, inflammatory breast cancer carries the worst prognosis, as it rapidly grows and spreads throughout the breast and lymph nodes under the arm. The cancer cells also quickly invade the tiny lymphatic channels of the skin overlying the breast, causing it to become hot, red and swollen....like an inflammation, from which the term for this type of cancer derives.

---

103 In 1999, the FDA finally approved epirubicin for the adjuvant (early) treatment of breast cancer in patients with spread to lymph nodes, but did not approve it for treatment of late stage, metastatic breast cancer. I continue to be amazed at such a narrow ruling.

The process is usually so diffuse that aggressive chemotherapy is almost always given first (so-called "neoadjuvant therapy"), in an attempt to shrink the tumor sufficiently to allow a mastectomy and removal of the lymph nodes.[104]

This neoadjuvant approach would also provide a unique opportunity to assess, first-hand, the killing effect of the DPPE, epirubicin and Taxol combination on the cancer since, after their removal, the breast and lymph nodes would be closely examined by the pathologist for residual malignant cells. I knew from the recent literature that, under the microscope, only about ten to twenty percent of mastectomy specimens showed no residual cancer after this type of aggressive chemotherapy. Would there be a better result with DPPE, epirubicin and Taxol? That is what I hoped to find out.

Initially, I had been told that as soon as the company's own version of DPPE was approved for human use, they would be happy to supply it to me for my local trials. This was followed by a flip-flop. After much hemming and hawing, word came from Renzo that DPPE would only be supplied for official, company-approved studies. I assumed that some legal eagle raised a scare that Bristol-Myers could be sued if any patient treated on my unofficial, unapproved study had an adverse outcome. I was peeved by the decision but did not really care. I had lots of my own Canadian-approved DPPE. To add to the hypocrisy, Renzo and his colleagues were anxious to see how the new treatment combo would fare.

It didn't take long to recruit patients for the new study. Because the Taxol portion of the treatment had to be given over three hours, we prescribed additional lorazepam and DPPE, and used a dark, quiet room so that patients could snooze undisturbed. Although it was demanding of her time, Susie was more than up to the task and got everyone through the treatment without difficulty. The patients then spent the night in an outpatient hospital

---

104 More limited procedures, such as lumpectomy, are not favored in the surgical treatment of inflammatory breast cancer.

ward and were discharged home first thing in the morning. Most
had only a hazy recollection of the event. This was due to a well-
known side effect of lorazepam called "retrograde amnesia", in
other words, a "hole" in the memory around the time of the chemotherapy and for a few hours afterward. Nonetheless, like the
humorous hallucinations, this was often regarded by the patients
as a "plus".

It soon became evident that the degree and rapidity of tumor
shrinkage with this new combination was greater than anything
I had seen before. Almost everyone improved dramatically after
the first cycle of treatment, including several women with inflammatory breast cancer. Equally important, the patients appeared to
tolerate it very well.

Highly enthusiastic, I called Renzo to tell him. He was happy
with the apparent safety of the treatment, but gently threw cold
water on my excitement about the responses. Some of his Italian
colleagues in Milan were now reporting to him that nine out of
ten patients treated with doxorubicin and Taxol had complete or
partial responses after four to six cycles of the treatment. "You
can't do much better than ninety percent," he said. Maybe, but
having treated breast cancer for twenty-five years, I suspected that
the profound responses after only one or two treatments with the
addition of DPPE were above and beyond anything that was being
observed with Taxol and doxorubicin alone, whether in Milan
or elsewhere.

Moreover, the results in several patients with inflammatory
breast cancer provided an important new clue: the most aggressive cancer cells were the ones that were being killed by the DPPE
combination. Where the initial biopsy showed only wildly-grow-
ing malignant cells, called *high grade,* the pathologist found no
residual cancer in the breast and lymph nodes after treatment and
surgery. Where, in addition to the more malignant high-grade
cells, the initial biopsy also showed a proportion of less malignant
cells, called *intermediate grade,* the post-treatment surgery specimens showed that all the high-grade malignant cells were gone,

leaving only pockets of intermediate-grade malignant cells. In other words, our DPPE-based treatment appeared to selectively kill the worst cells in patients with inflammatory breast cancer. When all the cells in the tumor were high grade, the tumor was wiped out entirely. When the tumor had a mixed population of cells, we did not eliminate the cancer completely but altered its composition, leaving only less malignant, slower-growing cells behind[105]. The future implications of this observation would prove enormous.

---

105 Pathologists assign a grade to breast cancers, based on the appearance of the cells under the microscope. Low-grade (Grade 1) tumors tend to be the least malignant in their appearance, and are usually slower growing. Intermediate-grade (Grade 2) tumors are more variable in their appearance and generally grow faster than low-grade tumors. High-grade (grade 3) tumors are highly malignant in appearance and grow the fastest. As might be predicted, the prognosis is best with Grade 1 tumors and worst with Grade 3 tumors. However, to complicate matters, breast cancers often contain mixtures of cells that can vary from low to high grade. The prognosis in such cancers may depend on the relative proportion of cell types present in the tumor.

CHAPTER FIFTY-FOUR:

Countdown

By the fall of 1997, the new phase three study, officially designated "MA.19", was hammered out and ready to fly.[106] However, "ready to fly" must be distinguished from "takeoff". There still remained the long, arduous process of regulatory approval, not only in each country where patients were being treated, but in every participating hospital or cancer centre as well.

Many trees were sacrificed during this time; the paperwork was staggering. Part of the reason was that the NCIC was partnering in this trial with the European Organization for the Research and Treatment of Cancer (EORTC), a clinical trials group made up of a consortium of western European countries. On top of that, Bristol-Myers was setting up its own independent sites in Russia and various eastern European countries, including Hungary, Croatia, Serbia and Romania. Medical monitors, specially picked by the company, oversaw the management of the trial there.

---

106 At my request, Len Reyno agreed to be chairman of the study. Dr. Lesley Seymour, an oncologist working full time at the NCIC Clinical Trials Group head office at Queen's University in Kingston, Ontario, was the trial's coordinator.

Although not members of EORTC, all were acceptable to the FDA. Indeed, Bristol-Myers had used a similar "third-world strategy" when testing Taxol for approval. "You would be amazed at some of the excellent facilities in places such as Croatia," David Lebwohl assured me.

The more I thought about it, the more it made sense to go to these poorer countries because patients with breast cancer often did not have access to drugs like doxorubicin in the early or even late stages of their disease. Clinical trials were a lifeline, allowing them to receive modern drug therapies otherwise not available. For that same reason, patients in Russia and Eastern Europe were much more likely than patients in affluent countries, such as Canada, Western Europe and the United States, to agree to being entered on a study.[107] Their participation would swell the number of women in the study and ensure that the results would come in earlier than otherwise possible.

One of the most important parts of any protocol is the "patient information/consent" page. *Pages* would be the more appropriate term. *Many pages.* The document outlined the nature of the trial, the possible benefits and risks of the treatments, the voluntary nature of any participation, the right to withdraw from the study at any time, and on and on. It was not unusual for each centre to request changes to the consent form to conform with institutional policies. Invariably, the modifications were made.

The entire study protocol "package", well over one hundred pages in all, had to be approved by a series of committees at each participating centre. This would include, among others, the ethics committee (to determine whether the proposed study was acceptable, morally and in every other way, and whether the information supplied to the patients in the consent forms was sufficient), and a resource impact committee (to determine whether the staff, budget, and overall physical facilities were sufficient to carry out

---

107 Amazingly, only about 3-5 percent of patients go on clinical cancer trials in North America.

the trial in any given institution). On average, it took four months for a centre to get the final "nod".

Of course, ours was one of them. Our very able group of protocol nurses and data managers, led by Erna Stiles, would make sure that the rules were strictly followed and the all-important case report forms properly filled out. By agreement, I would be allowed to participate and treat patients on the study, but had no other role. After all, as the drug's inventor, it was now important for me to remain at arm's length from any study that could lead to its approval by the regulatory agencies.

Sadly, nurse practitioner Kerry McDonald, who had been with Susie and me from the very beginning, would not be among those involved locally. For family reasons, she had decided to move back to her native Australia just after the trial got underway. In a touching goodbye letter, Kerry wrote, "My memories of you go back a long way and being the 'colorful' personality you are I will never forget you. I will check out the Sydney oncologists running MA.19 to see if any of them are as energetic, enthusiastic or brilliant as you. My experiences with the development of DPPE have been very educating and exciting for me although your enthusiasm tends to be exhausting for us mortals. Thanks for the memories and here's hoping DPPE continues to prove you right."

Finally, an investigators' meeting to launch the trial was held in Toronto in January, 1998. Each participating centre sent a delegation made up of a mix of doctors, nurses, pharmacists and data managers. I brought Susie along as my special guest.

David Lebwohl opened the proceedings by stating that Bristol-Myers considered MA.19 an important, pivotal study. A positive outcome would have great implications, not only for patients with breast cancer, but for those with other types as well. I was pleased to hear him say this, as it was the first time that anyone from the company had made such a statement in public. I assumed that it had been approved by Renzo.

Following remarks by trial chairman, Len Reyno, Lesley Seymour, the study's coordinator, explained how the trial would be conducted. The plan was to treat three hundred and fifty patients. Half would be randomized by chance to receive doxorubicin alone and half to receive DPPE plus doxorubicin. The main aims of the study were to look for significant differences between the two treatments in the number of patients who had major tumor shrinkage, and in the time to progression.[108]

Differences in survival would also be measured but, based on all the previous drug treatments that had failed to have an impact on this most important of parameters, there was no great expectation that DPPE and doxorubicin would fare any better. Put another way, failure to increase survival would not have a negative impact on DPPE's future as long as it significantly helped doxorubicin to increase the time to progression and shrink breast cancer. Side effects of the treatments would also be closely monitored, and detailed questionnaires would be given to patients for them to fill out. This would allow a comparison of the effects, positive or negative, of each of the two treatments on their quality of life. After all, what good is a more effective treatment if any extra months gained are a living hell?

Lesley then explained that what is called an "interim analysis" would be carried out after the first one hundred and fifty patients had been followed for at least three months. Its purpose was to allow the study to be ended sooner than planned if there was no evidence that adding DPPE to doxorubicin increased, by at least five percent, the number of patients with tumor shrinkage. The trial would also end early if the interim analysis showed an "extreme" difference in time to progression in favor of one treatment or the other.

I had mixed feelings about this approach. Although intended to protect patients from continuing on an inferior treatment, there was always the danger of coming to a wrong conclusion when the

---

108 Actually, the end point being measured in the trial was called "progression-free survival (PFS)". Although slightly different from "time to progression (TTP)", discussed by Renzo during my visit to Princeton, for practical purposes, the two are similar.

followup time was brief and the data "immature". The medical literature is rife with reports of treatments that were deemed to be significantly better (or worse) over the short term, only to reverse course over the long term. Given my recent insights into the machinations at Bristol-Myers, I suspected that the company pushed for the interim analysis so that it could cut bait as quickly as possible if there was no "instant gratification" with DPPE in this trial.

Luckily, I didn't have a lot of time to ruminate over this possibility as it was now Susie's turn at the podium. Although she eschewed public speaking, I had convinced her to present a talk on how to administer the DPPE treatment. After all, having given over six hundred treatments, she was the world's authority on the subject…a very nervous world's authority, but the world's authority nonetheless.

"Don't worry. If you faint, I'll quietly step over you and finish your talk," I whispered as she got up to go to the microphone.

"That's very reassuring," she quietly hissed.

Not to worry. She did just fine and didn't need my assistance.

To augment her oral presentation, Susie also handed out an authoritative guide she had written, called *"DPPE for Nurses"*. A masterpiece, it covered the subject from every conceivable angle. There was a unanimous decision to distribute her manual as part of the "package" to all chemotherapy nurses involved with the study. I was very proud of her.

Later, during a coffee break, I was introduced to some of the chemotherapy nurses who had participated in the IND.97 trial. Among them was Janet Cormier, Len Reyno's nurse.

"Len tells me you are impressed with DPPE," I said.

"I am," she answered simply, and without hesitation.

"Well, let's hope that it works in MA.19 as well as it did in IND.97," I replied, Agnes Klein's admonition still fresh in my mind.

"I really think it will," she said.

As I gave her a thankful hug in appreciation for her confidence, I realized that the fate of DPPE was now firmly in the hands of the gods. I had taken it as far as I could. Like those people in the movie, *Casablanca*, there was nothing for me to do but wait... and wait....

CHAPTER FIFTY-FIVE:

How It Works...Really?

I received a call from Renzo early that spring. He wanted me to come to Wallingford. The Oncology Discovery Group had dissected out, to quote him, "how DPPE was really working". Ana Menendez and her colleagues wanted to share their data with me prior to presenting it at a meeting of the American Association for Cancer Research. Renzo, Alice Leung and Bill Rose would also attend Ana's talk.

Two weeks later, we all met....all, that is, but Rob Kramer. He did not bother to show up. I did not bother to ask why. For the next hour we sat around a table in a small, narrow conference room as Ana presented data showing that DPPE was indeed overcoming chemotherapy resistance by inhibiting the P-gp pump. For example, it increased the concentration of Taxol in MDR-positive cancer cells that otherwise would kick the drug out. There was more. DPPE also poisoned cell components called mitochondria[109], decreasing adenosine triphosphate (ATP), a vital

---

109 Mitochondria are oval-shaped structures, crisscrossed on the inside by many membrane "walls". Present in all cells, they are miniature "power plants", producing energizing substances, such as ATP, needed to drive chemical reactions essential for the cell to survive.

fuel substance that they made. As a result, the ATP-starved cancer cells weakened and died. In this way, DPPE appeared to increase the natural rate of death (apoptosis) of cancer cells.

"That should make you happy," Ana observed, looking over at me as she finished her presentation. I nodded politely but was less than convinced that her findings held water. My misgivings stemmed from the fact that the concentration of DPPE required to do these things was much higher than the level that could be achieved in the blood stream. For example, the decrease in ATP occurred at DPPE concentrations twenty-five to fifty times the blood levels we measured in our patients. Add the same "industrial strength" of orange juice to the cells and the same thing would probably happen. In my opinion it was a non-starter.

Even the ability to inhibit the P-gp pump required five times higher concentrations of DPPE than we could achieve in the blood. Rob Warrington's tests, based on Keith Simons' estimation of DPPE levels in patients, led him to conclude that DPPE was overcoming drug resistance by some other mechanism. Previously, using MDR-positive cells, he had observed that histidinol acted in the same, apparently novel, way as DPPE. Although I tended to side with Rob, I remained open-minded about Ana's pump data because we now knew that DPPE inhibited CYP3A4, the P450 enzyme whose level and activity was closely tied to that of the pump. Moreover, in the women with inflammatory breast cancer, the DPPE/epirubicin/Taxol combo appeared to selectively kill aggressive (high grade) breast cancer cells, the very ones that are most apt to have too many P-gp pumps.

Any misgivings about the doses Ana employed did not appear to be shared by Renzo. He looked on, apparently pleased with what he had heard. I thought I knew why. He needed to be able to tell his clinical bosses, and the Bristol-Myers marketing mavens, that DPPE was working in some understandable, conventional manner to increase the killing of cancer cells by chemotherapy. Histamine, shmistamine…nobody cared about that aspect of the story. Not necessarily that it was untrue, just that it was off everyone's radar and not "sellable". Tell oncologists that DPPE was inhibiting the well-accepted Pg-p pump, or starving cancer cells of ATP, and everyone would be happy. Tell the same oncologists that DPPE appeared to be a novel antihistamine drug that prevented Professor Kahlson's "nascent" histamine from binding to growth-regulating P450 enzymes and...Professor who? Histamine what? It was a problem that would continue to haunt the development of DPPE for years to come.

Irrespective of how DPPE was "really working", the company paid attention to my latest clinical trial. Shortly after the Wallingford meeting, David Lebwohl called to say that, based on my results with DPPE, epirubicin and Taxol in patients with metastatic and inflammatory breast cancer, Renzo had decided to sponsor a new phase two trial to more fully assess this approach. However, DPPE would be teamed up with the more worrisome doxorubicin/Taxol combination because epirubicin was not yet on the U.S. market (the one that really counted as far as Bristol-Myers was concerned). Apparently Renzo had been reassured by the Italians, who reported to him that combining doxorubicin with Taxol was safe for the heart if the two drugs were not timed one right after the other. Therefore, the DPPE/doxorubicin combination would be administered over the usual eighty minutes. Then, after a two hour hiatus, the Taxol would be given by itself over three hours.

Franco Muggia and his group at New York University, and José Baselga and his team of oncologists in Barcelona would be among the investigators testing the treatment. I was especially pleased about Franco's involvement, given his long interest in DPPE stemming back to the Sparta days. On the other hand, my learning of this new trial made Bristol-Myers' refusal to supply me with DPPE for the original study all the more galling.

As the spring meeting of the NCIC was coming up in Montréal, David suggested that we could all meet there to review the new plans. Renzo had been invited by the Clinical Trials Group to present a major overview of Bristol-Myers' portfolio of oncology drugs under investigation. Naturally, I assumed he would use the occasion to discuss DPPE and was quite excited by the prospect. After all, who wouldn't be proud to have their discovery given its just due in front of their peers? Brent Schacter, who was also going to the meeting, had never met Renzo and hoped to learn, first hand, the company's development plans for DPPE. I promised to arrange for him to speak with Renzo after the talk.

The morning of my arrival, I bumped into Bob Phillips in the hotel corridor. He had replaced David Beatty as NCIC director. "It looks as though we may have been premature in cutting off funding for your research," he told me candidly.

"Which time?" I replied, reminding Bob that he had chaired that unforgettable 1985 site visit when my block grant-funding was first terminated. We were both able to laugh, but the memory remained a painful one.

After listening all morning to a slew of clinical trial reports, including Lesley Seymour's review of the newly-opened MA.19 study, I looked forward to Renzo's talk that afternoon. What would he say about DPPE? As it turned out, very little. Actually, "very little" would be a vast overstatement. After putting up his first slide showing all the compounds in the pipeline, he stated, "You all know about DPPE, so I am not going to say anything more about it." *What?? That was it??* Yes. That was it. *If this was not the time and place to talk about DPPE, when and where would be more opportune?*

He immediately launched into a review of other promising oncology drugs under development. His major emphasis was on an oral platinum agent and a new Taxol derivative. Early studies suggested that this second-generation "Taxol" molecule was considerably more potent than the parent drug to kill cancer cells. I sat there, embarrassed and angry, trying desperately to act as though his glaring snub of DPPE was no big deal. I searched my mind for a reason, finally concluding that by saying nothing, he spoke volumes: from Bristol-Myers point of view, it was still all about Taxol.[110]

Later that afternoon, I met up with Brent in the large conference hall. He too had been caught off guard and was amazed by the short-shrift given to DPPE. Despite wanting to avoid Renzo lest I speak my mind, I kept my promise to Brent and introduced the two, asking Renzo if he could spend a few minutes filling in our CEO on the big picture for DPPE. His reply was only slightly longer than his comments in the talk. Looking at Brent, he replied, "As you well know, we are supporting the development of DPPE and await the results of the new trial. That's all I can tell you. *Silence.* Sorry, but I really have to go. I'm late for another meeting." He then turned away and headed for the door leaving Brent and me looking like a couple of dopes.

"So much for the big picture," I sighed. Brent just shook his head in disbelief at Renzo's rude response.

"I think the Renaissance missed Renzo," Jeff Usakewicz had once told me about his boss, complaining that Renzo was often impervious to the feelings of others. Despite Jeff's managerial involvement in important company projects such as DPPE, he found that Renzo often ignored him, preferring to communicate only with more senior medical people in his employ, such as Bill or, now, David. I had not seen this side of him before, but now understood what Jeff had probably meant. On all counts today, I felt that Renzo had been insensitive to the occasion. That said, I decided that there was no point in telling him as, at least on this issue, he seemed to lack *seychel*, Yiddish for "smarts".

It was time to forget about the incident and move on. With the breast cancer sessions now over, I looked forward to attending a much anticipated talk. Harvard's Dr. Judah Folkman had been invited to lecture about his pioneering research on the blood vessels that nourish the growth of cancer. A brilliant scientist and engaging speaker, I had heard him present Grand Rounds at our

110 The oral platinum compound was dropped by the company a year later. The new Taxol derivative also eventually faded away.

medical faculty in Winnipeg some years earlier and was highly impressed with what he had to say. I also suspected that, like me, he marched to his own drummer.

Bucking the skepticism of his peers, Folkman had spent twenty years researching how, early in the game, cancer cells stimulate small blood vessels to sprout around them. He reasoned that without developing this vital new blood supply, the cells could not grow into actual tumors. His team then identified various natural body substances that block the formation of these new blood vessels. Forget about treating the cancer cells. By simply targeting a tumor's blood lifeline,[111] cancers melted away in mice. A recent flurry of publications from Folkman's lab, especially a paper in *Nature*, had everyone excited.

The gist of the *Nature* paper was that, by combining "angio-statin" and "endostatin", two anti-angiogenic protein substances discovered during the research, even advanced mouse tumors completely regressed. Moreover, unlike tumor cells that often became drug-resistant, the targeted blood vessels were made up of normal cells that did not. Stop the treatment and the tumors re-grew. Start injecting angiostatin and endostatin again and the tumors once again headed south. The implication was that inhibiting blood vessel growth could shrink and keep the cancer cells at bay permanently ....at least in mice. Was this the long-sought-after magic bullet?

As he reviewed all of these findings, one could hear a pin drop in the room. It was positively electrifying. At the end, Dr. Folkman announced that phase one human clinical trials of his two compounds would begin within a few short months. He had licensed the development rights of his discovery to EntreMed, a small Maryland-based biotech company. In turn, EntreMed had sub-licensed angiostatin to none other than.... *Bristol-Myers Squibb!*

---

111 Blocking blood vessel growth is called "anti-angiogenesis". "Angio" means *blood vessel* and "genesis" means *formation*, or *coming into existence.*

Dr. Folkman envisaged his anti-angiogenic treatment as an adjunct to surgery, radiation and chemotherapy. However, given the impressive mouse data, many in the audience, including me, were left wondering whether these other therapies were even necessary. If angiostatin and endostatin worked as well in humans as in mice, cancer treatment would instantly change radically and for the better. As we filed out of the talk, our collective response was, "*W-o-o-o-w!!!*".

Incredibly, that was exactly the sentiment following a front-page splash in that Sunday's *New York Times*! Written by reporter, Gina Kolata, the news about Folkman's research results rapidly spread around the world, helped in large measure by a quote in her story from none other than James D. Watson, who shared the 1961 Nobel Prize in medicine with Francis Crick and Maurice Wilkins for discovering the structure of DNA. Watson may have unwittingly planted the seed for the story by allegedly telling Ms. Kolata at a dinner party that, "Judah is going to cure cancer in two years." That definitive statement, made by a scientist of such renowned stature, was pretty hard to ignore.

As a result, the public response to this impending breakthrough quickly reached such a frenzy that, within days, Watson was compelled to send a letter to the paper, setting the matter straight. "What I told Ms. Kolata at a dinner party six weeks ago was that [angiostatin and] endostatin should be in ... clinical trials by the end of this year, and that we would know about one year after that whether they were effective," he wrote. Whatever James Watson had really said to Gina Kolata over a martini, shares of EntreMed stock went through the roof and Judah Folkman's picture appeared (deservedly, in my opinion) on the cover of many weekly news-magazines. In interviews, Dr. Folkman low-balled his findings. "If you are a mouse with cancer, we can take very good care of you," was his humorous and widely-quoted comment.

Quite frankly, I too was caught up in the potential enormity of the story, but at a more personal level. If Dr. Folkman was right, almost every other cancer treatment, past and present, mine included, could be passé. Why should Bristol-Myers care about DPPE when they had an incredibly exciting drug like angiostatin in their stable of candidates? Could that explain Renzo's blah attitude at the NCIC meeting? I decided to call him for clarification.

"Given all this news about angiostatin, is DPPE still a contender?" I asked, à la Marlon Brando in *On The Waterfront*. Renzo seemed taken aback by my question.

"Lorne, where is angiostatin in development?" he asked slowly and didactically.

"Preclinical, going into phase one," I answered.

"Yes. And where is DPPE?"

"In phase three."

"Exactly. So why do you ask me this crazy question?" He then burst out laughing. More out of relief than anything else, I followed his lead. Whatever his perceived deficiencies, Renzo also could be charming and obviously had a sense of humor.

Everything was clear again. Swayed by all the media hype, I had temporarily forgotten Bill Slichenmyer's "up escalator" analogy. In his own way, Renzo was reiterating exactly what Bill had told me. In the rigidly-structured world of drug development, whether or not anyone knew how it "really worked", DPPE was now midway up that moving staircase, possibly heading for the top. Despite all that had been written, and the strong scientific evidence that it targeted cancer by blocking its blood supply, angiostatin was on the bottom rung, just beginning its long journey.[112]

---

112 In February, 1999, Bristol-Myers abruptly announced that it was dropping its development of angiostatin, citing difficulties in making the substance and in reproducing its effects on tumors! In a February 10, 1999 interview with the *Wall Street Journal*, Robert A. Kramer (of, "So-o-o, you're here to tell us all about your new histamine receptor" fame) stated, "At this time, angiostatin protein in its present form does not meet our criteria for molecules that advance to clinical trials." To date, neither of Dr. Folkman's "statins" have been commercialized. Moreover, although human trials of some other anti-angiogenic drugs have demonstrated efficacy, none have remotely approached the "w-o-o-ow!!" results in mice. It has always been easier to cure laboratory rodents of cancer than to achieve this goal in humans.

CHAPTER FIFTY-SIX:

What The Angels Foretold

Our family often discussed religion and the nature of God. I always believed that creation was no accident, but that the Creator was beyond human understanding. "What's it all about, Alfie?" was my sixty-four thousand dollar question. Jason was non-committal, perhaps unsure of what he believed. On the other hand, Jill and Carolyn were very spiritual. Jill once told me she believed in the existence of angels, often regarded in Judao-Christian belief as divine messengers, or purveyors of God's will. Her admission reminded me of my own bar mitzvah, where I chanted a section of the Old Testament in which Jacob wrestled with an angel.[113] Moreover, every Passover we read about how God sent the Angel of Death to smite the Egyptian first-born males. Even then, I didn't give the concept of angels, or their messages, any credence. That all started to change in 1998.

---

113   (Genesis, Ch. 32) Actually, there are different versions of whom Jacob was wrestling. The text actually refers to "a man", but other interpretations are that the man was actually God, or an angel of God.

December of that year was a time of encouraging news and nervous expectations. Thanks mainly to the Eastern European sites, the MA.19 trial was accruing patients much faster than predicted. The interim analysis almost certainly would be carried out by mid-1999, just six months away. Moreover, the new phase two Bristol-Myers prostate cancer trial testing DPPE plus mito-xantrone and prednisone was already showing the same kind of promise that we had seen with our original study testing DPPE and cyclophosphamide. Just a week earlier, David Lebwohl had called to tell me that Derek Raghavan was highly impressed by what he was seeing with his patients in Los Angeles, and was now trumpeting the virtues of DPPE to his colleagues.

On the home front, Winnipeg was having a mild winter. The white stuff had only recently fallen. Christmas lights adorned the tall evergreens and twinkled in the window panes of the large, comfortable homes that were nestled along the quiet bay where Ernie and Diane Ramsey lived. Over a glass of wine and Diane's highly alcoholic rum cake, Ernie and I discussed the latest news on DPPE during a break in the singing at their annual Christmas music and food fest. "That calls for a round of *Back In The Saddle Again*," my dear friend replied in response to my positive assess-ment. Our performance was gre-e-e-yat!

A week later, toasts to everyone's health and to the success of DPPE were made around the beautifully-set dining room table at the Russell's Christmas/Anniversary dinner. Tony had carved an extra-big turkey that year, in part because Carolyn and husband, Jan, had been married the previous July. "And what would the good doctor like?" Tony always asked when it came time to serve me. It was the type of silly formality that only close friends could conjure up as a joke. Jill and I always addressed Tony and Susan as "Mr. and Mrs. Russell", while we were "Dr. and Mrs. Brandes". For reasons I never fully understood, Susan also often referred to me as "the delicate scientist".

Every year, the accoutrements adorning the Russell's table included an antique candle holder. The flames from four candles caused brass angels suspended above them to turn.

When this happened, a thin length of brass hanging from each angel would strike two small bells anchored below, causing them to chime. On this night, however, the angels refused to revolve despite the rich glow from the candles. "This could mean bad luck," I muttered as futile attempts were made to get them to spin. Despite my generally non-superstitious nature and previously-stated disregard of angels, I felt a bit concerned this time around. The situation deteriorated when we pulled the "crackers" and a nondescript fortune emanated from mine. *After all, DPPE and I needed every bit of help we could get.*

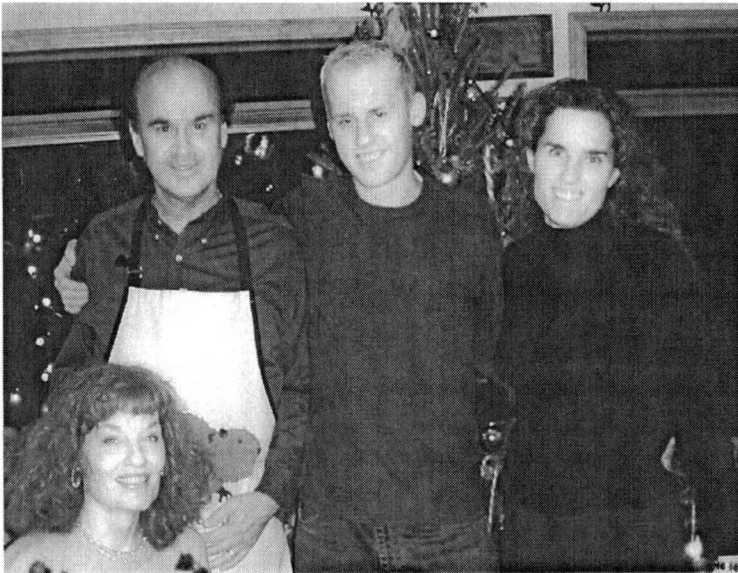

The Russells: Tony, Peter, Carolyn and (seated) Susan (Personal photo collection)

"Don't worry, Dad. I have really good vibes about DPPE," Carolyn whispered. I gave my highly-spiritual daughter a fatherly hug and kiss but continued to fret. Why did the angels suddenly pick this year to go on strike? Were they sending me a bad message?

"Dessert time. Have some Figgie pudding," Susan chirped, trying to distract me with a generous piece oozing with her special sauce. The diversion worked temporarily.

"The best Figgie pudding ever," I declared. The meal now at an end, we cleared the table. The candle flames in the holder had long since flickered and burned out. The stationary angel wings were dark with soot. As my eyes remained fixed on them, I told myself that it was all much ado about nothing...or so I hoped.

Needing to get away for a rest, a week later Jill and I headed down to Florida. Each year we rented a lovely one-bedroom condo, nicely situated in Pompano Beach, on Florida's intracoastal waterway, two blocks from the ocean. The floor to ceiling windows and an outside balcony just one storey above a beautifully land-scaped pool made for a happy, carefree existence as we watched luxury yachts ply the intracoastal water, just fifty feet from our door. Other Winnipeg friends and family stayed, or lived, nearby. The January weather was just right, sunny and mid-seventies most days. It was easy to forget about MA.19 there.

Unfortunately, mom and dad, who had been a major part of our Florida experience, no longer spent the winters in nearby Hallandale. Although in generally good physical health, dad had recently suffered a couple of mini-stokes from which he appeared to fully recover. Nonetheless, the episodes scared him and he now stuck close to home where he felt more secure. Even the prospect of missing his favorite pastime, betting on the ponies at Gulfstream, did not change his mind. Loss of confidence and diminished interest are all-too-frequent occurrences as many people age. I hated to see it happen to him.

Mom still fought the good fight. Two years previously, a mam-mogram had detected another primary cancer in her left breast, near the site of the initial lumpectomy. A few months earlier, she had stopped taking tamoxifen on the advice of her oncolo-gist. This recommendation was based on the then-widely-held consensus that tamoxifen was of no further benefit beyond five years. Clinical decisions are often based on statistics, but what is deemed best for the group does not necessarily apply to the individual. I believed that, in mom's case, stopping the tamoxifen likely led to a reawakening of dormant cancer cells.

When confronted with the recurrence, she opted to have both breasts removed. "I don't want to have to go through this thing a third time," she told me and her surgeon. I thought this decision was rather drastic....until the pathologist also detected a focus of cancer in the right breast after the double mastectomy. Trust mom's intuition to lead her in the right direction. "I'm just fine," she told everyone as she declared herself cured and resumed playing tennis. Knowing it was not necessarily that cut and dried, I worried but said nothing. After all, who could predict the future? Those who claimed they could, never seemed to win the lottery.

The month in Florida passed all too quickly. For the rest of the winter, I tried to keep my mind off the fate of DPPE as best I could. According to Jeff, over two hundred women were already on the study, with more being added every day. The interim analysis of the trial would now take place in late May or early June at the latest. *Que sera sera.* Visits to Frank's office usually helped quell my angst. We still have fire in our bellies as we talked, argued, pursued our research and prepared our latest findings for my presentation at the yearly meeting of the European Histamine Research Society to be held in mid-May.

Jill and I had already packed our bags for Lyon, the site of that year's histamine meeting, when David Lebwohl called. "Could you come to Orlando?" he asked on short notice. He was taking advantage of the large annual American Society of Clinical Oncology (ASCO) meeting to arrange an informal meeting of investigators involved with testing DPPE in the company's phase two breast and prostate cancer trials. José Baselga and Derek Raghavan, among others, would be attending the international meeting in just over a week's time.

David had reason to believe that, from their early observations, the investigators were favorably disposed towards further studies with DPPE and wanted to discuss "impressions and future directions". Unfortunately, his meeting was to be held the very day we were flying back from France. It would not be possible for me to attend. "Why is everything always a last-minute affair with them?" Jill asked, annoyed. It certainly did seem to be a recurring theme. Nonetheless, I was pleased that David had asked me to go and that, with or without me, important people would be discussing my drug.

We arrived in Lyon, considered the gastronomic capital of France, two days before the start of the meeting. Jill had already obtained the names of a few small family-run restaurants that, over the years, had received rave reviews from the critics. Our modern hotel was located in a pleasant residential area of the city, about three miles from the downtown dining establishments we wished to visit. Avid walkers, we immediately liked the idea of traveling by foot along the bank of the Rhône river…a great solution to eating rich food without gaining weight. The best part was that it really worked.

Many old friends, including Börje and Ingrid Uvnäs, turned up for that year's conference. At the final banquet, I confided to my tablemates that this might be our last histamine meeting for a while. If DPPE was successful, I would likely have to attend the competing ASCO meeting. On hearing this, Börje turned to me and said, "Then I hope it fails so you come back." His words shocked me. My eyes widened with horror at the very prospect. "Börje! Nej, nej, nej!" Ingrid immediately admonished him in Swedish. A sly smile was followed by a quick, "I kid you." As he apologized, his eyes twinkled like an angel. *Angel? Be careful of what you wish lest it come true, Börje.* We threw our arms around one another and promised to keep in touch. Among all the people there, I loved Börje the most.

Nonetheless, his jarring attempt at humor unnerved me. "Börje! Nej, nej, nej!" I kept repeating to myself.

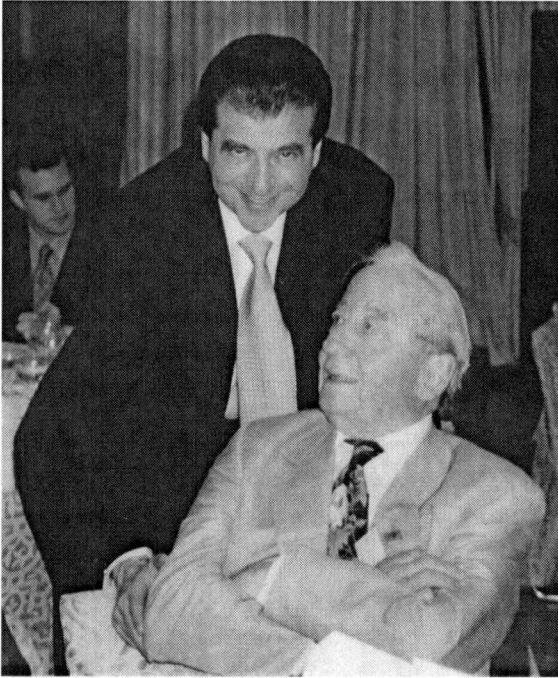

With Börje Uvnäs in Lyon, 1999 (Personal photo collection)

We returned to Canada to find Winnipeg in early bloom. The mild, relatively snow-free winter had quickly given up the ghost for spring's early arrival. The tulips had already been and gone and the trees were well on their way to being leafy and green. That first Friday back, I decided to come home early to enjoy the warm sunny weather that was forecast for the entire weekend. As Jill and I walked up and down our River Heights neighborhood, my cell phone rang. It was David Lebwohl calling from his car while driving through upstate New York on his way back to Connecticut. He had recently bought a sporty BMW and was enjoying breaking it in.

As I listened, he enthusiastically recounted the investigator meeting in Orlando the week before. The general consensus among those present was that DPPE-based chemotherapy appeared to be very active to shrink breast and prostate cancer.

Potential new protocols were discussed. David would be reporting all of this to Renzo on his return. Enthusiasm or not, everything would depend on the interim analysis report. "Are you optimistic that we will be okay?" I asked him.

"I think so....yeah," he replied.

Not knowing whether David was involved with the analysis, I chose to believe that his generally upbeat mood was a good sign that something positive was brewing. Jill squeezed my hand as we walked and I recounted the conversation for her.

Any optimism was short-lived. The following Monday I called Jeff, who told me that he was up to his eyeballs in case-report forms, the documents used to assess the interim results. The trial numbers were now approaching the three-hundred mark, far past the one hundred and fifty originally expected at this point in the trial. He figured that the task would take until the first week in July to complete.

"Have any obvious differences emerged yet?" I asked, point blank.

"No," he answered.

I let out an audible gasp and my mouth went dry. Sensing my distress, Jeff immediately tried to soften his reply.

"You know, we're just at the beginning of our analysis. I wouldn't read anything into that at this juncture. We only have to show a five percent difference in tumor response in favor of DPPE. That should be pretty easy to do."

"I sure hope you're right," I replied. My pulse remained noticeably high.

"Just hang in there," Jeff counseled.

"What else *can* I do?" I replied. Drug development was not for the faint of heart.

After hanging up the phone, I sat quietly at my desk for a long time. Given the rapid and robust nature of the responses we had seen with DPPE and doxorubicin in the phase two IND.97 study, I would have expected an early favorable trend to emerge. So far it had not. A red flag was raised. For the first time, I seriously entertained the possibility that DPPE might fail. "Try to put it out of your head," I told myself. There was absolutely nothing I could do to change the outcome, good or bad. Why fret until I knew that there was really something to fret about? That was easier said than done. I continued to fret.

A palpable silence pervaded the first two weeks of June. I was not-so-slowly going nuts and decided to take a chance on phoning trial chairman, Len Reyno. As I dialed his number, I knew he might not be comfortable hearing my voice on the other end of the line. To his credit, he accepted my call.

"Len, *I* know that *you* know how difficult this whole business is for me," I began. "Is there anything you can tell me without breaking the rules?"

"All I can tell you is that it is very close," he replied.

"Do you have any sense of whether we're going to be okay here?" I persisted.

"It'll be tight, but I'm hoping…I think… we will. That's all I can say."

I thanked him and hung up. All we needed was a lousy five percent difference and the trial could continue. Was that so much to ask?

No matter the outcome, Jill and I had firm vacation plans for early July. We had booked the Shaw Festival in beautiful Niagara-on-the-Lake, Ontario and would be staying at a "bed and breakfast", popular with devotees of the yearly productions of the plays of George Bernard Shaw. I left word with David and Renzo that I could be contacted on my cell phone if the verdict came in while we were away. They promised to call me as soon as they knew the outcome.

"Soon" came earlier than expected, on the afternoon of June twenty-fourth. I was kibitzing with the secretaries in the physicians' business office at the medical school when my pager went off. The hospital operator was holding an outside call from Dr. Seymour from NCIC. I told her to put it through. *Lesley Seymour? What was this about?*

"Hello."

"Hi. It's Lesley Seymour. Renzo Canetta has asked me to call you. Have you already received the fax?" *Renzo Canetta? Fax?*

"What fax?" *She's about to tell me.*

"You haven't seen it? Good. We wanted you to hear the news first-hand. It's about MA.19. The interim analysis detected no difference in the response rates or time to progression. The study has been stopped. Everyone has been sent a fax telling them to switch any patients receiving DPPE and doxorubicin to doxorubicin alone." *Ohmygod.*

"There was *absolutely* no difference at all?" I asked softly, trying to maintain my composure as four sets of eyes watched me.

"No. Sorry."

The Angel of Death had just smitten DPPE, toppling it off the up escalator.

CHAPTER FIFTY-SEVEN:
A Burden No More

Whether it happens to a person or a dream, sudden death is always a terrible shock...a life, or years of hard work, wiped out in an instant. Telling my family was the toughest thing I ever had to do. Jill was devastated, as were mom and dad when I called them. Carolyn rushed over to the house, threw her arms around me and cried as she whispered in my ear how proud of me she was and how much she cared. On hearing what happened, Jason was suspicious. Had Bristol-Myers hatched a plot to steal my drug? My dad and brother, Ken, had the same take. I assured them that their concern was unfounded. It was a simple equation. The drug had failed. A business decision had been made.

To me, the most upsetting aspect of having failed was how I learned the news. I had no issue with Lesley Seymour. She was only the messenger. No, I was sad and angry *because* she was the messenger. That fateful call should have been made by one person and one person only: Renzo Canetta. He finally contacted me at home after dinner in response to a message I had left with his secretary. The excuse given was that he had been in meetings all day deciding the fate of DPPE. When he suddenly realized that a fax was being sent to all the centres announcing the discontinuation of the trial, he contacted Lesley in a panic and requested that she phone me immediately. *What a piece of Swiss cheese. If he had time to call Lesley, he had time to call me.*

I quickly changed the subject. "What about the promising prostate cancer data? Isn't that still worth pursuing?"

"The market for prostate cancer isn't big enough for us to consider the drug for that indication alone," he replied. *That was an interesting turnabout. The company's original interest in DPPE was solely as a treatment for prostate cancer. During the licensing negotiations, I was the one who had to push them to recognize its potential in breast cancer.* There was nothing left for either of us to say, except that we were both sorry that things had ended this way. As Agnes Klein had warned, the landscape was littered with promising drugs that had failed in phase three. This was but the latest example.

An e-mail soon arrived from David Lebwohl. Since the results of the trial were "definitive" that DPPE added nothing to doxorubicin, he felt that everyone should be confident that stopping the study was the right thing to do. The response rates and "time to progression" curves for each treatment arm were virtually identical. As a result, based on their prior experience in such instances, the NCIC statisticians were positive that nothing would change down the road. The chance of observing any future difference in survival was as close to zero as could be predicted.

The "morning after" was spent emotionally thanking my wonderful staff for their years of hard work on my behalf. Of all those involved, the end was hardest on Susie, who just could not come to terms with what had happened. She poured her heart out to me in a quickly-penned three page letter. "I never for one moment thought DPPE would ever fail," she wrote, pointing out all the patients she believed had benefited over the years. She then blamed the negative outcome on some minor changes that had been made in the administration of DPPE and doxorubicin in the protocol.[114] When I called her up to my office to talk things over, she started to cry. I hugged her for a long time as she sobbed. She had worked her heart out and was left totally bereft.

Later that day a fax arrived from Alice Leung. Although not unexpected, it was still hard for me to read. Bristol-Myers had immediately terminated the licensing agreement and was returning DPPE to the University of Manitoba. What had taken well over a year to acquire took only minutes to give back. Any and all costs, such as patents, would immediately revert to us. "Isn't that a shame," was all Arnold Portigal could say on learning the news. Like everyone else, from Lyonel to Ernie to Frank, he was speechless.

After reflecting on the contents of the fax, I contacted Brent and Janet. "I would certainly understand if you decide to let the patents lapse," I told them. To their credit, and my surprise, neither was willing to do that. Both felt that Bristol-Myers had acted rather precipitously. They wanted time to reflect and consider the next move. Each would cover the cost of the patents for at least a year while we tried to find another partner.[115] "The debt was wiped clean when we received the milestone payment eighteen months ago," Janet explained. Any costs for the next year were no big deal as far as the administration was concerned.

As it turned out, I was extremely thankful that Jill and I had planned that July vacation and could get away for ten days. It helped to take our minds off the catastrophe that had befallen us. Not that we didn't talk about it. We did. But at least we had the distraction of going to the theatre, eating at some fine restaurants, drinking wine indigenous to the Niagara peninsula, driving

---

114 In our initial trials, DPPE and doxorubicin had been given through separate i.v. lines because we didn't know whether they were compatible with each other. Bristol-Myers had determined that they were. As a result, the two drugs were given through the same i.v. line in the MA.19 trial. I saw no problem with this.

115 That decision turned out to be an important one. Had the patents been allowed to lapse, there would have been no further possibility of commercialization. They saved the day!

through the countryside, and riding the Maid of the Mist to the very edge of the thundering Niagara Falls. A wonderful weekend stay with cousins Bob and Sandi Laine at their lovely summer home near Lake Simcoe capped off our time away.

A flashing red light on the telephone answering machine greeted our return home. The very first message was from Derek Raghavan. Please call him as soon as possible. In very blunt and direct terms, Derek stated his belief that Bristol-Myers had acted stupidly. Based on his experience with DPPE in the prostate cancer trial, he believed the drug had great potential. He had gone to the very top of the corporate ladder, asking CEO Peter Dolan to reverse the decision. It was to no avail. As a result, he angrily resigned from the company's drug advisory committee. Together, we decided to try to carry on with the study. Even though Bristol-Myers was no longer involved, Renzo had agreed that the company would continue to supply DPPE for the trial.

A few weeks later, I had occasion to call Kathy Pritchard about an unrelated matter. She soon brought up the topic of MA.19. "How do you feel about the decision to stop the trial on the basis of the interim analysis?" she asked.

"I'm okay with it, I guess. Any differences in tumor response or time to progression were apparently so minuscule that it must have made sense to everyone to stop at that point. I mean, you and your colleagues are supposed to be the experts on when to start or stop a trial. Who am I to second-guess your decision?"

"Well, in the absence of a compelling reason, such as unacceptable toxicity or a highly significant difference in outcome between two treatments, I think it is always dangerous to stop a 'close' trial prematurely, before all the data are in," she answered without hesitation. Little did I know how prescient those words would turn out to be.

The next few months were spent making up for the time I had neglected to give my family. There were occasional periods of sadness and depression, but I worked through them with Jill's help and understanding. During that time, a lot of the fire went out of me. For many weeks, I couldn't bring myself to write a paper or read a journal. It was probably part and parcel of being depressed. Then, slowly, slowly, everything righted itself. A weight lifted from my shoulders. When it did, Jill told me that I had fundamentally changed and had become a better, more attentive husband and father. She was right, and I now knew why. I no longer had to go through life bearing a burden called DPPE.

PART 2

"It ain't over 'til it's over."

Yogi Berra

C H A P T E R   F I F T Y - E I G H T :

Back In The Saddle Again

A ripple in the calm waters of my life occurred almost a year later when I received an unexpected phone call.

"Dr. Brandes?"

"Yes."

"My name is David Harper. I'm the licensing director of YM BioSciences.[116] We are an oncology drug development company located near Toronto. I would be interested in talking to you about DPPE."

"How interested is 'interested'?"

"Very interested. We have done our due diligence and spoken with a lot of people who believe that Bristol-Myers dropped DPPE prematurely."

---

116   The company's name at that time was actually York Medical, but it soon changed its name to the more high-tech moniker, YM BioSciences, and went public. Their board of directors included Henry Friesen and, later, Julius ("Now if only vee knew vat it vas good for") Vida !!! What goes around comes around.

Remembering my conversation with Kathy Pritchard, my ears pricked up. "You realize that DPPE was deemed to have failed in a phase three trial in breast cancer," I reiterated.

"Yes, we know that, but from reading your *JCO* publication on DPPE and cyclophosphamide, and from speaking to Dr. Raghavan, we believe that the drug still has exciting potential in the treatment of prostate cancer," he countered. "I wonder whether I can come out to Winnipeg to meet with you at your earliest convenience," he continued.

"I guess next Friday would be okay," I replied with no great degree of enthusiasm.

Quite honestly, I had very mixed feelings about resurrecting DPPE. I had finally managed to refocus myself, effectively putting the hurt and disappointment over its crushing failure behind me. When I wasn't busy with my clinical responsibilities or jousting with Frank over the meaning of our latest lab data, I was enjoying a more leisurely, less stressful existence. Rather than attending the annual EHRS meeting at a converted monastery near Rome, we and another couple had booked a twelve-day cruise from Lisbon to Istanbul. Later, Börje Uvnäs wrote to express his disappointment at our absence, but filled me in on what I had missed. I think he instinctively understood that I just wasn't ready to discuss the events of the last year with my histamine research colleagues.

A week later, David Harper sat across from me in my office. A large, bearded teddy bear of a man with a ready laugh and English accent, he spent an hour outlining his company's business plan. It was basically the same as Sparta's. YM did no in-house research, but acquired potentially promising oncology drugs discovered in university labs like mine. It then worked to advance them in clinical trials with the hope that they would eventually be licensed out to a major drug company for big bucks.

YM already had three drugs, licensed from Cuba, under development. That was somewhat problematical because, although the rest of the world was open, the U.S. market was still closed to anything Cuban. DPPE presented no such dilemma. The immediate plan would be to underwrite the cost for Derek Raghavan and me to continue the phase two trial of DPPE, mitoxantrone and prednisone in patients with advanced prostate cancer. If the results were positive, given the relative lack of effective chemotherapy in that disease, the company hoped to receive early regulatory approval from the FDA.

On hearing what he had to say, I had no doubt that David was sincere in his desire to make a deal. However, one thing was glaringly clear. No matter how much grief my former partner had caused me, YM BioSciences was a giant step backward from Bristol-Myers Squibb. Yet there had been no other interested party. Maybe Harper and his YM colleagues saw something that the others had not. What did we have to lose?

After he left, I spoke with Brent and Janet. Assuming the lawyers did not uncover anything that would be a deal breaker, I recommended that we give the company a chance. YM could have DPPE for no up-front payment provided that they agreed to fund my research for three years and pay me a consultant fee to help them in the venture. If the drug was successful, we would share in up-front payments and royalties. The administration, and David Allan, a former investment banker who was YM's CEO, agreed with the terms.

By the end of November, the attorneys for both sides were satisfied with the details of the contract, the provincial government approved, and the new licensing deal was signed. This time, at my request, there was no local press coverage of the event. Personally, I thought that YM BioSciences had acquired DPPE on a wing and a prayer and, given the history of its failure in MA.19, was probably wasting its money. Nonetheless, I decided not to look a gift horse in the mouth, especially one that restored my research funding.

I called Ernie Ramsey about this latest development. He was delighted to hear that the prostate cancer study would not be a casualty of Bristol-Myers' pullout. As YM had negotiated to secure the company's full supply of DPPE and would underwrite the costs of monitoring the patients in Los Angeles and Winnipeg, the FDA and Health Canada approved the switch in sponsors and gave their blessings for the trial to continue. "That's a really gr-e-e-yat Christmas present," Ernie replied enthusiastically. He promised to remain involved and to continue to send patients my way.

Speaking of Christmas, I had to give Ernie some bad news. For the first time in years, Jill and I wouldn't be attending the Ramsey's annual sing-along party. A musical version of Dicken's *Christmas Carol* was scheduled for the same evening at the local live theatre. We had been unable to exchange our tickets. He was clearly disappointed but very understanding. "Oh, that's really too bad. We'll especially miss Jill's singing," he lamented.

"What about me? Won't you miss accompanying me in *Back in the Saddle Again*?"

That produced a laugh. "We'll do it next year for sure," he replied, as we wished each other the best of the season.

CHAPTER FIFTY-NINE:

No Next Year

A few days after our yearly feast at the Russell's,[117] I received a chilling call from Susie. To supplement her income, she worked evenings in the CT scanner in the hospital's radiology department. "Have you talked with Dr. Ramsey?" she asked, her voice quavering.

"A week or two ago. Why?" I answered

"He was just in tonight for a CT scan. It doesn't look good."

"Susie, he was just fine when we spoke. What *are* you talking about?" I asked, a feeling of panic washing over me.

"It looks like he has a tumor in his pancreas and there's a spot on his liver. I'm sorry. I thought you would want to know." *Oh, God. Oh, God. This can't be happening. First Wayne. Now Ernie? Not Ernie. Not Ernie.*

I can't recall much of what was said after that. I do remember the horrible, hollow feeling in my stomach as I lay down, shaking, on the bed. I had to pull myself together and call my dear friend

---

117   The angels turned 'round and 'round over the candle flames that year. What had changed? Absolutely nothing that anyone could identify!

immediately. He answered the phone himself. Nothing seemed amiss. Maybe this was all a big mistake.

"Hi Ernie. Is everything okay?"

"I knew it would be you. I guess you've heard the bad news," he replied.

My heart sank. I told him about Susie's call and assured him that she had not told anyone but me. He understood.

"I'm glad you know," he sighed. "I don't think I could have called you. I'm still trying to come to terms with this."

"Then it's really true?"

"They're doing a needle biopsy of my liver tomorrow to know for sure, but things don't look good," he said, his voice breaking.

After learning what the scan had shown, he had immediately gone home, called his family into the bedroom and told them. They all hugged and cried. This was a force majeure….the worst of all random events.

The story he told was all too familiar. He had developed some heartburn a couple of weeks before the Christmas party, but at first didn't pay much notice. He had been taking an anti-inflammatory drug for chronic elbow pain that had resulted from years of playing squash and thought that the medication was the likely culprit. An H_2 acid blocker seemed to settle things down, but the symptoms came back when he tried going off it. He then stopped the anti-inflammatory drug, but the symptoms persisted. He had some blood work which indicated the possibility of a mild inflammation of the pancreas. He had probably drunk a little too much wine over the holidays, that was all. But that wasn't all. Neither the symptoms nor the blood tests improved when he refrained from drinking alcohol. He became concerned and requested a CT scan. We now knew the rest.

The next day, a thin needle was inserted into his liver where the CT scan showed a "spot".

The verdict came swiftly from the pathologist. He had pancreatic cancer and it had spread. Ernie was sixty-two years old. Based on the same terrible statistics that had faced Wayne Beecroft, he likely would not reach his sixty-third birthday. At Ernie's request, Lyonel and I huddled with one of the oncologists in our department. Always the fighter, Ernie wanted to try chemotherapy. There was a relatively new drug, called gemcitabine, that helped some people with pancreatic cancer live a little bit longer. Our colleague wanted to combine it with an experimental drug that he was able to obtain.

The night after the biopsy, Ernie and I talked on the phone for almost an hour. He had decided that he needed to conserve all his strength for the fight ahead and would not be going back to work. The impact of his leaving would be immeasurable. At one and the same time we were losing the head of the University's urology section, the head of urological oncology at the Cancer Foundation, the director of the kidney transplant program at the Health Sciences Centre, and the visionary who was planning the Foundation's new prostate centre.

"If it were any other cancer, I might have a chance....but this....?" He couldn't finish the sentence. I listened silently, nodding in agreement, tears in my eyes. "The crazy thing is that my symptoms have settled right down and I feel well," he said. We decided then and there that we would get together at his home that weekend. We had to enjoy life while we could....while Ernie could.

Ernie then made a request. He wanted me to call several of his colleagues to give them the bad news. He was too emotional to do it himself. I wasn't far behind him in that department, but agreed. My first call was to Al Downs, Ernie's former boss who had retired as head of the University's surgery department a few years earlier. Al had a reputation as a tough guy. On hearing about Ernie, he burst into tears. That was the reaction of almost everyone who learned the story. It was beyond terrible.

Our get-together that Saturday night was bittersweet. Ernie looked as well as I had ever seen him. "I love you, Ernie," I whispered as we hugged each other for a very long time.

"I love you too," he replied softly.

That evening we all tried very hard to act as if everything was normal. After a lot of small talk, we went into the living room where Ernie sat down at his beloved shiny black Yamaha grand and started to play his favorite Andrew Lloyd Webber show tunes. It was hard not to have a lump in your throat. He was as magnificent a musician as he was a person.

Later, over coffee, I made a suggestion. Ernie should consider recording his music and putting it on a CD for his family and friends. It would be a wonderful project, and good therapy. In fact, he and Diane had recently discussed just such a venture. One of the operating room assistants at the hospital worked as an audio engineer in his spare time and had access to state-of-the-art digital recording equipment. Ernie would talk to him following his return from Belfast; he and Diane were leaving shortly to visit with family.

A month later, Ernie's living room was turned into a miniature recording studio. Despite being on chemotherapy, he spent the next several weeks recording a wide range of selections, ranging from *Les Miserables* and *Phantom of the Opera* to his favorite Irish repertoire, including *Danny Boy*, to the second movement of Beethoven's *Pathetique* sonata.

One Saturday night in March, a bunch of us gathered around the towering stereo speakers in the Ramsey's big downstairs family room. Ernie inserted a shiny CD into the player and cranked up the sound. For almost fifty minutes we were treated to a musical tour de force. As we clapped and shouted our "bravos" after each piece, Diane sat on the floor in front of the fireplace, legs crossed under her, often lost in her own private thoughts. I knew what they were. We all did.

When it was all over, Ernie announced that he wanted to make a second disc of music. There was so much he wanted to record. I knew only too well how little time he had left to accomplish his goal. His strength was now rapidly diminishing, and he was much less robust than just two months earlier. The chemotherapy had not produced any slowing of his cancer and had been stopped.

Worse, he became jaundiced. A small tube, called a stent, had been inserted to open his bile duct, but became infected. He was taking hefty doses of antibiotics to combat the high fevers.

The second recording session took much longer to complete. He would often start to play a song, his fingers would stumble during a passage and he would stop. Then, resting with his head on his arm at the piano, he would find "the zone" for long enough to do what had to be done. While his first CD showcased his tremendous talent, the second was a testament to his incredible inner strength and courage.

By late May, unseasonably warm, summer-like weather prevailed. The Ramsey's downstairs family room opened onto the patio and swimming pool in the back yard. Ernie loved to lounge by the pool but was now too weak to go down the steep staircase that led there from his first floor bedroom. Diane called me with a plan hatched by the family to obtain a wheelchair so that Ernie might be transported out the front door and around a side path to the back of the house. It sounded like a good idea but, because of his increasingly frail condition, I suggested a dry run with me as the "test passenger".

The next day, as daughter Clare tried to ease me down the front step, I suddenly shot forward as the wheelchair tipped wildly before the front wheels could hit the sidewalk. Grabbing the arm rests and using all the strength in my legs and feet, I was just able to keep everything upright. "I think your dad would have been on the ground at this point," I observed. Clare nodded grimly. We tried the manouvre a second time with only slightly more success.

Things got even worse as we proceeded down the path at the side of the house. The front wheels kept jamming as they dug into the dirt between the uneven paving stones. "Stop before you kill me!" I gasped as the sudden stops and starts violently tossed me up and down, front to back and side to side. By this time, Diane and Clare were aching with laughter at the sight of me. I looked like a limp rag doll. It was clear that Ernie would not make it outside to his beloved pool by this means. True to form, he smiled as the girls described to him what had just taken place, and accepted, with calm resignation, the negative verdict on the wheelchair.

Ernie's life on earth came to an end very peacefully in early June, less than six months after his diagnosis. He died in his own bed, surrounded by his loving wife and children. Most of his siblings had been to Winnipeg to see him. The last was Cameron, a Belfast physician. When not at Ernie's bedside, he was at the computer, lovingly compiling the piano tracks for the CDs and designing a jewel case cover entitled, *For Diane*. He had just returned home a few days before Ernie died. They had tearfully said their goodbyes, knowing that they would never see one another again.

Jill and I, along with family and close friends, attended a small private service in the funeral home chapel. At the end, as we filed past Ernie's photograph placed beside a small mahogany box containing his cremated remains, I broke down. A memorial celebration of his life was held in a large downtown church a week later. My composure regained, I was given the honor of reading to the hundreds of people present, a personal letter from Ernie's six brothers and sisters. At his request, they did not travel back to Winnipeg, but held their own evening service for him in Belfast to coincide with the late morning hour of our memorial tribute in Winnipeg.

In the memorial program printed for the occasion, a quote from Yeats stuck with me: "*Think where man's glory most begins and ends, and say my glory was I had such friends.*" How true that was in Ernie's case. He had a wealth of friends. His death left a giant hole in my life….and in the lives of all of us. There was one last wish to be honored. After a period of mourning, Diane and the three Ramsey children travelled back to Northern Ireland to scatter his ashes over the water along the Antrim coast that he loved so much. He was home.

Ernie's contribution to the clinical development of DPPE in the treatment of prostate cancer cannot be overstated. His long experience in treating the disease was invaluable and he taught me a great deal. That he did not live to continue our work together constantly fills me with as much sadness as knowing that the two of us will never again enjoy a laugh. Yet, there is one soothing consolation. He, and his talent, live on in those two gr-e-e-e-yat CDs. I play them all the time.[118]

---

118 Ernie's was not the only tragic loss we endured. Two months before Ernie died, Arnold Greenberg succumbed after a courageous two-year battle with colon cancer. He was only fifty-nine and at the height of his career. With his passing, the Institute of Cell Biology and the world of cancer research lost a renowned and productive scientist. A fitting tribute in his honor was the naming of the Arnold H. Greenberg lecture theatre in the new facility that now houses CancerCare Manitoba. Jim Davie, who had collaborated with me to show that DPPE and histamine bind to DNA, succeeded Arnold as Director of Cell Biology.

CHAPTER SIXTY:

I'm Back!!!

The survival outcome of the MA.19 study was presented at the spring, 2001, meeting of the NCIC Clinical Trials Group. I was not there to hear the verdict. There was the greater concern to be with Ernie, who was still alive at that time, but failing rapidly. More to the point, why would I want to travel one thousand miles to sit in a room, surrounded by hundreds of people, listening to a final report about the failure of my drug? There was no reason to believe that the survival would be any different from what had been predicted by the statisticians at the time the trial was stopped. My colleague, David Bowman, would be attending the presentation. If there was anything to report, he would tell me on his return. I gave the matter no further thought.

Life is always unpredictable, sometimes astoundingly so. And thus it was with MA.19.

The final outcome of the trial proved everyone dead wrong! Despite having no effect to improve the ability of doxorubicin to shrink tumors, or increase the short-term "time to progression", an additional year and a half of followup since the study was stopped revealed that, compared to doxorubicin alone, the DPPE/doxo-rubicin combination increased overall survival by an amazing fifty percent. *It was just like those lab mice ten years earlier!* No matter how the data were analyzed (and they *were* analyzed…and analyzed….and analyzed….) the statistical significance remained. The Clinical Trials Group, spearheaded by Len Reyno, announced that the surprising findings would be presented at the upcoming ASCO meeting.

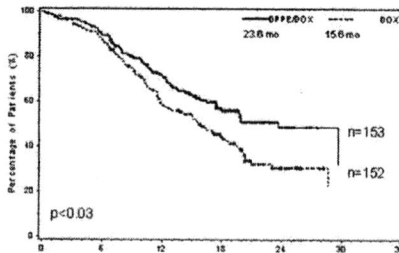

Figure 3: The median survival of 23.6 months in 153 women who received DPPE plus doxorubicin (top line) was 50% longer than the median survival of 15.6 months in 152 women who received doxorubicin alone (bottom line).

"It's a shame you weren't there to hear the reaction,"[119] David commented after giving me the astounding news. "People were really scratching their heads. There was a lot of speculation about how this could have occurred. They asked from the podium if you were in the room, hoping you could provide some insight."

"I would have, had I even remotely known about the findings," I replied grumpily. I realized it wasn't David's fault that I hadn't been contacted. He himself had only found out at the meeting. Nonetheless, salt had been rubbed in my wounds.

What I still find hard to believe all these years later, is that no one bothered to call me with a "heads-up". There is such a thing

---

119 David told me that when Lesley Seymour presented what Kathy Pritchard had dubbed the "Holy s—-!" slide, showing the improved sur-vival curve in the patients who were treated with DPPE and doxorubicin, a buzz filled the room. People were genuinely shocked by the result.

as common courtesy. What would it have taken for someone to pick up the phone, even at the last minute, to inform me of what had been found, thereby giving me a reason to be present for the surprising announcement? Several other suspects had now joined Renzo Canetta on my list of those who needed to enroll in an etiquette course.[120]

After David left, I closed the door of my office and sat quietly, gazing at the screen saver fluttering across my computer monitor. Truth be told, I had no idea why the survival had been so much greater in the group of women receiving DPPE. I was totally numb, afraid to believe what I had just heard. Maybe it was a fluke. Who could say? I thought I had buried the drug forever. Now it was back with a vengeance. The calmness in my life was shattered. The weight of DPPE was once more descending onto my shoulders.

My thoughts, or lack of same, were suddenly interrupted by the ringing of my phone. The Canadian Broadcasting Corporation was calling to ask whether I would do an interview for a popular country-wide evening radio news magazine called *As It Happens*. Apparently, a medical reporter had attended the NCIC meeting and tipped off the CBC news desk. "Tell them the answer is 'No,'" I instructed my secretary. It may have been all about my drug, but it was up to the NCIC Clinical Trials Group to tell the story. They, and those directly involved with the trial, including Bristol-Myers, should do the interview. Let them explain why the study had been stopped and what they were planning to do now that the survival data showed a benefit for DPPE.[121]

---

120 Over dinner at a restaurant in Winnipeg some years later, I took Kathy to task for not calling me ahead of time with the findings. Typical of her honesty and directness, she promptly apologized, saying that she was remiss in not doing so and was very sorry. I accepted her apology on the spot.

121 Contacted by a reporter with the *Globe and Mail*, an official in Bristol-Myers' Montréal office said that the survival increase was "great news", but denied that the company had anything to do with stopping the trial. Kathy Pritchard disagreed, telling me that Bristol-Myers was definitely behind the decision.

One thing was certain. I had to inform YM BioSciences about this stunning bit of news. I placed a call to Dr. Niclas Stiernholm, recently hired by David Allan to manage the company's scientific affairs. Nic, originally from Sweden, was a very bright young PhD with a background in laboratory research. David Harper had brought him to meet me over dinner in Winnipeg shortly after he had joined the company. We took an instant liking to one another, helped by the fact that Nic proved good fodder for my humorous asides.

"Nic, you'd better be prepared for what I'm about to tell you," I warned. After assuring me that he was all ears, I recounted everything that David Bowman had told me and then informed him that the national news media already had the story. Nic had not expected anything like that. Stunned, he remained silent for several seconds. "Wow. This changes absolutely everything for us," he finally said, his voice almost a whisper. We quickly agreed that he would inform the others, including medical director, Dr. Paul Keane, a pathologist and former professor at the University of Calgary and, later, McMaster. Before joining YM, Paul had directed clinical research at Miles Pharmaceuticals, now Bayer Canada. I would contact Kathy Pritchard, request a copy of the trial data that were presented at the meeting, and forward the findings to Nic and his colleagues.

The ball was now firmly in YM BioScience's court. As Paul Keane later confided to me, they all met around the corporate table after my call to Nic. "I don't know if any of you really understand the magnitude of this news. I mean to the company itself. If we don't handle this properly, YM might not survive," Paul wisely told his colleagues.[122] At that moment, the decision was made to proceed cautiously. Dr. Mark Vincent, the company's medical oncology advisor, would be brought in to spearhead a forensic analysis of the results, aided by statistician Judy McDougall of

---

122 A few years later, at a dinner he gave at his house, David Allan told me of his reaction to the news. "What the [expletive] do we do now?" he asked his staff as he threw his arms up into the air.

the University of Toronto, and a U.K. firm, Hesperion.[123]. Mark, a graduate of the University of Cape Town and, like me, an alumnus of London's Royal Marsden Hospital, was now affiliated with my alma mater, the University of Western Ontario. He had a cancer expert's grasp of the issues as well as a good knowledge of statistics.

Over dinner that night, Jill and I listened to the radio as Len Reyno and NCIC Clinical Trials Group director, Joe Pater, were interviewed on *As it Happens*. Len told the audience that he felt very strongly about giving DPPE a second chance in a new trial. The survival advantage was of great potential importance, but needed to be verified in a new phase three study. I nodded my agreement to Jill. Joe Pater then threw cold water on my growing hopes that the NCIC would mount such a study by saying that any new trial would have to be carried out by another clinical trials group. The NCIC would not do it. When asked, "Why?" by the interviewer, he suggested that if a second NCIC study again showed a positive outcome, it would not have as much credibility as a positive confirmatory study carried out by a totally different group.

If ever I heard a lame excuse, this was it. While he probably didn't intend it, Pater actually seemed to cast doubt on the credibility of his own organization. *The widely-respected NCIC wouldn't*

---

123 People involved with clinical trials generally believe that statistical analysis can only be justified on a pre-planned basis, requiring the entry of enough patients to allow clearly-defined, predetermined statistical comparisons. On the other hand, they argue that "after the fact" analysis is to be avoided. The term "data dredging" refers to post-hoc analysis of various subgroups of patients in a negative trial in an attempt to find something "positive" in the study. Nobody usually pays attention to the results of this type of exercise. However, as it turned out, MA.19 was a *positive* study with respect to survival. In that case, the statistical analysis was performed to see whether the survival benefit applied to all women or only certain groups. One prominent statistician has stated that not only is "subgroup analysis" justified, but imperative in positive-outcome trials like ours. The findings can then be used to generate hypotheses that can be tested in the next clinical study. As will become apparent, that is exactly what happened with DPPE.

be believed if it found the same increase in survival in a new trial? His response was both ingenuous and complete balderdash. My belief was that, unlike Elizabeth Eisenhauer, Joe Pater had never been a great supporter of me or DPPE and was now taking the opportunity to punt.

Avis Favaro, CTV's senior medical reporter, put together her own report on the MA.19 trial for the network's national newscast two weeks later. By that time, Len Reyno was less certain about DPPE's future.

Lloyd Robertson (anchor): "In medical news tonight, a promising new Canadian-made weapon in the battle against breast cancer, and a compelling story of persistence. The drug is called DPPE and [new] results showed it helped women with advanced breast cancer live up to fifty percent longer than patients on standard treatment. Yet, despite these impressive findings, DPPE was almost derailed in early testing. CTV's medical specialist, Avis Favaro, tells us why in this exclusive story."

Avis Favaro: "It's called DPPE, a Canadian-developed anticancer drug with an interesting story...a story with a question mark."

Dr. Leonard Reyno: "I cannot speak to exactly what will happen to this drug."

Favaro [voice-over]: "Dr. Leonard Reyno has given DPPE to women with advanced breast cancer, hoping that the compound makes standard chemotherapy even more powerful. Halfway through the study, researchers measured what they usually look for. Did DPPE slow or stop the cancer's growth? To their dismay, it did not."

Reyno: "In fact, it did not appear to have any difference in response rate or progression-free survival."

Favaro: "The results worried one of the drug's key developers."

Dr. Lorne Brandes: "I was very concerned when the trial did not show any difference in the early endpoints. In fact, the pharmaceutical manufacturer that supported [DPPE], dropped us within twenty-four hours."

Favaro [voice-over]: "Bristol-Myers Squibb dropped the drug and so ended the study. But Dr. Reyno decided to follow the patients for another two years to see what happened. The results were a surprise. Breast cancer patients on standard chemotherapy lived on average fifteen months. Those who had also taken DPPE lived just over twenty-three months. The drug may not have had an effect early on, but in the end it bought patients nearly a year more of life."

Reyno: "And that difference is of a size that's big enough to warrant further investigation and thought."

Favaro: "But DPPE is now a pharmaceutical orphan. Who, if anyone, will sponsor it? And should we consider changing how studies are funded to avoid drugs being abandoned?"

Pat Kelly (patient advocate): "Clinical trial reform would be about ensuring that there's sufficient investment from public money so that we don't have clinical trials which are only driven by pharmaceutical interests."

Brandes: "The real downside to the story is that drug development has really been derailed for almost two years because of what happened."

Favaro: "The moral of this story? Never judge an experimental drug too quickly. Even a long shot can surprise researchers and possibly win cancer patients the gift of time."

A few days after the CTV report aired, I received a late-night call from David Lebwohl. He had just heard Len present the MA.19 survival data at ASCO and was calling on his cell phone to congratulate me. "You must feel vindicated," he offered. My response was decidedly guarded. "David, why are you *really* calling me?" I asked, thinking that he might be doing Renzo's bidding to determine the chance of Bristol-Myers getting back in the door. "I really just wanted to say that I'm happy for you, that's all," he replied. I thanked him. As it turned out, David really was talking for himself. Subsequently, the company whose television commercials[124] feature its commitment to finding new drug treatments for cancer, showed not the slightest interest in reacquiring DPPE.[125]

---

124 In addition to now-disgraced perennial Tour de France winner, Lance Armstrong, the other "star" of those Bristol-Myers commercials was none other than Renzo Canetta, shown in a white coat doing "research" at the laboratory bench.

125 Bristol-Myers soon had other things on its mind, with little resources left to reconsider DPPE. The company had recently coughed up *two billion* dollars to license a high-tech "targeted therapy" drug called Erbitux from a company called ImClone that had developed it. However, the deal ended up causing the Bristol-Myers massive corporate heartburn and a huge loss of market capital when its shares plummeted following a financial scandal of international proportion. The saga was highlighted by the incarceration of ImClone CEO, Sam Wachsal, for insider trading, and celebrity, Martha Stewart, for obstruction of justice. Both dumped shares of Imclone prior to an FDA decision against approving the drug because of deficiencies in clinical trial data involving patients with colon cancer. With its champion, Wachsal, behind bars, Erbitux was ultimately successful for ImClone and Bristol-Myers, and is now licensed to treat advanced colon cancer. This was the ultimate example of selling a stock too soon!!!

CHAPTER SIXTY-ONE:

Not A Fluke

Two months into his analysis of the MA.19 trial results, Mark Vincent called to discuss the early findings. An important distinction had emerged. The drug did *not* improve survival in everyone. Rather, when added to doxorubicin, it caused women to live longer in two specific instances: when the cancer recurred within three years of the original diagnosis; and where the pathologist, performing a widely-used test, had identified that the tumor was not driven by estrogen, so-called "estrogen receptor (ER)-negative" breast cancer.

"In some way, DPPE appears to make ER-negative tumors act as though they were ER-positive," Mark observed. By this, he meant that adding DPPE to doxorubicin increased the survival of women with non-estrogen-driven cancer so that they lived as long as women with better prognosis ER-positive tumors.

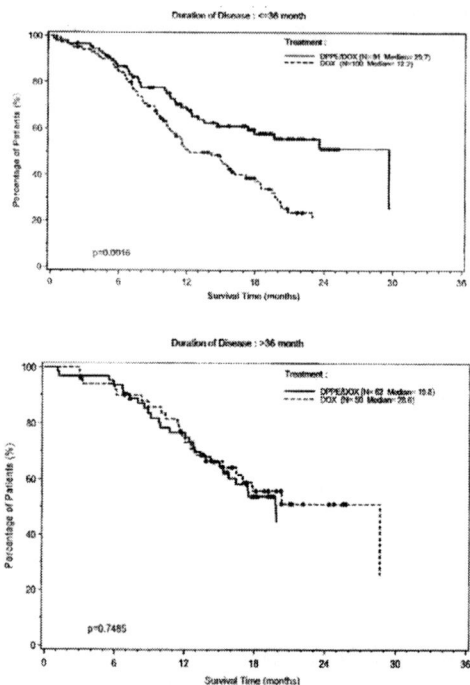

Figure 4: *The subgroup analysis of MA.19 revealed that, compared to doxorubicin alone, DPPE plus doxorubicin increased survival in women with aggressive breast cancer that recurred within 3 years of the original diagnosis and treatment (top graph), but not in those with less-aggressive breast cancer that recurred after 3 or more years (bottom graph).*

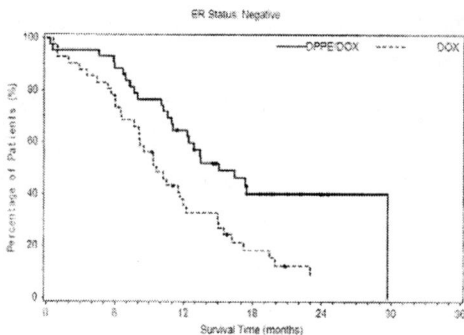

Figure 5: *As compared to doxorubicin alone (bottom curve), DPPE plus doxorubicin (top curve) increased the survival of women whose breast cancer was not driven by estrogen (ER-negative).*

Suddenly a light went on in my head. These findings were no fluke!
"I think I can explain the results in MA.19," I told my colleague.
"How so?" he asked.

"I believe that what we are observing is the ability of DPPE to improve survival in women with aggressive, rapidly-growing tumors.[126] But it only helps doxorubicin kill the fastest-growing cells, not the less malignant, slower-growing ones."

Having gained Mark's full attention, I then recounted my clinical experience in patients with inflammatory breast cancer, where adding DPPE to epirubicin and Taxol before surgery selectively took out the "high-grade" cancer cell populations when the tumor was examined under the microscope. The selective destruction of more aggressive cells would be predicted to influence the natural history of the disease (e.g. survival) but not necessarily to shrink tumors significantly.

"For example, let's assume that a patient's cancer consists mainly of high-grade, aggressive cells," I continued. "In that case, my hypothesis would predict that DPPE plus doxorubicin would have a powerful effect, both to shrink the cancer and significantly increase survival.

"In contrast, let's assume that a patient's cancer consists mainly of low- or average-grade cells, with only a minority (say, twenty percent) of high-grade, aggressive cells. Since only the high-grade tumor cells (in this example, twenty percent of the total number of cells) would be eliminated, the treatment would not shrink the cancer enough to qualify as a 'response'.[127] Nonetheless, with the aggressive cells elimi-

---

126 It is widely agreed that the time between diagnosis of cancer and recurrence [disease-free interval (DFI)] is a good surrogate of aggressiveness. Women whose breast cancer recurs within three years generally have more aggressive tumors than women with a longer DFI. A similar correlation has been shown in women whose breast cancer is not estrogen-driven (i.e., who have estrogen receptor-negative tumors).

127 The rules say that a tumor must shrink by at least 50% to be considered significantly smaller. In the second example I gave Mark, the tumor would shrink significantly less than that. Yet the nature of the cancer would have been altered by the treatment to make it slower growing and less aggressive, i.e., a qualitative rather than quantitative change.

nated, the cancer would now consist of lower-grade cells that grow more slowly, so once again the patient would live longer."

Yet why did the addition of DPPE to doxorubicin not increase the earlier "time to progression" endpoint? If, as I believed, the aggressive cells were being killed off, the cancer should have started to slow down early, increasing the time to progression. "Apparently that did not happen," I observed.

"That's not totally correct," Mark replied. In fact, the statisticians found that the "time to progression" curves started to diverge in favor of DPPE/doxorubicin much later than usual, at about seven months after treatment started. At exactly the same time, the DPPE/ doxorubicin survival curve started to exceed the doxorubicin survival curve. *Incredible!!!*

Something out of the ordinary was going on. Although further statistical analysis would be needed, Mark believed that the findings supported my hypothesis. In a subsequent report to YM, he wrote, "….I believe now much more strongly that DPPE is responsible for the major portion of the survival difference…Dr. Brandes believes DPPE acts by eliminating the more aggressive clones; this is consistent with the fact that only patients with more aggressive disease seem to be helped by DPPE….The likelihood is that [DPPE] is doing something during the period of co-administration of doxorubicin, perhaps assisting the latter in killing the more aggressive types of cancer cell[s]."

No matter how it happened, DPPE appeared to increase the ability of doxorubicin to improve survival in patients with the most malignant forms of advanced breast cancer. Since this included women whose tumors were *not* estrogen-driven, one thing was clear: as predicted from our binding experiments all those years ago, DPPE was not working like tamoxifen!

CHAPTER SIXTY-TWO:

Outside The Box

Somebody once said, "Build a better mousetrap and the world will beat a path to your door." YM's CEO, David Allan, now believed that the drug he had acquired only a few months previously could be the best cancer-fighting mousetrap ever invented. Forget what had happened previously with MA.19 and Bristol-Myers. What drug company wouldn't want to get their hands on DPPE now? As it turned out, none....at least not immediately.

It wasn't that there was a lack of interest. The problem was that DPPE did not fit into a neat little box. First of all, it was an "add-on" drug with a reputation for some "weird" side effects but no apparent antitumor activity of its own. Therefore, from a drug company perspective, DPPE had some problematical toxicity on the one hand and efficacy that had to be linked to a chemotherapy drug on the other. Secondly, how could a drug that didn't increase the ability of doxorubicin to shrink tumors or increase the time to progression, end up increasing survival? It was counterintuitive. How could one occur without the other?

What drove me, and YM, nuts was that the "accepted" paradigm for chemotherapy drugs was equally counterintuitive. Despite putting the brakes on tumor growth, the vast majority of such drugs, including doxorubicin and Taxol, did not significantly increase survival in metastatic breast cancer trials. Why was that? Shouldn't one lead to the other?[128] Nonetheless, new drugs that were "active" to improve the early endpoints, but did not increase survival, continued to attract the interest of drug companies and to win regulatory approval. *Here we had DPPE, a drug that accomplished exactly the reverse, and no one was willing to buy in.*

Not accustomed to inaction, David Allan announced to his YM colleagues that, drug company or no drug company, he intended to go for broke and ask the FDA to approve DPPE on the basis of the increased survival in MA.19. David Harper and Paul Keane, who had experience with drug regulators, were alarmed by this approach, fearing that it might backfire and create a bad karma for the company. "Maybe you can talk some sense into him," an exasperated Harper suggested to me during a phone call. Although I had very little to do with his boss, a sixtyish businessman blessed with youthful good looks, I knew from Nic and the others that once Allan made up his mind about something, it was very difficult for anyone to get him to change his opinion.

"I'll speak with him," I answered, undaunted. My own encounters with the regulatory world had recently widened from developing DPPE to carrying out external reviews for Agnes Klein and her colleagues at Health Canada. I had come to know first hand the volumes and volumes of clinical trial documentation required for successful oncology drug submissions. While no one wanted to see DPPE approved more than me, I knew intuitively that the

---

128 One explanation is that clinical trials usually allow patients who progress on a treatment to "cross over" to the other arm of the study, and/or to receive additional therapies after they go off the trial. As a result, any survival benefit of a drug in a clinical trial may be hard to measure as a result of the confounding effects of crossovers and subsequent treatment(s).

response to Allan's request would be negative. Given the upside-down findings in MA.19, the FDA would do nothing without confirmation in a second trial. While there was nothing wrong *per se* with asking the question, I and the others believed that the best way to move DPPE forward with the FDA was to establish credibility with them. That would *not* include a request for immediate regulatory approval of DPPE based on the outcome of a single, prematurely-ended trial that had failed to meet its primary targets. Why risk a "Rejected" stamp on your file that could bias future consideration?

Unfortunately, when I called to put my views to him, Mr. Allan was less than happy with my intrusion into his affairs. He made it clear that he ran the company and, my opinion notwithstanding, would proceed with his plan. A heated exchange followed. It was not the finest moment for either of us. However, a few weeks after the dust settled, Allan decided to adopt the more prudent approach. YM would submit its dossier to the FDA along with a series of written questions as to what would be required for DPPE to win regulatory approval from the agency. A collective sigh of relief followed his decision.

While all of this was going on, David Harper continued to flip his Rolodex, calling or e-mailing each and every licensing director in the pharmaceutical world. Over the next months, many "sweet nothin's" were exchanged. Finally, he made headway with someone called Hooshmand Sheshberadaran. The owner of that tongue-twister of a name was the oncology licensing director of New Jersey-headquartered Pharmacia.

As with most drug companies, Pharmacia's pedigree was complex. Although it began in Sweden as Pharmacia Aktibolaget in 1911, its modern-day iteration began with the 1951 merger with Milan's Farmitalia Carlo Erba, developer of both doxorubicin and epirubicin. In 1995, Pharmacia merged with Upjohn (originally founded in 1886 in Kalamazoo, MI as the Upjohn Pill and Granule Company); the combined company, known as Pharmacia and Upjohn, had the ignominious New York Stock Exchange symbol,

PU. In 2000, the Upjohn part of the name was dropped in favor of Pharmacia and a less odorous stock symbol, PHA.

After sending Hooshmand the dossier on DPPE, a meeting was set up between YM and Pharmacia. Paul Keane and David Harper flew to the company's corporate head office in Peapack, New Jersey, where they made a formal presentation on the results of MA.19 to Oncology VP, Dr. Langdon Miller, his colleague Dr. Franzanne Vreeland and various representatives of the marketing and finance departments. There was some additional good news to report at that meeting. In response to YM's submitted questions, the FDA ruled that, even though MA.19 had been prematurely stopped, it was acceptable because of the significant survival advantage. Only one more phase three study would be required; if again positive, a New Drug Application (NDA) could be filed.[129] Good news, indeed!

Although the reception to their presentation seemed positive, weeks went by without a response. Finally, Hooshmand called to say that, while the clinicians were very supportive, the bean counters in marketing and finance were concerned that doxorubicin was "losing market share", and epirubicin was soon to come off patent. Therefore, the prospects for DPPE as a money-maker were diminished. They would have to pass on the opportunity.

When Nic called me to explain the reason for the turndown, I became furious. "What do a bunch of people in marketing and finance know about the treatment of breast cancer?" I sputtered. "They're just plain nuts when they say that doxorubicin or epirubicin won't continue to be important drugs in fighting this disease. Do they know that DPPE can be combined with other drugs,

---

129 Two positive phase three studies are normally required for drug approval. Therefore, only one more phase three study, with survival as the primary endpoint, would be needed. Filing an NDA (New Drug Application) is the final step along the regulatory road to approval. ODAC (the Oncology Drug Advisory Committee) then reviews the data and advises the FDA on whether to accept or reject the application. Although not obligated to do so, the FDA usually follows the advice of ODAC.

including taxanes? They obviously don't understand anything about this whole concept. Why don't they talk to someone who works in the trenches every day, like me? I'll straighten them out in a hurry!" I was getting more steamed by the minute. Once again, it seemed to me that the primary issue for the drug company was profits, with patient welfare taking a back seat. Worse, the equation they had used to arrive at their so-called "business decision" was all wet. I could only shake my head in disgust.

Nic agreed, sharing my disappointment. As luck would have it, he was soon off to Tucson to meet with the head of the Arizona Cancer Center, Dr. Daniel von Hoff, a member of YM's scientific advisory committee. During their discussions, the Pharmacia affair came up. "Langdon Miller was a student of mine. I'll call him," von Hoff announced to a startled Nic. Not long after, Hooshmand was back on the line to David Harper. The company wanted one more kick at the can. This time they wanted to talk with me. *Well, well, well!*

A conference call was set up for the afternoon of February 21, 2002. As David Harper was on business in Singapore, Nic filled in for him. While I sat in my warm office waiting for the others to come on the line, poor Nic joined in from a cold phone booth outside the Waldorf Astoria in New York.[130] Langdon Miller was running late, but expected shortly. Perhaps as a result of his absence, the other Pharmacia officials seemed to lack direction and started off with such vague and simplistic questions about DPPE that alarm bells went off in my head. *Did these people read any of the scores of reprints of my lab and clinical papers they were sent by David Harper?*

Finally, Langdon came on the line and offered his apology. Just as he did, his oncologist colleague, Franzanne Vreeland, launched into her very negative assessment of the hallucinations, nausea

---

130 "Why did you spend two hours in a freezing phone booth rather than make the conference call from the hotel?" I asked Nic a few years later. "To save fifteen dollars a minute," he replied. I forgot how expensive it is to make long distance calls from a New York hotel room.

and vomiting associated with DPPE. I countered that the so-called hallucinations were pleasant, transitory and usually enjoyed by the patients; they did not cause any problems in the clinical trials. "If the drug fails in cancer therapy, it might do well on the street," I suggested. Laughter followed, but not from Franzanne. Then, after reviewing the successful protocol modifications that had been made to prevent, or markedly reduce, nausea and vomiting, I took the offensive: "Look. We are treating women with very serious metastatic disease, here. Taking the worst case scenario, a small excess in nausea or vomiting is rather a small price to pay for the increase in survival that was found in MA.19." *No response from Franzanne.*

One of the marketing people then spoke up. "Dr. Brandes, we have a problem in that nobody here seems to have any idea how DPPE works." *Yes, I've already figured that out for myself.*

"Perhaps you should be more focused on *that* it works, rather than *how* it works," I replied testily. At this point, feeling I had nothing to lose, I continued my aggressive stance. "Why can't everyone just be excited about a drug that, for the first time, appears to markedly increase survival in women with metastatic breast cancer? That's certainly the name of the game for the patients I treat."

"We understand and respect your position. We are also intrigued by DPPE. That's why we are having this call," the marketing manager replied. "It's just that for us to determine what new drugs to develop, we need to have some rationale on which to base our decision. We don't have that for DPPE."

"As an oncologist, and the only person on this conference call who battles this disease every day in the clinic, I can tell you that the mechanism of action of many of the approved chemotherapy drugs we use is poorly or incompletely understood," I quickly retorted. "That doesn't keep us from using them. Moreover, I have yet to have a cancer patient refuse treatment with DPPE because its mechanism of action is not well understood." *Touché.*

I don't know why, but as I was answering his question, I clicked my mouse to bring up the CNBC financial website, looking for any news from Pharmacia. Scrolling down the computer screen, my eyes opened wide as I came upon the previous day's announcement from the company. I couldn't believe my good fortune. The gods were smiling on me.

"Now here's something relevant to our discussion," I added. "It appears that yesterday, Pharmacia dropped a late-stage, high-tech 'anti-angiogenesis' drug that failed in a phase three cancer trial. Obviously its mechanism of action was well-understood and yet, despite high expectations for success, it didn't work. Now here we have a fifty percent increase in survival in a phase three trial with DPPE, a low-tech, small-molecule drug whose mechanism is debatable from your point of view. Which would you rather have? A drug that works according to a well-defined mechanism but flops, or a drug whose mechanism may be open to question but succeeds?"[131] That comment stopped him in his tracks. *Did I hear some nervous laughter?*

Perhaps my "from-the-lip" remarks shook things up. Suddenly the tone of the discussion turned more positive and upbeat as Langdon Miller finally engaged in the conversation and the marketing people retreated into the woodwork. "I want to assure you that, from my perspective, we are very excited about the clinical potential of DPPE," he stated. For the next hour, the conversation centered on how, together, we could move the drug forward.

By the end of the conference, I felt much better about our chances, but still wondered whether much of the information we

---

131   In a subsequent e-mail summary of the conference call, Nic wrote as follows: "Brandes and I hook up on a mega-teleconference call with eight people from Pharmacia.... Brandes tells Pharmacia that they have crap for products and reminds them that they just failed in a phase III trial! He also points out that it's easy for them to sit in an office and make decisions when it is people like him who actually fight in the trenches where people are dying every day. He also answered their questions for two hours!"

had supplied to Hooshmand had been read. Then again, was it possible that he had not been given a full dossier?

Concerned, I e-mailed David Allan: "As you know, Nic and I had a conference call today with various representatives of Pharmacia. Although it went reasonably well, based on the questions that were asked it quickly became evident to me that much of the basic information, including previously-published clinical studies and the prostate cancer data, appeared to be largely or completely unfamiliar to these people. Were all the data supplied to Pharmacia in the YMB package?" I soon heard back from him, telling me he assumed so, but didn't know for sure and would investigate the matter. He ended his reply with, "I gather from Nic that you did an excellent job under the circumstances." *Some job! Some circumstances!*

A few days later, I received a call from an annoyed David Harper. *Of course he had sent them absolutely everything!!* It was obvious from the tone of his voice that his boss had grilled him vigorously about the issue. The two were like oil and water at the best of times, and Harper's blood pressure often suffered accordingly. "You know, Lorne, you can lead a drug company to water, but you can't make it drink," he said in exasperation.

The more I thought about it afterwards, the more I believed that David had done his job and was sorry that I had cast doubt on his thoroughness. *Sure. Why spend a lot of time reading all the informative documentation you are sent when you can be spoon-fed the answers in a conference call?* Was that how important decisions were made by drug companies? I hoped not, but past events led me to be cynical.

C H A P T E R   S I X T Y - T H R E E :

Tod Und Verklärung

The verdict came quickly. We had prevailed with help from Kathy Pritchard who, in a separate conference call, had been very supportive. Pharmacia was now definitely interested in DPPE. However, prior to making any final decision, the company needed to carry out its due diligence. I happily e-mailed the following message to Brent, Janet and the others: "I received word today from Dr. Niclas Stiernholm of YM BioSciences that DPPE passed an important hurdle at Pharmacia, who have decided at their Licensing Review Committee meeting to take DPPE to the next level. This will take the form of their regulatory people meeting with YMB.....The decision to proceed followed conference calls over the last month with me, with Dr. Kathy Pritchard (Toronto, who was involved with the NCIC MA.19 trial), Dr. Derek Raghavan (USC, who is involved with the prostate studies) and with Dr. Daniel van Hoff...."

As part of the decision-making process, Pharmacia performed its own statistical analysis of MA.19, while asking Janet McDougall to look at survival patterns in additional subgroups of patients.

Every morsel of information pertaining to how, when and why, DPPE increased survival would be examined under the Pharmacia microscope. In addition to Mark Vincent's original findings, this methodical fishing expedition provided some potentially stunning information.

Revelation number one: the McDougall analysts estimated that approximately two-thirds of the three hundred women in the trial had the more aggressive type of breast cancer, based on the identification of patients whose tumors came back or spread within three years of initial diagnosis and treatment, and/or whose tumors were not estrogen-driven. The remaining one hundred women had slower-growing, less aggressive tumors that are often active over many years and usually estrogen-driven.

When these two groups were compared, the increase in survival in women with aggressive breast cancer who received DPPE was not fifty percent, but a mind-boggling *one hundred and forty-three percent!* Put another way, whereas the average woman with aggressive cancer lived for about one year after receiving doxorubicin alone, she lived almost one and one-half years *beyond that* after receiving DPPE with doxorubicin. On the other hand, not only did women with slower-growing tumors *not* derive any benefit from DPPE, there appeared to be a trend towards decreased survival, and an increased risk of what is called "progression on treatment".[132]

Here was the progression breakdown: in the group with slow-growing cancer, four women who received doxorubicin alone had to have the drug stopped because tumor growth increased significantly on the treatment. However, *over four times that number* (seventeen women) receiving DPPE and doxorubicin had to be taken off treatment for the same reason! In contrast, in the

---

132 Progression on treatment means that the tumor grows by more than twenty-five percent on measurement, or new tumors are detected. In both instances, the patient is deemed to have progressed on that particular therapy and it is stopped. Alternative drugs or other treatments may then be considered.

group with aggressive breast cancer that had a survival benefit with DPPE, eighteen women on doxorubicin alone had progression on treatment; that number *dropped* by one-third, to twelve, in women who received DPPE and doxorubicin.[133]

Because the total number of patients who progressed on treatment was relatively small, no statistics were applied. However, seventeen to four in the group with slow-growing tumors, a lopsided score by any measure, seemed to fit the known facts: as compared to aggressive, more rapidly-growing cancers, slower-growing cancers are the ones that tend to be innately less sensitive to the DNA-damaging effects of chemotherapy. *Just as the mice and rats had predicted, and as I had warned my patients early on, there now appeared to be evidence in the MA.19 study that DPPE had the potential to stimulate cancer growth when tumors were not sensitive to doxorubicin!* If we were lucky enough to get a second shot at a clinical trial, women like my mother, with slower-growing breast cancer, would be excluded.

These findings also rekindled my longstanding concerns about antidepressants and antihistamines. I now believed more than ever that our previous reports, dismissed by the FDA as "creating a stir where a stir should not have been created", were indeed valid. After all, had we not conducted that research based on my initial concerning observations in those depressed patients with cancer, and with the knowledge that chemically-similar DPPE stimulated tumor growth in rodents?

Revelation number two: the McDougall group also discovered that better survival with DPPE and doxorubicin in women with aggressive cancer depended on the number of treatments the patients received. Up to seven could be given in the study. That

---

133 As compared to slower-growing tumors, aggressive cancers would be expected to progress more often on treatment, correlating with the higher overall number of treatment progressions in the latter group (thirty in total: eighteen on doxorubicin vs. twelve on DPPE/doxorubicin) than in the former (twenty-one in total: four on doxorubicin vs. seventeen on DPPE/doxorubicin).

maximum number was mainly governed by the risk of doxorubicin damaging the heart if the dose went any higher. However, there were two other major considerations that determined whether or not patients received the full seven treatments of doxorubicin alone, or doxorubicin plus DPPE. The first was whether their tumors were shrinking or, at least, stable, on treatment; if either applied, treatments could carry on to the maximum of seven. The second was side effects; as long as the treatment did not cause unacceptable toxicity, the full seven cycles of treatment could be given.

Here was the grabber: a survival benefit for DPPE occurred *regardless* of whether tumors shrunk or were merely stable, *but only if patients received more than four cycles of treatment.* My first thought was that the finding was a red herring. Then I remembered Mark Vincent pointing out that adding DPPE to doxorubicin actually *did* result in a delayed trend, after six or seven months, to increase the early "time to progression" endpoint. Now I realized that this observation correlated with the time it took for patients to receive more than four treatments. It also coincided with the point at which the more important survival curves then started to diverge, strongly and significantly, in favor of the patients who had received DPPE with doxorubicin!

What was the explanation for all of this? Suddenly, the ability of DPPE to overcome so-called "multiple-drug resistance (MDR+)" came roaring back to life. Whether it inhibited over-active P-gp pumps (as suggested by the Bristol-Myers experiments), or worked by some other novel mechanism (according to Rob Warrington's experiments), it was likely that DPPE targeted emerging MDR+ cancer cells. Although some particularly ugly cancer cells can be resistant to chemotherapy drugs from the very start, the weight of laboratory evidence and clinical experience suggests that drug resistance almost always develops after several cycles of chemotherapy have been given. Invariably, that is why drugs almost never cure most types of metastasized adult cancer.

So here was my hypothesis: for the first few treatment cycles, when the number of resistant cells was likely to be relatively low, doxorubicin alone, or doxorubicin plus DPPE, would be equally effective to kill breast cancer cells. This meant that no difference in the two treatments would be seen during that time. However, bit by bit, doxorubicin would be predicted to lose steam as sensitive cells were killed off, leaving more aggressive, drug-resistant cells to emerge with each subsequent treatment....*that is, unless DPPE was also given to prevent them from escaping its clutches.* With DPPE on board, and resistance tamed, doxorubicin could continue to effectively kill cancer cells in later treatments. This would result in a positive impact on survival that would become increasingly apparent with time. Now the late-breaking improvement in "time to progression", accompanied by a significant separation of the survival curves in the group of patients that received the two drugs together, was starting to make sense.

The more I studied the data, the less I could contain my enthusiasm. For the next two weeks, anyone unlucky enough to pass my open office door was pulled in for a look at the various graphs generated by the latest McDougall analysis. Others, who by good fortune escaped the initial snare, were accosted in the hallway and subjected to a verbal précis of the new findings. My spirits were lifted when both Lyonel and Frank agreed that the findings looked real and that my hypothesis might go some distance in explaining them. "So what are they waiting for?" asked Frank in his usual no-nonsense way, referring to a new clinical trial.

"It should happen very soon if Pharmacia signs a licensing agreement," I replied hopefully to my colleague.

If there was one person I absolutely had to call about this new development, it was Georgie Hogg. When things fell apart with Bristol-Myers, my calls to Georgie diminished for some time. "After all, what is there to say?" I would ask myself, trying to justify the fact that I had not kept in touch with her as a good friend should. Now that things were looking up, who more than Georgie deserved to know why? I dialed her number.

"Hi Georgie. It's Lorne," I proclaimed enthusiastically when she picked up the phone.

"Who?" *Her hearing must be going. Well, what do you expect? She is almost eighty-five.*

"It's Lorne, Georgie," I said more emphatically.

"Yes?" Silence. *Oh, oh!* Choosing to ignore the warning signal, I started to tell her the exciting news. However, after a few minutes went by with no response from Georgie, I stopped short.

"So what do you think about what I'm telling you?" I asked.

More silence, then, finally, "Uh, huh." *Georgie didn't know who I was or what I was talking about.* I was devastated, all the more so because I immediately felt great pangs of guilt that I had been remiss in not calling her all along the way.

"It's been downhill quite a bit lately," Colin Merry confirmed the next day when I visited him in his hematology lab office to tell him about the call. Ever the good samaritan, Colin had continued to keep a close eye on Georgie. She had apparently suffered a recent series of small strokes, little by little erasing her memory. Mercifully, she slipped quietly away two months later. In a eulogy at the funeral, her niece observed that Georgie was physically small but cast a giant shadow over the landscape. Everyone nodded. *That, she did.*

Our long years of friendship aside, without her enthusiastic support and brilliant expertise in pathology, I could not have obtained the rodent toxicology data needed to bring DPPE into the clinic. Georgie had singularly helped to make that possible, no doubt about it.

Listening to the oration, I smiled through my sorrow as I saw her, clear as day, sitting at the dining room table in her little apartment, peering through the microscope, frequently stopping to dab her tearing eyes with a Kleenex. *She was a giant all right.* In life, she helped give birth to DPPE. Sadly, her illness and demise prevented her from learning of its amazing transfiguration[134] from "dead drug" into a potential blockbuster treatment for patients with the most malignant of tumors.

---

134 The word is used here in its non-biblical sense to mean "metamorphosis". The German "tod und verklärung" means "death and transfiguration". In choosing it as the title of this chapter, I was inspired by Richard Strauss' epic tone poem of the same name (the 1981 Philips recording by Bernard Haitink and the Concertgebouw Orchestra, Amsterdam, is strongly recommended).

CHAPTER SIXTY-FOUR:

The Salivating Statistician

Finally....finally...in late June, Hooshmand contacted David Harper. Pharmacia had completed its due diligence. Having apparently found everything in order during their visit to YM, they wanted to proceed.[135] It was time to talk business. The company was also very interested in my clinical data combining DPPE, epirubicin and Taxol in women with metastatic breast cancer and wanted me to present my findings in person to Langdon Miller and his oncology group.

Paul Keane, David and I converged at Toronto's Lester B. Pearson International Airport for the early morning flight to Newark. Paul and I had not met previously, although I knew from our many phone discussions that he was quite erudite and gentlemanly in the English tradition. He also had a very personal interest in seeing DPPE succeed; his first wife had died of breast cancer. In his late sixties, and slightly short in stature, he carried

---

135   One of the visitors to YM from Pharmacia was Hooshmand's boss, John McBride....the same John McBride who had been with Sparta and visited Winnipeg with Bill McCulloch.

himself like a much younger man. His short grey hair was cropped in a way that somehow added a youthful look to his rugged face. To keep in shape, he golfed regularly and exercised daily.

After landing in Newark, we rented a car for the ninety-minute drive to Peapack. As we hummed along the turnpike that knifed through the pastoral New Jersey countryside, David and Paul took great pains to impress upon me the importance of this meeting. *Gee, I didn't know that!* David was still smarting over the "dossier affair" and both had heard from Nic about my acerbic comments during the conference call. They were nervous lest I get testy over any less-than-brilliant questions or comments that might emanate from the other side.

Nothing was to come between them and a deal. I assured both that I would "think Yiddish but act British", all the while silently believing that, during that contentious call, what I said, and how I said it, was the very reason we had got this far.

Arriving at the company gate, we parked the car in a huge lot and proceeded to one of two almost identical modern, low-slung buildings. We impatiently cooled our heels for several long minutes at the front reception desk until Hooshmand suddenly swished through a pair of tall glass doors, introduced himself and whisked us down the hall past someone on a cell phone leaning against the wall. My previous exposure to drug company executives had not prepared me for Hooshmand's appearance: late thirties, short buzz cut, black T-shirt with color-matched pants, sport jacket, socks and shoes, complemented by an earring and other assorted bling. He definitely stood out.

Awaiting us in the conference room were the company statistician, a youngish studious-appearing fellow in a bland suit, and Franzanne Vreeland. We shook hands with each and then took our seats at the opposite side of the table. As the chronically-behind-schedule Langdon Miller was not yet there, we passed the time by exchanging small talk with Hooshmand while he hooked up the laptop computer to the projector for my presentation. Franzanne, who appeared to be in her early fifties and was pleasant looking in a rather nondescript way, preferred to sit quietly, her face showing little expression. Looking at her, I kept having flashbacks of her negative assessment of DPPE during the conference call. *Was she going to give us the knife again today?*

Finally, after what seemed an eternity, Langdon rushed into the room, sounding somewhat breathless as he apologized for his tardiness. He was a nice looking man, somewhat stocky, with a full head of dark hair. On shaking hands, I realized that he was the one leaning against the wall, talking into his cell phone[136] as we had passed. After a few pleasant introductory remarks from both sides, it was time for my presentation. Lights dimmed as I flipped on the first Powerpoint slide.

By way of introduction, I explained that when DPPE had been prematurely declared DOA two years earlier, I felt morally obligated to terminate this latest phase two study after only twenty-two patients had been enrolled. "Nonetheless," I continued, "it appears that the survival with DPPE, epirubicin and Taxol was even better than with DPPE and doxorubicin." All eyes were riveted on the numbers on the screen. Whereas the median survival of the patients receiving DPPE and doxorubicin in MA.19 was approximately twenty-four months, the average survival in the women receiving the new combination was an even more impressive *thirty* months. That information seemed to give everyone a comfortable feeling. Since I was using a stronger combination of drugs along with DPPE, anything less than parity with the MA.19 result likely would have cast doubt on the survival advantage in that trial and thrown cold water on our cause.

To add to the "comfort zone", I then compared the results of my new study to five other published phase two studies that reported survival data in similar groups of women with metastatic breast cancer treated with epirubicin and Taxol alone. On average, despite receiving almost twice as much epirubicin as my patients, the women in those studies lived only twenty months, while the

136 During our meeting, it rang so often that he looked as if the device was growing out his ear.

higher doses of epirubicin resulted in more side effects than I had encountered, especially the risk of fever and serious infection resulting from very low blood counts.

"That is an important comparison, and the only valid way to assess your results," Langdon interjected just as his cell phone chimed to once again interrupt his concentration. I nodded in agreement. His point harkened back to Agnes Klein's sage observation that drugs almost always look better in phase two trials than in the more stringent and randomized phase three studies. When presenting phase two data, the results are best compared to other phase two trials. If compared to phase three studies, where the outcome is likely to be less robust, the phase two data would look better than what actually might be the case. By being aware of that fact, I had obviously scored points with Langdon. My talk now over, Paul and David sat back in their chairs, appearing pleased with my performance.

Then, as if we were not in the room, Langdon and his group debated at length the merits of the data among themselves. About five minutes into their discussion, as I was about to interject with a comment, Paul, who was seated next to me, shook his head, gently put his hand on my sleeve and surreptitiously passed a note that he had quickly penned. "They are very interested!" it said. Deferring to his experience, I remained silent, continuing to think Yiddish but acting British.

Langdon next turned to the statistician, asking him to comment on the various subgroup analyses of MA.19 that had been carried out at Pharmacia's request. "I've been reviewing the data during the presentation. This survival advantage is *very* significant and will likely *continue* to be significant over time. The only way for it *not* to continue to be significant would be if, from this moment on, *every* single patient who received doxorubicin *lived*, while *every* single patient who received DPPE plus doxorubicin *died*. I think we would all agree that the likelihood of that occurring is *zero*," he proclaimed exultantly.

As he waved one graph after another in the air, the young analyst became more and more animated. From my experience, this was definitely a first. Very few things beyond Kaplan-Meier plots[137] excite most statisticians. As a group, they would have trouble making the D list for a cocktail party. Now, holding up the *actual* survival curve for patients who received DPPE and doxorubicin, this guy was almost salivating. Paul, David and I exchanged smiles and nods. There was no doubt about it. This statistician *l-o-v-e-d* what he saw. DPPE was now in the statistical equivalent of paradise.

Apparently impressed with what he had just heard, Langdon peered over at us. Question after question followed. Many of them rattled me by their implied skepticism and my concern eventually started to show. "Sorry if I sound a bit unsure or even negative, but if I am to sell DPPE to senior management, I need to anticipate their every question before I go into that room," he explained apologetically. Once again I settled down. It had just become as clear as the prominent nose on my face that Langdon Miller was definitely on our side. *Ask away, my friend.* And ask he did.

Langdon's inquiries continued endlessly. Looking around the room, I could see that the silent Franzanne was now consulting her wrist watch. Finally, he repeated himself once too often: how could he convince the executives that the increased survival in MA.19 was for real? *"Oh, for God's sake, Langdon, it was a large phase THREE trial, not some small phase two study!"* she exclaimed forcefully, her exasperation evident. It stopped him cold.

"Yes....I guess you're right," he agreed after a split second of silence. At that moment I could have leapt over the table and given Franzanne a big hug. She had come a long way!

---

137 Kaplan-Meier plots are projected, rather than actual, survival curves. They are based on a mathematical model that calculates future survival outcome based on the current data. Rather than relying on Kaplan-Meier analysis to predict the outcome, the statistically-significant curve for DPPE and doxorubicin represented actual survival out to just under two years.

"Could we have a terms sheet by next week?" Hooshmand suddenly asked David Harper.

"Absolutely," David answered triumphantly as Langdon nodded his approval. *Terms sheet?* "What's a terms sheet?" I whispered to Paul.

"They want us to make them an offer. You know…up-front payment, milestones and royalties. I told you they were very interested." He gave me a wink.

CHAPTER SIXTY-FIVE:

Storm Clouds

Our mission a roaring success, the three of us walked out of the building into the parking lot without touching the ground. Who cared that the sky, previously a bright summer blue, was now extremely ominous? A large expanse of dark black storm clouds obscured the sun as far as the eye could see. The temperature appeared to have dropped several degrees and the wind was now starting to rustle the leaves on the trees. "Looks like we are headed for some bad weather," I brilliantly observed. No matter. Nothing could rain on our parade after that meeting. *Or could it?*

The closer our Ford Taurus sedan got to the Newark airport, the darker the sky became. Bolts of lightning started to arc across the heavens. Just as we entered the terminal building after returning the car, there began a torrential downpour of gigantic proportion. Almost continuous thunder rattled the terminal's large plate glass windows. Travelers who were unfortunate enough to be caught out in the open were drenched in a millisecond. The wind was now roaring mercilessly. Baggage carts, and the people pushing them, were being blown across the airport roadways and parking lots. *Yikes!*

The overhead television monitors at the arrival and departure gates told a much bigger story. Almost the entire east coast, from Boston to Atlanta, was in the middle of the deluge. No planes were taking off from Newark or anywhere else in the path of the storm. Flights from as far north as Montréal were hurriedly cancelled or diverted. Could we get back to Toronto? As they say in New Jersey, "*Fuggedabuddit!*" While Paul and I looked on, David calmly worked his trusty cell phone, first calling home to pass the word that we would not be flying tonight. "Not to worry. We have rooms at the Hilton," he informed us after a second call to his travel agent.

An hour later, as the storm continued unabated, the three of us, warm and dry, dined in the hotel restaurant just off the lobby. Toasting our impending deal, we recapped the day's discussions over red wine, Caesar salad, and tenderloin steaks, cooked rare and smothered with large fresh mushrooms. Langdon had departed from the meeting in a very hopeful mood that he would win company approval for DPPE. Once a license was negotiated and in place, he wanted us to work with Pharmacia on the design of a new phase three protocol. The company would then provide expert advice to help YM shepherd it through the bureaucracy of the FDA.

"Are we talking potentially big bucks here?" I asked my two companions.

"No doubt about it," David replied. Paul grunted his agreement through a mouthful of food.

"Okay, then. Give me a ballpark figure," I prompted.

"For a drug like DPPE, in late final-stage development, we are likely to ask mid-seven to low-eight figures up front, nine figures on approval, and somewhere around twenty-five percent royalties on sales which, after subtracting development costs, as per our agreement, will be shared proportionally with you and your colleagues at the Cancer Foundation and the University of Manitoba. Funds are payable in U.S. dollars, of course," he rattled off.

At those words, U.S. dollar signs floated in front of my eyes. If the drug succeeded, I would have to hire a financial consultant. *Maybe we all would.*

"With that happy prospect to dream about, I think I'll turn in early," I announced, wishing my friends a good night. In reality, another, less happy, prospect was starting to compete for my thoughts. On entering my room, I immediately went to the window, pulled back the floor-to-ceiling curtain and peered out at the airport. It was in easy sight, about a half-mile directly in front of me. The rain and wind were now dissipating. Off in the distance, I could see a myriad of small trucks, their revolving blue roof strobes flashing, driving up and down, back and forth, checking the runways for debris. Air traffic was starting to pick up. Every few minutes, the piercing landing lights of an arriving jet broke through the low cloud hovering just a few hundred feet off the ground. Things were slowly returning to normal. It appeared we would definitely get off in the morning.

Continuing to glumly gaze at the wet scene outside, I remembered the term "pathetic fallacy". It means "nature in sympathy with man", a literary technique used by writers. Why was it raining in my head? Was this storm another bad omen? *Nonsense. All the signs at that meeting were so positive. Just remember Paul's note. And that salivating statistician. Didn't Franzanne perfectly state the case for DPPE? Didn't Hooshmand ask for a terms sheet? Didn't Langdon look happy at the end? It's a summer thunderstorm, that's all. They happen all the time. Don't be so paranoid! Forget the angels and Bristol-Myers. How often does lightning strike twice? Now go to sleep.*

The next morning dawned muggy and mildly overcast. The storm had petered out in the night. Evaporating puddles and assorted broken twigs and leaves strewn here and there across the hotel parking lot marked its passing. Planes were now taking off left, right and centre to clear the backlog of stranded passengers. After a quick breakfast, we boarded an Air Canada flight and were in sunny Toronto an hour later.

"We'll be in touch with you right after the long weekend," David promised as he and Paul went out the arrivals door. He was referring to the three-day break over the July 1st Canada Day holiday. As soon as they were back to work, he and his colleagues would bang heads to come up with the terms sheet. It would be ready to go as soon as Pharmacia reopened after the extended July 4th holiday south of the border. With that prospect, and the sun now warmly shining outside, any gloomy thoughts of the night before vanished as I headed to the departure gate for Winnipeg.

Jill was waiting for me at the airport later that afternoon. "I think this could be the big one," I told her during the drive home, recounting everything about the meeting including David Harper's calculation. "I'm really pleased, but I don't think we should get our hopes up until the cheque's in the bank," she replied cautiously. Although Jill shared my excitement, after what we had been through with Bristol-Myers, she was reticent to get caught up in another round of "what if?". Carolyn, very pregnant and expecting our first grandchild any moment, was less constrained on hearing the news. "I always told you things would work out," she crowed. Wisely, I said nothing to her about my worrisome thoughts during the storm.

Let's all keep our fingers crossed on this one," I told my colleagues at the Cancer Foundation and the University on Tuesday morning. They said they would.

"Are you making progress on the terms sheet?" I *noodged* Nic two days later. He had been sequestered with David Allan, going over strategy and playing with the numbers.

"We'll be finished this afternoon. I'll e-mail a copy so you can have lots of time to read it over the weekend before we send it to Pharmacia on Monday," he promised. A few hours later, it arrived. There were no surprises. The terms were very close to those that David Harper had suggested over dinner in Newark. From licensing to approval, YM was asking for just under nine figures with subsequent royalties on sales of twenty-five percent, all in U.S. dollars.

While actually seeing the amount in print took my breath away, I believed that it was a realistic appraisal of the drug's current and future value. For that matter, YM's terms sheet actually paled in comparison to other recent drug company licensing deals. Hadn't Bristol-Myers' deal with Imclone for Erbitux totaled *two billion dollars*? If the new breast cancer trial was again positive for a survival advantage, DPPE would almost certainly receive accelerated FDA approval. Add to that the likelihood that it had great untapped potential to help chemotherapy drugs more effectively treat other forms of aggressive cancer. All told, Pharmacia was acquiring the drug without having invested anything in R and D up to its final confirmatory trial. Moreover, that entire study would probably cost a lot less to conduct than the company's monthly marketing or advertising budget. I quickly sent back my approval and copious good wishes for success.

Nic called me the following Monday, July 8th. He had faxed Pharmacia that morning. Hooshmand contacted him at noon to say that he had received the document. He and his colleagues were discussing the offer. He hoped to get back to YM within a week, telling Nic that he was not surprised by the "bottom line" of the terms sheet and that Pharmacia definitely wanted DPPE. As I learned this, I realized how silly I was to worry during that stormy night in Newark. Not only that, we now had a beautiful new grandson, Jack Willem Lindner, the first baby to be born in Winnipeg on Canada Day. With a good omen like that, how could we lose?

CHAPTER SIXTY-SIX:

Lightning Strikes Twice

One week later, on Monday, July 15th, I awoke, went downstairs to gather the newspaper from the front step and turned on the coffee maker to percolate some brew for Jill and me. As part of the ritual, I turned on CNBC to watch *Squawk Box*, my favorite early morning TV entertainment. The show's quirky cast of characters could be counted on to provide a knowledgeable, but refreshingly irreverent, overview of the U.S. and world financial markets. The program was also a good source of information for anyone, like myself, who was interested in the goings-on in the pharmaceutical industry. Joe Kernan, one of the "regulars" with a science background, expertly handled developments in the medical field.

"Our big story this morning is the just-announced takeover of Pharmacia by Pfizer," droned veteran host Mark Haines. "More on this from Joe Kernen." *What did he just say???* My jaw hit the floor. As Kernen reported at length on the proposed merger, I sat transfixed, not believing what I was hearing. "....and Pharmacia's board of directors has approved the Pfizer offer, calling it a good deal for their shareholders....however, before becoming final, the merger will need both Federal Trade Commission and stockholder approval….."[138] *If this takeover was like any other, our pending business deal with Pharmacia was dead in the water. Lightning had just struck twice!!!*

I ran upstairs to tell Jill what I had just heard. Still lying in bed, she reacted with tears and shock. "I'm just numb. I'm so sorry. I don't know what I can say. It's just so terrible," she sobbed.

"I know. I know," I sighed. *What had we done to deserve this?*

The minute I got to my office, I called David Harper. He and his colleagues had already heard the bad news. David had immediately

---

138 Robert Frank and Scott Hensley of *The Wall Street Journal* summed up the deal this way: "In the biggest corporate combination in more than a year, Pfizer Inc. agreed to buy Pharmacia Corp. for stock valued at $60 billion, giving what is already the world's biggest drug company full rights to one of the industry's crown jewels, the blockbuster arthritis drug Celebrex. [a] The deal will create an industry behemoth [b] with over $48 billion in revenue and a research-and-development budget of more than $7 billion. The new combination will be the world's largest drug maker by far and the leading pharmaceutical company by revenue in every major market around the globe."

[a] Just two and one-half short years later, Pfizer's acquired "crown jewel", Celebrex, was severely sideswiped after Merck pulled Vioxx off the market amid fears that it, and other COX-2 inhibitors, doubled the risk of heart attack and stroke. Sales of Celebrex plummeted and Pfizer's stock took a huge nosedive. It didn't end there. In April, 2005, the FDA ordered Pfizer to remove its Celebrex successor, Bextra, from the market.

[b] This was the latest in a long line of Pfizer acquisitions that changed the pharmaceutical landscape. Here is some genealogy: in 1955, The William R. Warner Company (also famous for Chiclets and Dentyne gum) merged with the Lambert Pharmaceutical company (also famous for Listerine mouthwash) to become "Warner/Lambert". After acquiring Parke-Davis in 1970 and Agouron in 1999, Warner/Lambert disappeared from the scene when, in 2000, it merged with Pfizer. Also in 2000, Pharmacia and Upjohn (which had merged the two entities into one company in 1995 and then acquired Sugen in 1999), took over Monsanto (which had previously merged with G. D. Searle in 1985) to become, simply, "Pharmacia". Finally, in 2003, Pfizer swallowed Pharmacia to reign alone as "Pfizer". And you thought that understanding your family tree, with all those second and third cousins twice-removed, was hard?

contacted Hooshmand who confirmed that Pharmacia's hands were tied. Everyone at YM, from David Allan to Paul to Nic, was devastated and at loose ends, not knowing what to do. Not that there was much they *could* do. Of one thing we were all sure: this was one terrible random event.

Somehow, I got through the day. Brent, Janet and Lyonel all commiserated with me. I ran into the Dean of Medicine, Nick Anthonisen. Over the years, Nick had a lot of dealings with drug companies. "Mergers can kill things for a year or more," he counseled. *Thanks.* That night was one of restless sleep. The next morning, bleary-eyed, I once again went through the ritual of getting the newspaper, making coffee and turning on CNBC. As the screen came to life, Mark Haines was in the middle of an introduction. "....and our guest this morning is Hank McKinnell, CEO of Pfizer. Welcome, Mr. McKinnell.....". Once again I sat transfixed as McKinnell was grilled by Haines. Question: What strengths would Pfizer inherit from Pharmacia? My eyes widened when McKinnell singled out Pharmacia's oncology pipeline as one example. That would be a very important addition, given that Pfizer's representation in the area of cancer therapies was weak, he responded. *He said that? Maybe there was yet hope for DPPE.*

Late that night and into the early-morning hour, I hatched a plan. Since oncology was on his radar, I had to get through to McKinnell personally. Maybe I could save the day. He was the only one who might be able to help us out of this mess. Telephoning him would be useless, though. "What did you say your name was? Can you spell that?" someone low down in the chain would ask. But e-mail....if he were like most of us, he would read his e-mail. Even if incoming messages first went to his secretary, I might have a chance.

There was one minor problem. I didn't know his e-mail address. Actually, that wasn't entirely true. From the company website, I knew the last part: @pfizer.com. But what was the first part? I tried sending a couple of test messages: no text, just address iterations: mckinnell@pfizer.com; then, h_mckinnell@pfizer.com.

Both bounced back within a couple of minutes as "undeliverable". I then tried hank.mckinnell@pfizer.com. *Bingo.* For the next hour, I poured my heart out in the following e-mail:

> "From: Lorne J. Brandes
> "Sent: Wednesday, July 17, 2002, 1:01 AM
> "To: hank.mckinnell@pfizer.com
> "Cc: Nic Stiernholm; David Harper; Paul Keane; David Allan
> "Subject: Your personal help urgently requested
> "Importance: High
>
> "Dear Mr. McKinnell,
>
> "My name is Lorne J. Brandes, MD. I am Professor of Medicine and Pharmacology at the University of Manitoba in Winnipeg. I am a medical oncologist and the inventor of tesmilifene[139] (DPPE), an extremely promising new cancer chemotherapy-potentiating drug that, in a recent prospectively-randomized phase 3 study in 300 patients, showed a highly significant effect to increase survival by 50% in women with metastatic breast cancer. In a written opinion, the FDA has stated that an NDA[140] can be filed if a second study confirms the significant increase in survival afforded by tesmilifene. Promising phase 2 survival data have also been generated in late-stage prostate cancer.
>
> "Following extensive due diligence, Pharmacia was involved in negotiations, and the development of a clinical strategy plan, with YM

---

139 YM always referred to DPPE by its assigned generic name, tesmilifene. However, all the published papers at that time referred to the drug by the acronym, DPPE, that I had originally given it.

140 New Drug Application (the official application for approval).

BioSciences, the current licensee, to acquire tesmilifene; today, however, we (YM BioSciences and I) have been informed by Pharmacia that, as a result of the recent takeover by Pfizer, this process is now a casualty of the freeze in all new drug licensing.

"Since few, if any, drugs increase survival in metastatic breast cancer, I am sure you can understand the importance attached to the rapid development of this drug.

"Given these circumstances, I am taking the distinctly unusual step of appealing to you, as the CEO of Pfizer, to personally intervene and to help us get tesmilifene back on track with Pfizer/Pharmacia, especially as you have publicly stated your intention of supporting the oncology portfolio in the new Pfizer/Pharmacia organization.

"I am sure that Langdon Miller, Director of Clinical Oncology (Pharmacia) can provide you with any additional information you may need. I am also copying this letter to Dr. Niclas Stiernholm, COO, David Harper, Licensing Director, Dr. Paul Keane, Medical Director, and David Allan, CEO, of YM BioSciences, any or all of whom you may wish to contact directly as well. In addition, I am taking the liberty of attaching, for your information, the clinical data that we presented just 2 weeks ago when we met with the oncology and licensing group at Pharmacia in NJ.

"I thank you for giving this highly important matter your personal attention.

"Lorne J. Brandes, MD"

I must have stared at what I had written for at least ten minutes, reading it over and over. Finally, the moment of truth arrived. As I had not consulted them about this, I hoped my colleagues at YM would be understanding of my efforts. I also hoped that Hank McKinnell would read my message. Even more, I hoped that he would answer me. Most of all, I fervently hoped that he would help us. *Enough hoping already!* Without further delay, I clicked on "Send". The message, hopes and all, instantly shot into cyberspace.

"What were you doing all that time?" Jill sleepily asked as I climbed into bed.

"I e-mailed Hank McKinnell, CEO of Pfizer, about DPPE," I replied.

"Seriously?"

"Seriously."

"You're a gutsy guy," she said as she rolled over and put her arms around me.

"Let's hope Hank McKinnell and the others feel the same way," I answered, closing my eyes. I was exhausted.

CHAPTER SIXTY-SEVEN:

Feet Of Clay

Early the next morning, I gently slipped out of bed without waking Jill, tiptoed into the next room and turned on the computer. "You have new mail!" announced the window that popped up on the screen. *There it was. A reply from Hank McKinnell!*

"RE: your personal help urgently requested

"Dr. Brandes,

"I have asked our head of licensing to look into this opportunity. Pharmacia appropriately stopped all new business development work, but that does not stop Pfizer's work. If your project is as compelling as you imply, we could be interested. Thank you for writing to me.

"Hank McKinnell"

It was very carefully worded to give nothing away, but at least I had his attention. I quickly forwarded McKinnell's reply to my colleagues at YM BioSciences, adding these words: "We got through to the CEO of Pfizer!! Now let's play hardball. LJB"

"Good on you. Excellent move," David Allan e-mailed later that morning.

"Good work Lorne," echoed Nic, who then outlined some contacts he had at Pfizer and whom he intended to call. The atmosphere at YM was instantly transformed from gloomy to hectic as multiple calls and faxes were exchanged with people at Pfizer.

There was one small glitch. In addition to my e-mail, McKinnell had forwarded the attachment containing my Powerpoint presentation on DPPE, epirubicin and Taxol to his licensing people. David Harper was soon contacted by Pfizer's VP of licensing, Lisa Ricciardi, to expedite a confidentiality agreement within twenty-four hours. However, until it was in place, the contents of the attachment were not yet protected. They both agreed to trash it then and there. It could be resent once the agreement was signed the following day.

Although I was proud of myself for taking the brash initiative to send that e-mail, I was now pessimistic that it would advance our cause rapidly, as I had hoped. The reason? I had specifically requested that McKinnell intercede to allow Pharmacia to conclude the negotiation so that DPPE could move forward to help patients with cancer. His reply made it clear that any of Pharmacia's impending business deals were in suspended animation. Now it looked like it was back to square one with Pfizer, albeit with a foot firmly in the door. However, the foot in the door soon became one foot nailed to the floor, as we went around and around in circles.

An e-mail two days later from Nic best summed up the events that subsequently followed: "I [Nic] write the head of licensing at Pfizer and volunteer to interact with a director of licensing that I know from before, Dr. Knowles….[who] calls me (not remembering me!!). He asks for non-confidential info to begin with. I send everything I possibly can. Brandes and I realize that this is idiotic for Pfizer to start from scratch, since it will take them 12 months to make up their minds. Brandes tells me to call them back and explain that he wanted them to allow Pharmacia to complete the deal, not Pfizer starting all over again.[141] I call Knowles back and plead with him…..he says that they can't even speak to Pharmacia, but that as soon as the FTC hearing is over and they know what products they will keep,[142] everything will move quickly, maybe 3-4 months. I tell Brandes and we declare half a victory.

"Pharmacia calls YM later the same day and declares that they are very upset with having to sit around for 6 months doing nothing. They want to license and they are going to get a legal opinion on their ability to do so, despite Pfizer's request that they stop all negotiations. They are also involving their CEO, Fred Hassan, directly. They will get back to us in 2 weeks, and by the way, the terms sheet was in line with what they expected."

Despite Pharmacia's bravado, a subsequent e-mail from David Harper on August 1st was much more sobering: "Spoke with Hooshmand this morning. Their offices are deserted as most people take vacation that has been owing to them. This includes many of the senior management who are not going to have positions with Pfizer. Meanwhile the lawyers are very busy on other elements of the takeover. Subsequently they have not yet been able to get the necessary people together to make a decision about lifting the moratorium for tesmilifene.

"…We will unlikely hear anything next week but possibly after that when the team reassembles. Needless to say the Oncology group maintain their interest and desire to get moving but it is a decision that requires a legal view and management consensus. Will let you know when we do hear anything positive."

---

141   I actually e-mailed McKinnell again one day later, reiterating my request that Pharmacia should be allowed to finalize the deal, rather than our having to start all over again with Pfizer. This time, he did not reply.

142   One major issue with the merger was the need for divestiture of certain drugs or other assets by each company to prevent the possibility that their combined portfolio could corner the market and result in an unfair trade advantage over competing companies. This was not likely to be an issue with oncology drugs, given Pfizer's weak oncology pipeline.

And finally, this even darker assessment from David a month later: "Finally got to talk with Lauren Silverman today for an update on where they [Pfizer] are at. We spoke openly about the Pharmacia situation, but she explained that there are still official walls between the management groups of the two companies so they cannot communicate directly at this time. Bottom line is that the Pfizer team have the usual concerns about the opportunity—-patent coverage and life, any bias in the MA.19 stats and the clinical relevance of the CNS side effects of tesmilifene. However, the team is aware that Pharmacia were happy to proceed with a deal having spent considerable time to address all of these issues. The Pharmacia oncology team is held in very high regard.

"Rather than spend the next weeks and months repeating the due diligence and evaluation of the Pharmacia team, they would rather wait until the 'wall' is broken down and they can pick up where Pharmacia were forced to leave off. The opinion was that if we were to force the issue at this time, it would likely result in a rapid negative decision based on the heavy workloads on other projects already in hand. There is also the chance that the Pfizer team might not come up with the same positive decision as did the Pharmacia team! It looks, therefore, that an opinion would be forthcoming in January although, if the walls disappear earlier, the time might be shortened (December at best)."

It was now unhappily clear to me that whatever I had tried to put in motion with that e-mail to Hank McKinnell was firmly stuck in the mud. I did not share the general consensus that everything would fall into place by January, 2003, when it would be back to "business as usual". How could it be, when I had recently spoken with Hooshmand who told me that he did not expect to survive the transition? "There could be twenty-five thousand Pharmacia people out of a job by the time this is finished," he told me matter-of-factly when I called him on his cell phone. He was now easy to reach, a sign that there was nothing on his plate in the day-to-day business of Pharmacia.

Even more disconcerting was an e-mail from Langdon Miller, who implied that there was uncertainty about his own status in a merged organization: "Things are very much on hold here given the impending takeover by Pfizer. I remain very interested in tesmilifene as a prospect for further development. Assuming the timing would be right from your side and that of YM, I would hope to be an advocate for the drug here or wherever I may land in the next few months. I will probably have a better sense in early December," he wrote.

Was I angry about what had happened? You bet I was. That a boardroom decision made "for the good of the shareholders" had unwittingly blindsided the renewed development of a promising cancer treatment was, you should excuse the pun, a bitter pill to swallow. As for Hank McKinnell, who, when push came to shove, was unable, or unwilling, to go by anything other than "the book" to help us in our hour of need, I penned the following verse:

"Why did he not rise to the challenge I threw his way,
Rather than to show that he had feet of clay?"

CHAPTER SIXTY-EIGHT:

Slick Talk

In late August, while the Pfizer/Pharmacia deal was still in limbo and they were not talking to one another, there appeared an unexpected glimmer of hope. It all started with a phone call to Jeff Usakewicz. We had kept in touch even after he left Bristol-Myers in 2002, during the dark days of the Imclone/Erbitux fiasco, and moved over to AstraZeneca to be project manager for the company's new lung cancer drug, Iressa. Jeff was, and is, the kind of person I could trust to keep a confidence. One afternoon, I called to tell him about the latest calamity to befall DPPE. "That's terrible," he exclaimed as I spared no details. "You know I always believed that you and DPPE got a raw deal at Bristol-Myers," he added. With those words, we traded some memories of the "good old days" when hopes for my drug ran high after it was licensed to his former employer. The conversation then segued to our mutual friend, Bill Slichenmyer.

"Jeff, do you ever talk to Bill?" I asked.

"No, I don't. I have to say I'm really disappointed that he never kept in touch with me after he left Bristol-Myers," he replied.

"I spoke to him once or twice in late 1999 when he had moved from that belly-up biotech company to Parke-Davis," I allowed.

"You know where he is now, don't you?" Jeff asked.

"No. I lost track of him," I replied.

"Well, he stayed on and became VP Oncology at Warner-Lambert after the company folded its Parke-Davis division. Then Warner-Lambert was taken over by Pfizer and...."

"Don't tell me he's now at Pfizer!" I half-gasped, cutting him off in mid-sentence.

"Yeah. You didn't know that? He's VP Oncology at Pfizer. I think he's at their Groton facility in Connecticut. Why? Do you think you should call him?"

I was floored by this news. "Maybe I should. Man, oh man. People just keep going around and coming around in this industry, don't they?"

"You've got that right," Jeff laughed, repeating one of his favorite phrases.

I thanked him and promised to keep in touch. *Well! That bombshell certainly explains why Langdon Miller is now uncertain about whether he has a future at Pfizer!*

After hanging up the phone, I called David Harper. As far as I knew, Bill's name never came up in any discussions with Pfizer. I needed to verify this for myself. "David, does the name Bill Slichenmyer mean anything to you?"

"Refresh my memory," he replied.

"He headed up the DPPE project at Bristol-Myers in the early days. He left the company just at the time DPPE was looking like a winner in IND.97."

"Okay. Can't say as I remember him."

"Well, guess what my friend? He's head of oncology at Pfizer!"

After talking over the implications for a few minutes, David said he had no objection to my getting in touch with Bill. At worst, we might learn something. At best....who knew?

I soon obtained his number from the operator at the company's Groton switchboard. "Do you want me to connect you?" she asked.

"Sure, why not?" I replied, hastily writing down the number as the phone started to ring.

"Bill Slichenmyer," a familiar voice answered. I couldn't believe my good luck.

"Hi Bill. It's Lorne Brandes."

"Hey! Lorne! Good to hear from you. How are things?" For the next ten minutes I told him. "You didn't know anything about this?" I asked at the end of my story.

"Absolutely nothing, I promise you," he confided. *Wait a minute! This guy was Pfizer's VP of oncology and nobody told him about the series of events my e-mail had engendered?*

"I definitely think it's time I get involved," he added, reassuringly.

Bill promised he would obtain the file and get back to me within one or two days. To back up what he had said, he immediately followed with an earnest e-mail: "Lorne, it was great to speak with you today. I'll give you a call later this week. Bill."

"Thanks," I replied. "Please lead me/us out of the wilderness!! All best wishes…LJB."

Sure enough, two days later I arrived in my office to find a message from Bill on my phone. He was sorry to have missed me. He was now fully engaged with the DPPE file. He would work hard with his colleagues to move things forward. There were specific people he wanted to involve. He would get back to me with regular updates. Hang in there and give him some time. *Good for you, Slick.*

I felt elated as I played back his message two or three times and then called David Harper and Paul Keane. "I really think Bill's our man," I told them. I then followed up with a suggestion. "I would like to put together an executive summary containing all the pertinent information that Bill will need. We can include the various survival graphs, our interpretation of how DPPE increased survival, and suggestions for the design of a new trial." Both men agreed with the plan as long as they could review the document before I sent it. "Of course," I said, initially surprised that they would feel it necessary to ask. Then again, I had taken some of the steam out of their sails by contacting Pfizer in the first place. Viewed from YM's perspective, I now understood their request.

I spent the better part of the Labour Day weekend putting the fifteen page summary together and e-mailed the draft to Paul who, as a physician, was the most able person in the company to pass judgment on the document. In a covering message to him, I wrote:

"As discussed, here is what I want to send Bill Slichenmyer at Pfizer for their upcoming high-level meeting. Please get back to me ASAP with your comments/criticisms."

Paul replied: "Lorne, I have been through this and it is very compelling."

With that, he gave me his approval to e-mail the summary to Bill. It was September 3rd.

As I had not heard anything from him since that initial voice-mail, I decided to first call Bill to give him a heads-up that the summary was on its way. This time a woman answered. "Dr. Slichenmyer is tied up in a meeting. I'm his executive assistant and usually handle all his calls," she informed me. *Obviously I was lucky to get through to him that first time.* I told her about the executive summary that I was about to e-mail. "I'll make sure he gets it," she cooly assured me.

"Great. Perhaps you can tell him I called, and that I was hoping he might get back to me."

"I will definitely give him the message," she replied. *Hmmm. We'll see.*

There was no further word from Bill. The weeks stretched into months. I e-mailed him on several occasions, requesting that he contact me, but he did not. I then resorted to calling, but he was never in and my messages were not returned. Something had fundamentally changed since our first communication, but I didn't know what or why. Now Jeff's words kept creeping into my mind: "*I have to say I'm really disappointed that he never kept in touch with me....*" It seemed that Jeff wasn't the only person Bill had disappointed by not keeping in touch. I was now on that list. Given his initial enthusiastic response, it wasn't fair. He owed us the courtesy of a decision. Another e-mail and two calls went unanswered.

Finally, in April, 2003, the Pfizer/Pharmacia merger went through, almost ten months after the takeover was first announced. Enough already. Bill needed to be pressed for an answer. I took the bull by the horns and, putting on my "business hat", wrote one last time:

> "Dear Bill,
>
> "I e-mailed you last week on behalf of YMB and have called your office twice, but so far have not had a reply. Langdon Miller, who had previously championed acquisition of DPPE by Pharmacia, suggested we contact you directly about the future of DPPE with Pfizer, as he is leaving the company at the end of June.[143]
>
> "Given that negotiations were 'on hold' for over 10 months, now that the Pfizer/Pharmacia merger is complete we believe it reasonable to request an early indication of interest (or non-interest) in moving forward with a licensing deal. We firmly believe that DPPE is a low-risk business opportunity; it is in late-stage development and requires only 1 more clinical trial [in metastatic breast cancer] which, if positive for a survival benefit, is almost certain to receive accelerated FDA approval.

---

143 Langdon and Hooshmand did not survive the merger with Pfizer. As for the rest, I have no idea.

"Bill, I would be very appreciative if you would
call or e-mail me. LJB"

This time, he replied within a day. His words were painfully
short and not sweet: "Lorne. Thanks for your note. Pfizer has
concluded that we are not interested in pursuing DPPE as an in-
licensing candidate. Bill."

Of the several people who had disappointed me along the way,
Bill now took first place as he exited the stage for good. Once
again, it wasn't so much *that* he let me down, but *how* he did it.
He had handled this whole matter incredibly badly, taking a page
from Renzo, rewriting it, and doing his old boss one better in
the process.

Given his previous championing of DPPE when he was at
Bristol-Myers, Bill's terse two sentence response was especially
hard to take. Why didn't he have the decency to explain the
reasons for the negative decision? Some time later, David Harper
called one of his contacts at Pfizer. She told him that Bill's analysis
of the information I had provided led to the conclusion that, even
if it was successful in the next trial, the market for DPPE would be
fairly small. After all, it only helped patients with aggressive breast
cancer. *Only?? Patients with aggressive disease don't count??* Yet,
despite everything, given our past relationship, I could not bring
myself to dislike him as a person.

*Me: "Hey! Bill! I thought we were friends. How could you be
so cold-hearted?"*

*Bill: "Come on, Lorne. We're still friends. It was strictly a busi-
ness decision."*

Me: "Really? Tell that to the patients with cancer."

There was a post-script to this unhappy episode. Remember
David Allan's e-mail to me the morning after I had contacted
Hank McKinnell? *"Good on you. Excellent move,"* he had written. It
now seemed that he, and perhaps the others, had second thoughts
about what I had done, especially my contacting Bill and taking
the initiative to write that "compelling" executive summary. No

matter that David Harper and Paul Keane had approved of everything I did along the way, "someone" was to blame for Pfizer
going off the rails. That "someone" appeared to be me. I was now
regarded as a loose cannon, as David Allan soon let me know in
no uncertain, if less than grammatically-pretty, terms:

"Dear Lorne,

"Given some of the misunderstandings that have happened
in the past, I believe it is crucial to clarify lines of communication in respect of the people for whom we have responsibility in
the process of developing tesmilifene. It is imperative that the
people at YM get on with the job of communicating directly on
regulatory and clinical matters going forward as much as with
prospective partnering activities and as much as we will continue
to rely on your participation, it is difficult for us to move things
forward if you have direct contact with the people for whom the
YM staff have responsibility. I appreciate the enthusiasm you
bring to the process and, of course, your unparalleled knowledge
of the molecule as well as of many of the people we are interfac-
ing with. Notwithstanding, staff here cannot manage the process
for which we are contractually responsible if you, in parallel with
their efforts, communicate directly.

"While the enthusiasm is admirable, YM is the licensee and
I think that you should direct any comments only to YM staff
and not around its flank. That latter can be very confusing, both
to regulators and to prospective licensees. Let me reiterate our
appreciation for your input, but I must strongly urge that it be
channeled through this office.

"Best regards, DGPA"

I was tempted to respond to him with a line I have quoted
before in this story: "Success has many fathers; failure is an
orphan". The problem was that, in this case, YM's CEO believed
failure was spelled "B-R-A-N-D-E-S". In the end, I decided against
replying. While I felt that his blame was misguided, he was not
necessarily wrong in the larger context of what he said. Okay then.
I would leave all future contacts with drug companies to David

Allan and YM BioSciences. We would see whether doing it "their way" would be any more successful than it had been for me.

CHAPTER SIXTY-NINE:

Not Letting The Grass Grow

Lest anyone think that we remained paralyzed or in suspended animation in the weeks and months following the mid-2002 announcement that Pfizer intended to merge with Pharmacia, be assured that nothing was further from the truth. Even before my ill-fated contact with Hank McKinnell, I e-mailed my colleagues at YM BioSciences, urging that we not let the grass grow beneath our feet. We could write up the new breast cancer protocol ourselves and submit it to the FDA for approval. Based on the early comments of the regulators, we had already reached a consensus on the design of the trial. To be consistent and comparable with MA.19, the FDA did not want us to stray far from that original study. Specifically, YM was told that regulatory approval would most likely follow a positive trial that again combined DPPE with doxorubicin, or a doxorubicin-like drug. Jumping to a test of DPPE with the more current, but unrelated, taxanes was not encouraged. Clearly, reproducibility within the box would be the key to success with the FDA.

To comply with this suggestion while expanding the horizon to a slight, but acceptable, degree, I recommended to Paul and Nic that the new study use a two-drug chemotherapy combination with DPPE. This would consist of doxorubicin's cousin, epirubicin, and cyclophosphamide. By this time, my preference for epirubicin was no surprise to anyone, as the drug had already shown itself to be very active with DPPE in breast cancer and was less toxic than doxorubicin. There were two reasons for adding cyclophosphamide to the mix. First, the drug was already approved in both adjuvant (early) and metastatic breast cancer treatment, especially in combination with doxorubicin or epirubicin. Second, my early prostate cancer study had shown that the DPPE/cyclophosphamide combo was safe and, seemingly, quite effective.

Paul and I then used the original MA.19 study as a framework on which to write the new protocol, but changed the rules in two important ways: the primary endpoint was survival, not tumor shrinkage or "time to progression",[144] and women with the slow-growing form of breast cancer were excluded, leaving us to concentrate our efforts on those with aggressive tumors. In another twist, using the more "heart-friendly" epirubicin allowed us to increase the number of possible treatments from six to ten. Why did we do this? If the hypothesis was correct that DPPE worked by preventing the emergence of drug resistance over time, the survival advantage for women receiving DPPE might be further amplified with an additional four treatments.

Two additional decisions, made early in the game, proved extremely important. Paul contacted Professor John Whitehead at the University of Reading in the U.K., who had pioneered a new statistical method. Called "planned sequential analysis", Whitehead's approach allowed clinical trials in progress to be analyzed at pre-specified intervals without compromising statistical integrity. Simplistically-speaking, performing the usual type of interim analysis before a trial ends is assumed to add a degree of

---

144 If DPPE again conferred a significant survival advantage, this would trump any other endpoint.

bias, even if the actual results are known to only a few people on an external monitoring committee. To compensate for this, more patients are built into the study to reduce the chance of statistical error resulting from any bias introduced by the interim analysis.

In contrast, a planned sequential analysis circumvents the "numbers" problem while still able to declare an early winner. The tradeoff is that the bar for a successful outcome is set highest for the first planned analysis and then lowered progressively for each subsequent assessment. For DPPE to be declared an early success in YM's new study, a fifty percent or greater improvement in survival had to be evident in the first planned analysis, triggered when the first 192 patients died. This total, strange at first glance, was equal to the number of women with aggressive disease whose survival appeared to be so robustly increased by DPPE plus doxorubicin in the MA.19 trial. What better way for an early comparison of the two studies? If second and third analyses, each triggered by an additional 64 deaths, were required, the survival advantage needed for a successful outcome dropped progressively to a final required difference of thirty-three percent.

There was only one problem: this new approach had not been used before in FDA-approved cancer trials such as ours. Paul wanted to break new ground, to convince the regulators that the sequential method was a sound way to analyze the results.

The second decision, championed by Nic Stiernholm prior to his departure from YM, was to ask the FDA for a "Special Protocol Assessment" of the new study. By taking this course, YM worked closely with the FDA as the regulators scrutinized every aspect of the trial. Although the review took over six months to complete, it ultimately paid off when the agency approved the trial design, including the sequential analysis. YM's decision had been a very smart move. By receiving the blessing of the FDA *a priori*, the company could be assured that, if the trial outcome was positive, there would be no criticism of the study at the end of the day to derail an NDA application. Moreover, the FDA likely would agree to any request for an accelerated review of the NDA filing if the trial succeeded.

David Allan and his colleagues were justifiably proud of themselves when the decision came through. Not only was receiving the Special Protocol Assessment designation a first for any small Canadian biotech company developing a cancer treatment, the FDA approval should now attract big pharma to sign a licensing deal and put up the bucks needed to get this final trial underway! Back to the Rolodex went David Harper. Once again the three of us, this time with Mark Vincent in tow, travelled south for discussions with Berlex, a second-tier, but able, oncology-oriented drug company whose head office was in Germany. Its U.S. licensing director was none other than Alice Leung, who had also left Bristol-Myers around the time of the Imclone fiasco. Her subordinate, Leon Rubin, set up the meeting. I was to present my "Pharmacia" talk while Mark would concentrate on his subgroup analysis of MA.19.

Try as we might, neither of us seemed to make much headway, either with the two German company officials around the table or two oncologists who were sitting bolt upright on chairs somewhere in Germany, "participating" via a video link. I say participating in quotation marks because neither uttered a word for the entire duration. During my presentation, I could see over the television monitor that one of the two stood up and left the room. We were later told that he had to answer a call. Whether it was from a patient or mother nature, I never learned. Whatever the reason, his presence or absence made no difference. David Harper later learned from Leon Rubin that one of the main concerns of the company was that our use patents for DPPE might not be strong enough to prevent infringement in Europe were DPPE to be successful. *How many ways are there to say no??*

There was a further low point. On the heels of the failed Berlex visit, David Allan and his colleagues became very hopeful that a white knight, in the form of a company called Chiron, would come to DPPE's rescue. "Why would we be interested in them? They make flu vaccines, not cancer drugs," I exclaimed to Paul Keane on learning that a conference call was in the works. Apparently they wanted to speak with me. "Because, dear boy, they have loads of m-o-n-e-y and nowhere to spend it," Paul shot back, more than a hint of British sarcasm in his voice. Money or no money, for long-term development of DPPE, I believed we needed to attract a company whose primary expertise was in oncology drugs, not vaccines, and said so. Paul just sighed.

The conference call took place during a sunny, warm afternoon in Winnipeg. Shirtless and barefoot in shorts, I sipped a cold glass of beer as I talked from a portable phone while slouching on the comfortable cushion of a wicker chair, my feet up on an ottoman, in my back yard gazebo. Large mosquitoes buzzed and banged against the screened-in enclosure, attracted by my bare legs and torso. Paul and David Harper were on the line from Toronto, while an assorted group, including an oncologist/consultant, gathered around a speaker-phone at Chiron. After the obligatory introductions, we were underway.

"Dr. Brandes, how can you assure us that a new trial will be successful?" the consultant immediately asked.

"I can't. However, based on what we learned from MA.19, it has been designed to test patients with the highest chance of being helped by DPPE." *Pregnant pause.*

Apparently my answer did not satisfy him. He rephrased the question. "Dr. Brandes, you must understand that Chiron is very risk-averse. Our job in advising the company is to minimize any financial risks. In making any recommendation, we need to know that there is a very high likelihood that DPPE will be successful." *Now I see. It's kindergarten time.*

"The only way to find out if DPPE is successful is to license it and run the phase three trial. If the group receiving DPPE survives significantly longer, you will know that it is successful." *Did I hear people groaning?*

Suddenly Paul Keane interrupted in his most diplomatic tone. "What Dr. Brandes meant to say…."

The coup de grâce came with the final hackneyed question: "In the absence of an improvement in response rates or time to progression, why should we be excited about DPPE, especially in view of the fact that nobody knows how it works?" My patience at an end, I answered with thinly-disguised contempt, my voice rising with each word. "Well let me put it this way. If this drug and the research behind it...and believe me, there are many published papers on its possible mechanism of action.... came out of Harvard or Stanford, rather than some place in The Great White North called the University of Manitoba, I believe you would be much more excited about it.

"Second, no one *cares* about, or *should care about*, early endpoints. *I* don't care about early endpoints. Increasingly, *the FDA doesn't care about early endpoints.*[145] From your question, *you* seem to be the only one who *cares* about early endpoints. *What you should care about is SURVIVAL. That's all that really matters to patients with cancer!*" The last two sentences were enunciated slowly and emphatically, just in case he hadn't got my drift.

In a post-mortem the next day, David and Paul made their displeasure abundantly clear. My lack of diplomacy had let YM down. A great potential deal was now in jeopardy, or worse. "Nuts to that," I replied. "They were childish, stupid questions, plain and simple. The guy even wanted us to give him an iron-clad guarantee for goodness' sake! We would have to be desperate to hook up with a company like that!" Silence. *Oops! I guess they're desperate.*

---

145 Recently, the FDA had moved the bar even higher. Now cancer drugs that increased survival had a far better chance of approval than those that merely improved early endpoints.

CHAPTER SEVENTY:

Unanswered Prayers

One by one, drug company interest in DPPE dried up over the next few months. Try as they might, David Allan and his colleagues could not convince Chiron, or any other major player, to make a deal. Whether it was Novartis or Aventis, the result was *bubkes*.[146] Although the excuses for saying "no" varied, one, evoking past memories, repeatedly stood out: *we don't know how DPPE works.* Never mind that the drug appeared to dramatically increase survival or that our research had pointed to novel and potentially important targets for its action, nobody in big pharma seemed willing to give it the chance it deserved. David Allan was now forced to rethink his strategy.

Soon, Nic announced the hiring of Dr. Vincent Salvatori. It was a move designed to bolster YM's clout, but left David Harper in a precarious position. Vince was more well-rounded than David in terms of experience (and also, rather unfortunately, in waist circumference).

---

146 "Bubkes" is a Yiddish word that literally means "beans" and figuratively means "nothing".

A PhD by training, he had long worked in the Canadian pharmaceutical industry, most recently with QLT, a British Columbia company. Under his stewardship, QLT had successfully developed and marketed a new eye treatment, called "photodynamic therapy", a combination of a light-activated chemical and laser procedure for a serious vision-threatening condition called "wet macular degeneration".

Soon after joining YM, Vince called me. Gregarious by nature, with many Jewish colleagues in the pharmaceutical industry, he shared his belief that, religion aside, Italians and Jews were first cousins. He then enthusiastically vowed to his new "cuz" that he would use his considerable expertise to carry DPPE across the finish line.

Next, Allan engaged the services of a corporate head hunter in the hope that a professional agency with access to drug companies might accomplish what YM could not. Although I thought it was a good idea, Vince told me frankly that he was against such an expensive venture, feeling that it was unlikely to pay dividends, but was overruled by his boss. In the end, Vince proved to be right. The result was *"nada"*!!

With each licensing failure, my gloom increased. With it came anger, not at little YM, which was obviously trying as hard as it could to make something happen, but at the stiff-necked attitude of the big drug companies for not helping us out. How could they not see what we saw? Why were they so unwilling to put up a few million dollars, a spit in the bucket for them, really, for a chance to help humanity? Often, I would sit in my office and put up the survival graphs on my computer screen, staring at them for minutes on end. That just made me feel worse. Even if the difference in survival was only half as great as it appeared, there were so many women, young and old, who were being denied the chance of benefiting from DPPE. Seeing what I had seen with the drug, could I feel any other way?

One evening, in desperation, I contacted Kathy Pritchard. In the months after presenting the survival data at the NCIC meeting, she had done her best to put DPPE back on the table with Joe Pater and his colleagues in the organization, but to no avail. Recently, thinking it might jump-start the impasse, I suggested to Paul Keane that he send Kathy and Len Reyno the new "Pharmacia" subgroup survival analyses. Surprisingly, neither had replied. Wondering why, I decided to call Kathy at home.

"Have you had a chance to review the new survival graphs Paul sent you?" I asked, after first exchanging a few pleasantries.

"Yeah. I've looked at them," she replied without a hint of interest, let alone excitement, in her voice.

"Don't you find them compelling?" I replied, forging ahead.

"Compelling for what?" she asked.

I was shocked. "Compelling for a remarkable survival advantage in women with aggressive breast cancer who received DPPE. I really believe that the NCIC has to reconsider its position in light of this new analysis. We owe it to our patients," I shot back.

"I don't pay much attention to subgroup analysis. The MA.19 study was not designed or powered to look at survival in these various categories," she said, dismissively.

"Whether it was or wasn't, Kathy, just look at what these data are telling us. Despite the smaller number of patients with aggressive tumors, the survival difference in favor of DPPE and doxorubicin was statistically much greater than in the trial as a whole. How often does something like that occur? Virtually never, I would suggest.[147] It has to be telling us something important."

---

147 When breaking down a large group into smaller subsets for analysis (whether it be of survival or any other endpoint), the statistical significance of any differences usually decreases as the number of patients decrease. Although women with aggressive tumors made up only two hundred of the three hundred patients in MA.19, the statistical significance of the survival benefit in this subgroup of subjects actually *increased* by over thirty times. As Paul Keane later e-mailed me, "The next time someone expresses doubt about the subgroup analysis, tell them that if it walks like a duck.....". He and I appeared to belong to a small minority of people who believed that the findings were highly important.

"I don't happen to agree with you," she replied, matter-of-factly.

"Well, if *you* of all people can't see the *obvious*, what chance does *any* of us have?" My voice was rising rapidly.

"Don't yell at me or I will hang up the phone," Kathy scolded.

I apologized and immediately lowered the decibels, trying again to make the case. It was a lost cause. Dejected, I turned to a second issue that was bothering me. "Why hasn't the NCIC written up the MA.19 study? It's been over eighteen months since the survival data came out. Are the findings not important enough to publish?" I inquired.

"On that you are absolutely right. We should and we will. I'll contact Len Reyno. As trial chairman, it is his responsibility," she agreed. *Why do I need to be the one to bring this up anyway?* Kathy then tried to change the subject to less-charged matters, but by this time I was in no mood for small talk.

If I was depressed before calling Kathy, I was moribund after. How could she not see the light? How could she be so rigid in her thoughts? Or was it me? Was I reading too much into the graphs? "NO!" my inner voice commanded sternly. Sometime afterward, the discussion with Kathy prompted a new idea. Perhaps the U.S. National Cancer Institute could help us with the new trial. After all, this was the very same organization that had put Taxol into clinical studies before Bristol-Myers came along. Maybe the NCI could help us do with DPPE what its Canadian counterpart and drug companies would not. It was worth a try.

Paul Keane gave me his blessing to contact Dr. Richard Kaplan, director of the the NCI's Cancer Therapy Evaluation Program (CTEP). I did not know Dr. Kaplan personally and decided to e-mail him. "Could you contact me about an urgent matter?" I wrote, hoping to get his attention. After all, he probably received a lot of e-mail. My wording paid off. He quickly responded on his Blackberry from somewhere in Europe.

A few days after his return, we spoke at length. I pushed all the buttons when making my appeal: we owed it to women with metastasized breast cancer to see whether DPPE really increased survival; if DPPE worked late in the game, imagine how it might help adjuvant chemotherapy save thousands of lives every year in women with early breast cancer; the drug might have unlimited applications in other forms of cancer where chemotherapy is of benefit; DPPE appeared to fit the NCI's mandate to improve the outcome in patients with cancer. Listening to all I had to say, Dr Kaplan responded sympathetically. He suggested we meet at NCI headquarters in Bethesda, and proposed that it would be helpful if someone involved with the MA.19 trial could attend. When I mentioned Kathy's name, his interest peaked; as a result of her many years of clinical trial experience, she had a high profile with Kaplan and his NCI colleagues.

Paul was very congratulatory when I informed him of my success in contacting Dr. Kaplan and about his offer to meet with us. Having worked quietly behind the scenes to engender support from Kathy and MA.19 coordinator, Lesley Seymour, he leapt at the idea of both coming along. An early date was arranged. Despite the fact that contacting the NCI had been entirely my initiative, he, Kathy and Lesley were to make the presentations.

"I want you to promise to sit quietly and be on your best behavior at the meeting tomorrow," Paul admonished as we sat in the Toronto airport departure lounge waiting for Kathy to appear for our late afternoon flight to Washington. It was obvious from his comment that he had not yet forgiven me for my mishandling of the Chiron conference call. To add to his displeasure, Kathy had been peeved by our telephone argument and told him so.

Hurt by his words, I remained silent for some time, staring straight ahead. Okay, so I wasn't perfect. Sometimes, in my frustration to move DPPE ahead, I came on too strongly. Nonetheless, I felt Paul's judgment of me to be overly harsh. He himself was highly opinionated and at times could be chippy and quick-tempered. That said, he was a good and decent man; it was important that we repair our relationship. "You have nothing to worry about and I mean that," I finally responded. Satisfied, he gave my shoulder a fatherly pat.

Soon Kathy appeared. We bussed one another on the cheek, putting any disagreement behind us. Neither of us believed in holding a grudge. We had known one another for over thirty years and she remained very supportive of my work. Vivacious, with a quick smile, a good raconteuse with a sometimes kooky sense of humor and a hearty laugh, Kathy was also a compassionate physician. Over the years, she had cared for three of my relatives who were unlucky enough to need her services; all spoke highly of her.

This day, she came armed with welcome news. The MA.19 manuscript had been just reviewed by *JCO*. Some revisions were necessary, but the signs were promising that it would be published. Following my call, she and Lesley had taken the bull by the horns and written the paper when Len appeared unable to do so. Kathy wanted me to read it during the short flight.

After checking into a Bethesda hotel, the three of us met Lesley for dinner. Temporarily interrupting her mini-sabbatical, she had flown in directly from the U.K. Seeing her for the first time in over three years, my eyes bulged. Lesley had undergone a major makeover, complete with spiked blond hair. At first I didn't recognize her. She was now jogging religiously, had shed a lot of pounds and looked great. Over the next hour we all worked together to answer the *JCO* reviewers' questions and criticisms.

Following a strategy session the next morning, we headed to our meeting at NCI headquarters. Richard Kaplan was the first to enter the large boardroom to meet us. Short, bearded and professorial in appearance, he presented the same kind demeanor that had come through during our telephone conversation. He had arranged for several of his colleagues, including breast cancer trial chief, Dr. Jeff Abrams, to be at the table.

After the presentations and discussion, Dr. Kaplan gave an overview of the role of the NCI in clinical drug development. He agreed that DPPE deserved further testing. However, while his organization had a mandate to review and approve cancer studies, it could not force clinical trials groups to carry out the testing of a specific drug or protocol such as ours. He also believed that leadership in moving DPPE forward should come from the NCIC (exactly what I had been saying for over a year to all who would listen!).

At Kaplan's words, I fixed my gaze on Kathy and Lesley. Both nodded their agreement. After further discussion, it was decided that Kathy would present the issue to her colleagues at the next "Intergroup" meeting, a combined North American clinical trials group effort to test promising new therapies. She and Lesley agreed to have further discussions with Joe Pater at NCIC. That was all anyone could promise.

"Let's all pray that, as a result of today's meeting, DPPE finally gets the chance it deserves," I intoned as the session finally came to an end.

"I think we all agree with you that DPPE deserves a chance but, unfortunately, prayers are not always answered. I pray every day for world peace, but so far...." Dr. Kaplan replied somewhat pessimistically, raising his arms in a shrug as his voice trailed off. What a downer. Yet, I knew all too well what he meant. Suddenly my gloom was back.

CHAPTER SEVENTY-ONE:
That's Life

For a variety of reasons, 2003 is a year I would rather forget. Life's trials and tribulations are often best put into perspective after the fact, when the emotions of the moment give way to thoughtful contemplation. Still, all I can say about that twelve-month span is that a series of negative events, especially the loss of people so very dear to me, overshadowed any good that occurred.

For starters, like Richard Kaplan's prayers for world peace, mine for DPPE remained, in the main, unanswered. My forebodings at the end of our meeting with him and his colleagues were not without merit, as Dr. Kaplan soon left the NCI and moved to the U.K. When I tried to contact Jeff Abrams, he never returned my calls. So much for my hope that the NCI would help us.

Furthermore, Kathy garnered no interest from her colleagues in the Intergroup to carry out the new phase three study, FDA-approved or not. Nor, apparently, did the NCIC change its mind. DPPE was off their agenda. Despite this, and to his great credit, David Allan's commitment to DPPE continued to be resolute. He had given up on drug companies and was now knocking on the doors of financial institutions around the globe, trying to raise private capital. With enough money, he told financiers, he could hire a contract research organization (CRO), a professional FDA-approved outfit to provide the stringent oversight needed to conduct the clinical trial. Yet, it was a tough sell. Indeed, YM's very future was at stake. After a successful IPO on the Toronto Stock Exchange, the company's market cap slowly dwindled in the absence of any news that might entice buyers and prevent sellers.

YM's gyrations did not stop there. Nic called to say that he was leaving to join another company. I had known for some time that he was restless and that his patience was often sorely tested. He had often confided that working for David Allan was not easy. There was also tension in the office, fueled by ever-increasing shouting matches between the CEO and David Harper. Yet Nic's confirmation of something that I knew would happen sooner rather than later still hit hard. He had been a good friend and ally, and had worked tirelessly to promote DPPE. A bright young man with a promising future, his move, while difficult for YM and me, made perfect sense in terms of his career development. I could only wish him well. We promised to keep in touch.

Nic's departure was soon followed by agony over Lyonel. Athletic and trim, my friend and mentor had experienced tiredness and some mild shortness of breath after a strenuous workout on the tennis court the previous summer. "You are seventy-six and trying to keep up with guys less than half your age. Maybe it's time to slow down a little," Esther had counseled her jock of a husband. He followed her advice but the weakness wouldn't go away. Over the next few months he noticed that he was losing weight and that his once strong muscles were melting away.

Medical consultations and neurological exams followed. A chest x-ray showed some fluid around the heart, a sign of possible heart failure. What was going on here? Blood test after blood test came back normal. Soon he regularly came to discuss his health concerns with me in my office, just across the hall from his. "You know my biggest fear, don't you?" he said one day. I slowly nodded in the affirmative. Always the brilliant diagnostician, he believed that he might have a rare malignant blood disorder called amyloidosis, a condition that two decades earlier had killed his older brother, Monty. Amyloid,[148] produced by certain cancerous immune cells, fills the bloodstream. From there, it slowly but tenaciously accumulates in vital body tissues and organs, disrupting their normal function.

Not long afterwards, a biopsy confirmed that his diagnosis was all too accurate. Moreover, he had a particularly virulent form of amyloidosis that was attacking both his heart and nervous system. All of the symptoms were now explainable. "It is better to have a good disease and a bad doctor than a bad disease and a good doctor," was a droll "Lyonelism" that he had imparted to me during my training, and that I had then quoted to many others over the years. How ironic that this memorable dictum now applied to its author.

When chemotherapy and high doses of prednisone failed to slow the murderous progression of his disease, he became increasingly incapacitated, unable to walk more than a short distance without resting. Knowing he was dying, the Board of Governors of his beloved University of Manitoba bestowed upon him their highest honor, The Chancellor's Award, at the spring convocation. By then, Lyonel was much too weak to attend.

"I want to see him," I begged Esther over the phone one Saturday in early September. Among other reasons, I had a book of Einstein's essays that, ever the deep thinker, I hoped he would enjoy reading. Because of his poor stamina, visitors had been severely curtailed. "Let me ask Lyonel if he's up to seeing you," she replied. A few moments later she returned to the phone to say he was, but that I should limit my visit to thirty minutes. "I'm coming right over," I replied.

---

148 The term *amyloid* derives from the Latin word for *starch*. The suffix –*osis* means "a condition". However, the name resulted from mistaken identity. The abnormal substance is now firmly established as a protein, not starch.

An hour later, Esther and I quietly talked as we waited for him in the family room, its windows looking out on a forest of trees at the back of their large property that sloped to the edge of the Red River. It was from that very place that I had taken the call from *The Wall Street Journal* eight years previously. *Eight years? Where did the time go?* After a few minutes, Lyonel slowly made his way from the bedroom, finally settling into a chair next to the sofa where Esther was seated, opposite me. Having seen him just a month earlier, I was not prepared for the change in his appearance. His feet swollen, his voice too weak to speak more than a few words at a time, this once seemingly-invincible man struggled just to sit upright and listen as Esther and I carried the conversation about people and events that we thought might interest him.

After twenty minutes of bravely holding on, he apologized that he was tired and would have to go back to bed. Realizing that this was the last time we would be together on this earth, I stood, walked over to where he was sitting, bent down and gently hugged him. "I love you, Lyonel," I tearfully whispered into his ear. Whether too weak or simply startled, he did not respond. No matter. Nothing had been left unsaid. Two weeks later, the great man whose booming laugh could fill a room, the perpetual student whose love of knowledge framed his life, the remarkable physician and teacher who had shaped my career and those of countless others, was gone, his passing noted in major stories in local and national newspapers. "There are literally hundreds and thousands of people to whom he meant a lot," I told a reporter with the *Winnipeg Free Press*. Life would never be the same without him.

However, Lyonel's was not the only death with which I had to contend that year. Two months later came the sad news that Börje Uvnäs had died suddenly in Stockholm. Although I realized that he was ninety and had lived a long, full and productive life, his passing, like Lyonel's, hit me hard. Börje and I seemed to have a special bond that went beyond our mutual interest in histamine and growth. I respected his opinion and often sent him papers to read before they were published; he would always reply with a critique written in longhand. Yet, life and death balance out. Just a few hours before learning about Börje, Jill and I received the long-awaited news from Jason and daughter-in-law, Kathryn, that our second grandchild, Lily, had been born. Could their souls have passed in the night? To this day, when celebrating Lily's birthday, I am always reminded of my wonderful Swedish colleague.

Then there were my folks. On a visit the previous year, mom's stamina was noticeably lower, and she complained about "arthritis" in her back that hurt when she walked. Suddenly, she looked and felt much older than her eighty-one years. I was concerned and spoke to her oncologist. A bone scan subsequently revealed that she did indeed have a lot of arthritis in her spine. Unfortunately, she also had spread of the breast cancer to her bones. Naturally, she was devastated by the findings, as we all were. Dad was scared and very quiet.

I spent many an hour on the phone trying to reassure her that a new generation of estrogen blockers, called "aromatase inhibitors", might be very effective in combating the metastases, helping her to live for years rather than months. In reality, given the extent of the problem, I feared that her future was far less certain. However, as she tended to deal only in absolutes, I decided to play the game her way. "You are in no immediate danger of dying from this. There is no evidence of spread beyond the bones. I predict that you will outlive all of us," I told her forcefully.

"I don't want to outlive *you*. I just don't want to leave dad behind. He needs me. All my life, I was terrified that he would die first, leaving me alone. Now I don't want to leave him alone," she replied. It was hard to argue with her reasoning.

Despite a respite when her disease responded to treatment, recently life had taken a downward spiral for both mom and dad, she mainly as a result of depression, he from further small strokes and progressive loss of memory. Their golden years were now severely rusty. "What should we do?" my brothers asked. While there was little that could improve dad's infirmity, there was no doubt in my mind that mother needed psychiatric intervention, including antidepressant medication. Ironic, considering my research findings? Perhaps, but what choice did we have? "I would rather she live happily and possibly die sooner from her cancer than live longer in tortured misery because of untreated depression," I told my family.

It was the right decision. Slowly but surely she responded to psychotherapy and medication. Her depression and anxiety improved and the lights came back on in her life. Remarkably, dad had perked up when mom was so low. Suddenly the man who would sit in a chair all day, staring straight ahead at the TV, was on his feet tending to her needs and helping around the house. "I have to be strong for your mother," he explained in a moment of striking lucidity. Now that she was functioning again, he fell back into quiet passivity.

By the spring of 2003, mom had recovered enough for her and dad to travel to Winnipeg to spend two weeks with us. Her mood was much better and she was in no physical pain. Yet something was not right. "Oh dear, oh dear," she would continually repeat.

"What's the matter, mom?" we would ask. She didn't seem to know. In addition, her ability to understand and concentrate was deteriorating almost by the day. Was it due to her medications or something more sinister? I called her oncologist. A CT scan of the brain was arranged as soon as mom returned home.

"I'm afraid the cancer has metastasized to her brain," her doctor reported a week later. I was not at all surprised. What came first, the depression or the tumor in her right temporal lobe? Did the antidepressants play any role in the cancer suddenly spreading beyond her bones to her brain? Who could know? At this point it really didn't matter. Although a short course of radiation treatments, often prescribed in these circumstances, proved effective in shrinking the tumor, she was not able to regain the ground she lost. It was time for palliative care. Dad would stay home with hired assistants.

A few days before year's end, my brother Ken called. "I need your medical advice, doc," he lamented. I assumed it was about mother, who was sinking fast. A fighter to the end, she had stubbornly held on long after most people in her situation would have given up. However, that was not the reason for his call. Dad had developed a cold a few days earlier but seemed to be recovering. Now, he had suddenly developed a fever and become very confused. Just a month short of ninety, he normally had the constitution of a horse but something was very wrong.

"Take him to the hospital emergency room. It could be pneumonia," I answered. A few hours later, Ken called again. Dad had been admitted to the ward, apparently with a mild heart attack. "His blood work and cardiogram definitely indicate some heart damage but his blood pressure is good and there is no obvious pneumonia or heart failure," the consulting physician explained to me. Despite the encouraging medical report, dad did not rally. His balance was off. He just lay in bed with his eyes shut and refused any sustenance.

"Dad, it's important that you eat and drink to regain your strength," I urged over the phone. *No answer.*

"Dad?"

"Yes?"

"Do you hear me?"

"Yes." *Silence.*

"Dad, are you depressed?"

"Yes."

"Is it because of mom?"

"Yes."

"Promise me you'll hang in there. I'm flying home to see you and mom in two days."

"Okay."

"Dad, I love you."

"I love you too, doll."

Those were the last words he ever spoke to me. I arrived to find my parents in the final hours of their lives. Incredibly, they

both died on the same day, mother finally succumbing peacefully
to the inevitable, and dad....well.... obviously he didn't want to
stick around without his partner of sixty-two years. Although
unconscious, and lying in two separate hospitals at opposite ends
of town, somehow they must have signaled one another that it
was time to go. As tough as it was for our family to endure, their
leaving this earth together was the right thing to do....romantic,
really. They were a team in life and remained so in death.

That neither would be around to gush with pride if their
"Whaddat?" boy succeeded with DPPE, was one of many reasons
to mourn their passing. Their tears of pride the day we signed the
licensing agreement with Bristol-Myers and their distress when
the drug was dropped will forever remain fixed in my mind. They
so desperately wanted to be there if, and when, "it" finally happened. I could only hope that there really is a great beyond and,
if so, they would know. Of one thing I *was* sure: it was good rid-
dance to 2003.

CHAPTER SEVENTY-TWO:

Jekyll And Hyde

For the first three years of our association, my only contact with David Allan was by telephone. The first call was actually initiated by Nic Stiernholm several months after the licensing agreement was signed. "Are you serious?" he replied incredulously when I told him that YM's CEO and I had never talked, let alone met. David called me shortly thereafter, apologizing for not speaking with me sooner. He then congratulated me on my scientific achievement, promising that he would do everything within his power to bring DPPE to market. "You'll be nominated for the Nobel Prize if you're right," he predicted. *Nobel Prize?? Wouldn't that shock all those grants panels!!* I thanked him for his faith in me and we wished one another well.

Subsequent discussions were not always so pleasant. My next call to him, instigated by David Harper, ended in the shouting match over Allan's plan to ask the FDA to approve DPPE based on the head-scratching survival results of MA.19. Later, after cooling down, I concluded that I was not without sin, having contributed significantly to the acrimony. I called him back the following week to patch things up. Happily, his response was calmer, agreeing that we both had flown off the handle, and apologizing for his part in the verbal mêlée. "He's not such a bad guy," I thought.

Nonetheless, doubt about that conclusion resurfaced from time to time. For example, late one Friday afternoon, apparently working alone in his office, David e-mailed me an urgent request. Could I fax him several of my early journal articles right away? He needed them for a presentation he was preparing. Unfortunately, I was only able to come up with two of the papers and called to tell him of my limited success. Rather than a "thank you for your effort", he coolly brushed me off for coming up short. I was very upset, but said nothing.

"Try dealing with him *every day*," Paul Keane replied when I told him about the episode, adding that neither he nor David Harper ever received credit for contributing to YM's success. "And this is a man who got his start selling dodgy mining stocks to old widows," Paul commented derisively on more than one occasion.

"One moment he's Dr. Jekyll, the next, Mr. Hyde. You just never know which you'll get," Nic once told me. Within months of joining the company, Vince Salvatori came up with his own diagnosis: "David is a control freak. Even if you know he doesn't have a clue what he's talking about, you quickly learn not to argue with him or your job could be on the line," he confided. Yet, there could be a positive side to the man. "David Allan? He's absolutely brilliant and dynamic. I certainly would want him on the board of any company of mine," declared the usually insightful Henry Friesen who, coincidentally, sat on YM's Board of Directors.

So there you have it. There were no neutral opinions. In the years that followed, depending on whether I encountered Henry Friesen's "brilliant and dynamic" Dr. Jekyll, or Vince Salvatori's infuriating "control freak", Mr. Hyde, my feelings about YM's CEO fluctuated wildly. Dealing with him was akin to riding a bucking bronco. *Will the real David Allan please stand up?*

For example, almost exactly three years after licensing DPPE, the Jekyll in David Allan truly shone forth. In two separate deals, he raised forty million dollars from Wall Street and Canadian institutional investors.[149] The money was publicly earmarked to fund the phase three DPPE study. He no longer needed a drug company to move DPPE ahead. The accomplishment represented a truly large feather in his cap. Not that he did it entirely alone. By that time, the MA.19 results had been published in the ever-influential *JCO*, lending a degree of credibility to DPPE that potential investors could not ignore. Moreover, a series of slick presentations in New York and Toronto boardrooms by Paul Keane and Mark Vincent helped cement interest. "If the results you see in these graphs are confirmed to be true, tesmilifene will represent the greatest advance in cancer treatment we have seen in the last fifty years," Mark reportedly told the wide-eyed crowd of suits.

When I found out about the deals on the newswires (*given my track record with "heads-ups", does that surprise anyone?*) I left David a voicemail, warmly congratulating him on his marvelous achievement. In a phone message the next day, he apologized for not telling me personally. He had been out with his staff toasting success and neglected to call. *I could identify with that.* YM would now hire a contract research organization to run the study. As there were several in the running, interviews would start almost immediately. Was I a happy camper to learn all of this? Naturally.

However, the re-emergence of Mr. Hyde soon dampened my spirits. It all came about because my three-year consulting agreement and research funding were coming to an end. I assumed a continuation of the consultancy was a given, but was nervous about the research because, as Nic told me at the inception, David simply viewed the lab money as the cost of doing business to obtain the license. Business or not, the infusion of research funding by YM had been a godsend. Although Frank and I had published two further papers on histamine's role inside cells, prior to David Allan coming on the scene we were unable to attract any new grant money. Just a few months earlier, with the cupboard

---

149 U.S. investors included SDS Merchant Funds, OrbiMed Advisors, SCO Capital Partners and Xmark Funds.

almost bare, I had no choice but to say goodbye to Patty. She had been my faithful assistant for fifteen years and the parting was painful, to say the least. Now, aside from me, Gary Queen was the only "survivor" of that *U.S. News* table-top group picture from happier times.

Then, just as the first check from YM arrived, Frank reluctantly decided to retire and move back to the United States. Although nearing seventy, he was as sharp as ever and longed to continue our work together. The problem was that his wife, Arlyne, was having increasing problems with arthritis, made more unbearable by the long, cold Manitoba winters. The couple was hoping that the more temperate climate of Gainesville, Florida, would change things for the better. For years, they had maintained a large property, complete with ranch-style home, barn, pasture and several horses, in Oakbank, a thriving bedroom community situated in the country, twenty minutes from Winnipeg. Now, keeping up the property and tending the nags was getting to be a burden.

At a going away party, hosted in the gracious old home of one of our pharmacology department colleagues, I toasted my long-suffering research partner. Saying goodbye that night put a lump in my throat. Even though we had enjoyed a good run, both of us hated to see it end. Not given to great emotional outbursts, Frank played down the whole scene, although, over a beer, allowed that he would "definitely miss the heartburn". After all these years, I would once again carry the research ball solo, assisted by Gary.

Influenced by the continuing skepticism over how my drug "really worked" and the recent data suggesting that it only helped patients with aggressive tumors, I made the decision that we would reluctantly turn our attention away from histamine and use YM's money to further investigate DPPE's mechanism of action. For the first two years, our progress was painfully slow. Many leads were followed only to be abandoned. That's how it is with research. Finally, Gary and I appeared to hit on something potentially important. Remember how DPPE affected the level of prostaglandins? New experiments showed that it caused a related substance, abbreviated 12-S-HETE,[150] to go up or down in our trusty MCF-7 breast cancer cells.

Other researchers had shown that, when produced in large amounts, this particular chemical causes breast and other cancers to grow more rapidly and to spread. On the other hand, turning off the production of 12-S-HETE causes breast cancer cells to die. Since DPPE sped up cancer growth in mice and rats while increasing the killing effect of chemotherapy, maybe an up or down effect on this substance could explain its ability to help doxorubicin take out aggressive cells. And guess what natural substance was reported to potently stimulate cells to produce 12-S-HETE? That's right. Even then, we were never far from histamine!!

As I had heard nothing about a renewal of my consultancy, let alone research funding, I e-mailed David Allan directly in October, 2003:

"David, I have discussed with you previously my desire to maintain a consulting contract with you, as well as to receive further monies to continue to fund our laboratory investigations on DPPE mechanisms. Recently, I have spent considerable time reviewing YM's breast cancer patents and responding to patent reviewers' criticisms for Michael Stewart....I....believe that my advice and insights should continue to be remunerated. Even if you can't commit new monies towards my research at the moment, I hope you agree that my work for you is mutually beneficial, important to any success at the end of the road, and worthy of payment via a new consulting agreement. I look forward to your reply."

He did not answer me. Nervous, I contacted Vince, who e-mailed back that he would speak to YM's CEO on my behalf. It didn't seem to work. "He'll get back to you eventually," was all Vince could muster. The silence continued.

---

150 Forget the "S". HETE stands for "hydroxyeicosatetraenoic acid". Try saying the word rapidly ten times....or maybe just once. Now you know why the abbreviation is used.

Finally, in early December, David wrote to offer me a one-year extension, at no increase, of my consulting agreement. *One year? My previous contract had been for three.* As for research funding, I would have to precisely outline "timelines and deliverables". It was painfully obvious that he was speaking as a businessman who knew precious little about science. *Timelines? Deliverables? Who can guarantee timelines and deliverables in research??* Moreover, given YM's vastly-improved cash position, and with the new trial likely to take at least three years to complete, I viewed the offer of a one year renewal to be incomprehensible, an unwelcome irritant. In a long e-mail to Vince, I outlined my new research plan, complete with budget estimate, made what I thought was a strong case for a three-year consulting agreement, including a raise, and asked him to present the package to David.

"He won't go for it, cuz," Vince reported by phone the day after I got home from Florida. Jill and I had gone to Pompano Beach to recuperate from the trauma of burying my parents.

"What won't he go for?" I questioned.

"Well, for starters, he won't go for a three-year consulting agreement. In fact, he won't go for three years, period."

"Are you serious?" I asked in stunned amazement.

"I'm afraid so." *Nervous laugh*

"Vince, you tell him that I'll back off the raise, but my request for three years is non-negotiable."

"Lorne, why not just go with the one year he's offered?"

"And after that? What? Nothing??" I asked skeptically.

"Come on. I'm sure he'll renew it year to year. I mean…that's David. You know how he is. I told you before that he's a control freak. What can I say?" *Nervous laugh.*

"Look, Vince, as the inventor of DPPE and the guy who recommended that the University of Manitoba hand it over to YM for no up-front payment, I think I am owed a certain degree of respect by David Allan. I mean, if it wasn't for me, he'd have nothing. In view of the original three-year contract, a similar extension is only reasonable. In fact, I consider it *absolutely non-negotiable.*"

"Are you sure you want me to tell him that?" Vince asked, thinking I would back down.

"I said '*absolutely non-negotiable*' and I mean it," I replied. It was time to firmly stick up for myself.

"Okay. I'll talk to him, cuz. That's all I can do," Vince's nervous laugh was now more nervous than ever. "By the way, I should tell you that David Harper is no longer with the company."[151] *Why wasn't I surprised by this piece of news?*

"I know you are upset and still contending with everything that has just happened with mom and dad, but I think you have made a very big mistake," Jill warned after I hung up the phone. She was in the bedroom across the hall and had heard every loud word.

"Why? Because I stuck up for what I believe is right?" I replied, still agitated about the conversation. She shook her head.

"I know better than anyone that you deserve everything you requested, but using words such as '*absolutely non-negotiable*' with David Allan is like holding up a red flag to a bull."

"We'll see," I replied.

David Allan, a.k.a. Mr. Hyde, let me cool my heels for almost three weeks before writing a letter in which he pulled everything off the table. There would be *no* consultancy, let alone a one year renewal.: "...I must advise that we do not consider ourselves able to undertake such an extension," he wrote. I was welcome to bill by the hour for any work I did for YM.

And my research? "....we are advised that the remaining research which is required...must necessarily come from an independent source so as to allay the voiced concerns of prospective industry partners regarding validation. Accordingly, I do not see how a continued basic research role at Manitoba adds to the

---

151 I called David Harper at his home to tell him I was sorry to hear that he had left YM and to thank him for his efforts. "After all, you were the one who convinced us to license DPPE to YM," I reminded him. He laughed, sounding surprisingly relaxed for someone who had just received a pink slip (apparently he had been given a generous severance). "I haven't had to take my blood pressure medication since I left," he told me.

commercial value of the drug which is now dependent on clinical outcomes and independent validation….I recognize that this is a difficult moment…with my best personal regards…"

Jill had been deadly accurate in her assessment. The bull had gone straight for the red flag. I had been badly gored. *His best personal regards??* A cold fury spread over me as

I took the letter, tore it to shreds and threw the bits and pieces into the air. I would never dignify it with a response. Ever!!

Even if, as Jill suggested, I had committed a tactical error in my approach, what he had done, and how he had done it, was beneath contempt. *Why, that dirty rotten……! After all my hard work! Had he no decency? Had he no respect? How could he do this? And to what purpose?* Unless there was a radical change in his position, David Allan and I were through, pure and simple.

CHAPTER SEVENTY-THREE:
War And Peace (or, Money Talks)

Someone once said that countries do not have friends so much as they have interests. To some extent, the same can be said of people. Where there is a common interest, personal animosity is often put aside for the sake of the greater good. Despite our serious conflict, David Allan and I shared the same passion for DPPE to succeed. The basis for that passion may have differed somewhat but, in the end, we both wanted the same thing. Whether we liked it or not, we needed one another to accomplish our goal. Yet, it took the occurrence of another random event for us to break four months of icy silence.....

The decision to "cut me loose" had been hard on more people than me. The Monday after receiving Allan's letter, I phoned Paul Keane. He sounded horrible, his breathing wheezy. Covering the same ground as Jill, he became very emotional as he told me that this whole episode had been very hard on him. It was now clear to me what had triggered his asthma. After regaining his composure, he asked me to promise "not to make waves". In return, he would see what he could do to rectify the situation. It would take time. I called back later to check on him, only to be told that he had left the office to spend a day or two recovering at home.

Vince felt terrible about the situation, but was powerless to do anything. "It was like I told you on the phone, cuz...," was all he could say by way of explaining his inability to change the outcome. Perhaps to mollify me, he then confided that he had a similar problem with long-term commitment from YM's CEO that often left him dangling in uncertainty. "No matter what happens, there is one thing I promise you from the bottom of my heart, and that is my absolute commitment to DPPE. I will get that trial done," Vince declared on a more optimistic note. He and his colleagues had just hired a CRO called Pharm-Olam International.[152] "They are a very impressive organization, fully accredited by the FDA, with good people on board," he assured me.

Vince was right. Pharm-Olam was an excellent choice. Established only ten years earlier, the company specialized in running clinical studies in countries such as Russia and India, where they had identified a roster of excellent oncologists working in the very best facilities. India, alone, with a population of over one billion people, provided a huge reservoir of potential patients for clinical trials. More and more, the large pharmaceutical companies were turning to the Third World to test new therapies. Compared to North America, the results came in years earlier. Indeed, Bristol-Myers had used this same strategy with DPPE, rapidly accruing patients to the MA.19 study.

Even though the new trial, now officially designated YMB-1002-02 (and, unofficially, "the DEC study),[153] would include the United States and Canada, times had changed since the earlier MA.19 trial. Now, almost all patients requiring adjuvant chemotherapy after surgery for breast cancer received doxorubicin or epirubicin, making them ineligible for the new study. Even with patients who had spread of their disease at the outset, the

---

152 *"Olam"* is Hebrew for *"the world"*, designating Pharm-Olam's international presence.

153 DEC stands for DPPE/epirubicin/cyclophosphamide.

Americans, especially, were tempted to add taxanes to the mix. "I want to see DPPE work out and would love to help you, but we have too many competing protocols," Sloan-Kettering's Larry Norton explained by way of turning me down. I had worked hard for months to get him and his colleagues aboard, but to no avail.

Although disappointing, Norton's response was not a shock. While Kathy Pritchard had kindly agreed to lend her prestige to chairing the North American arm of the trial, YM and Pharm-Olam knew at the outset that they could not count on participation from many U.S. and Canadian centres and were gearing up to treat most of the patients in Eastern Europe, Russia, Georgia and India. An investigator's meeting was set to be held in Austria in March, 2004, to launch the European and Asian part of the study. There would be at least two hundred people in attendance.

"Am I invited?" I asked Paul Keane.

"No," was his short reply. Along with Vince, he would handle the presentations. It was clearly obvious that I was *persona non grata*, a sad reflection of the state of my non-relationship with David Allan and, by extension, YM. All but Vince, that is. He continued to stroke me, letting me know that he was embarrassed by my exclusion from the meeting. He promised to help smooth things over with David, but I knew it was a tough assignment. As badly as Bristol-Myers had treated me, the rift with YM hit me harder. That said, I decided to take the high road for the sake of DPPE and all those who might benefit from it.

A Texan, named Bruce Ross, was responsible for Pharm-Olam's recruitment and monitoring of North American centres for the study. "If Bruce has any questions about DPPE, he is welcome to call me," I told Vince. My offer was gratefully passed on. Soon after, Bruce e-mailed me. Within a short time we were having long phone discussions, ranging from the side effects of DPPE to the protocol itself. He obviously appreciated my help: "Isn't it the kingdom of Brunei where they pay their king each year by his weight in gold? I hope you are a very petite individual! Your support has been, and continues to be, invaluable and I appreciate it far more than my e-mails can say. I trust we will be able to meet at the [North American] investigators' meeting. It probably will be scheduled for mid-May in Toronto. If so, I owe you a quiet dinner - at the very least!" Bruce wrote on one occasion after he had called with some further questions.

"Thanks for your offer of dinner. I would be delighted to break bread with you...assuming that YM BioSciences sees fit to invite me. You had better check with Vince Salvatori on that one," I answered. He was startled by my reply.

"Why wouldn't you be invited? You're the guy who invented the drug. Who better to field questions than you?" he asked during a subsequent call. *Who indeed, my friend?*

"I agree but...well....let's just say I haven't received a formal invitation yet," I answered.

Shortly after, Vince e-mailed me, with a copy to Bruce: "Lorne, I personally want to thank you for the professional support you are giving Bruce. I know both Bruce and Paul have had great conversations with you and we do appreciate your ongoing intellectual input. As you know, they have expressed their warm welcome for your presence at the investigators' meeting on May 15 in Toronto. Our organizers will contact you in the near future and will make all of the necessary arrangements for your flights and hotel.

" I also personally look forward to seeing you at this meeting!

"Best regards,

"Vince" *Thanks, Bruce.*

A week later I was contacted from the U.K. by a young woman named Miriam Dervan. She was a professional meeting organizer who had run the Austrian session for YM and would now be doing the same in Toronto. I was instantly smitten by her Irish charm. "Oh, Dr. Brandes. I am *so* looking forward to meeting you. It's like....I've never met an inventor before, you know?" I assured her I would introduce myself.

"Now don't you be forgettin'. I'll be at the welcoming table as you come in the door," she added with that lovely Irish lilt of hers. *Ah, tut, tut, tut.*

Then, two days before the Toronto meeting, I received an unexpected call from Paul Keane. A series of technical questions had been posed to YM by an influential Canadian financial analyst, David Martin of Dundee Securities, that only I could answer. David Allan would be very grateful if I could provide the requested information. Paul's call was quickly followed by a list of Martin's queries attached to an e-mail from Vince:

"Lorne,

"We will need to send him the answers in writing. Can you please compile your answers to these questions and send them to Paul or I [sic].

"Obviously, we would be happy to pay for the time spent on this important information." *Really? Hm-m-m-m.*

By their very nature, random events do not occur by the clock. Luckily, this one could not have come at a more opportune moment. If ever there was a lever with which to renegotiate my consulting agreement, this was it. David Allan may not have appreciated *my* needs, but I certainly understood *his*. And *his* needs were the solution to *my* problem.

In the end, it was, indeed, all about money. More specifically, it was about market cap. The higher YM's share price went, the more bargaining power David had to make deals. Now, with a clinical trial underway that would cost him millions, he was desperate not to have his company's shares continue to languish at the two dollar (or lower) mark at which they had traded on the Toronto and London Stock Exchanges for most of the previous three years. He had recently filed papers with the S.E.C. as a prelude to having YM's stock trade in New York, preferably on the NASDAQ although, in the end, he would settle for the AMEX. If he could get the David Martins of the financial world to buy into the DPPE story and recommend an "outperform" rating on YM's stock, who knew how high it might go? David would be attending the Toronto meeting. It was time for us to finally meet.

"Cuz, when you get to the hotel, come over to the bar. I'm hard to miss. I'll introduce the two of you," Vince offered.

"Perfect," I replied. There would be no tactical error this time. *Fool me once, shame on you; fool me twice, shame on me.*

Sure as Irish spring, Miriam was at the meeting registration desk as I checked in. *Gads!* She was an absolute stunner!!! After warmly hugging the inventor, she pointed out where the bar area was located. Looking across the lobby, I immediately spotted Vince. He was right about not missing him. The bright orange short-sleeved shirt he was sporting on his robust frame made sure of that. Sitting with him at a table were three other men.

"Join us," Vince warmly greeted as he introduced me to John Hovre, Pharm-Olam's VP, and two other members of his team. Soon, a slim executive, well-dressed in an expensive suit and designer shirt with red stripes and open white collar, walked over to our table. His skin was tanned and his thick grey hair carefully coiffed. Having never seen me before, he didn't know who I was. I was under no such disadvantage. Over the years, David Allan's handsome face had appeared in the financial pages. "Hello, David. I'm Lorne Brandes. Nice to meet you at long last," I said with a smile, standing up to shake his hand. For a split second he rocked back on his heels, looking a bit unsure of what was to come next.

"Lorne," he repeated my name. "Would you like a drink?" he offered, quickly recovering as he sat down.

"That would be great," I answered, giving my order to the waiter.

For the next half hour we traded stories and had a few good laughs, each thinking that maybe the other wasn't so bad after all. Hopefully, the melting ice wasn't just in our drinks.

"I need to speak to you, Vince," I said as I caught him alone in the hallway just before dinner.

"Sure. What's up?" my friend inquired.

"I'll be happy to answer the questions that David Martin has submitted."

"Good. Good," Vince nodded, smiling but not really making eye contact as he kept looking around for any new arrivals. *He doesn't see what's coming.*

"However, I am not prepared to bill by the hour."

"Meaning?" he replied, now looking me directly in the eye.

"Meaning I want my consulting fee back....in full."

Suddenly, no longer smiling, his forehead beaded up with perspiration.

"Lorne, come on..."…..silence….then, "Geez, I just don't think David will go for it." His head was now shaking slowly from side to side to emphasize the point.

"Well, I guess he'll have to decide how important it is that I answer the questions," I replied evenly, not wishing to be the first to blink. "And Vince, tell him that as time goes on there will be more analysts with more questions that only I can answer. Capice?"

"Okay. I'll talk to him." *He blinked!*

The food and wine that evening were terrific. As a combo played jazz in the corner, the gorgeous Miriam, now in a shimmering long white strapless evening dress slit up the side for good measure, flirtatiously hopped from table to table, welcoming one and all to the meeting. Everyone enjoyed her "attention", including the inventor, for whom there was another hug. The smell of her sublime perfume lingered on my cheek. *Maybe we should have her organize the yearly histamine meetings!* From the fixed smile on David Allan's face, I also suspected that Vince was saving the less happy news of my demand until the next day. As soon as we met, Bruce Ross and I embraced warmly and, as promised, broke bread over dinner. David and other members of his YM team sat across the table from us.

During dinner, Paul Keane came to me with the news that Kathy Pritchard could not chair the next day's session; her aunt died and she had to attend the funeral. Would I be willing to fill in by presenting a talk and fielding questions about DPPE? "I'll be happy to help out in any way I can," I replied in full diplomatic mode. It had been a good day and, now, a good evening. Bit by bit, things were going my way. Sleep came easily that night.

The next morning, everyone got down to business as Bruce reviewed the protocol. Taking it all in from his seat near the front of the room was David Allan, looking like he should be on the cover of GQ. Bruce made it clear in his introduction that this study was possibly the most important with which he had been involved over the years. "If we have a positive outcome in this trial, as I hope and believe we will, the potential application of DPPE to many other forms of cancer causes me great excitement," he exclaimed. He clearly saw the big picture. *Now if only he was right!*

As the morning progressed, there were quite a few questions about the side effects of DPPE. Although Paul provided some of the answers, he deferred more and more to me. After all, in total, I had by far the lion's share of experience with the drug. When one of the investigators expressed some nervousness about the hallu-cinations, I quickly calmed her, explaining their transient nature and the cartoon characters that were often reported to us. "Believe me when I tell you that what the patients may see or hear during their DPPE treatment gives them a chuckle," I answered in a reas-suring tone of voice. Everyone, including David Allan, chuckled at my answer. And so it went.

The meeting finally wrapped up at four o'clock. As the last of our departing visitors shook hands with me, Vince came to my side. "I need you to come with me right away," he said somewhat tensely, immediately leading me away from the others into an adjoining empty ballroom containing many round tables that were being set up for an event that evening. Sitting quietly at one of them was YM's now tieless CEO. As Vince closed the double doors for privacy, David and I exchanged a few perfunctory pleas-antries about how well the meeting went. A few seconds later, it was time to address our "problem".

"I understand you have something you want to discuss," he said matter-of-factly. As he listened pensively, I wasted no time in telling him what I had told Vince. After I finished, he remained quiet for a few long seconds. Then, slowly nodding his assent, he capitulated. A new consulting agreement would be prepared for me to sign. It would not be limited to a year. Vince obviously had convinced his boss about what he must do before I came into the room. We were just going through the motions....pro forma, as they say. I glanced over at Vince, sending him a silent thank you. *Good work, paesan.* He just smiled, looking pleased with himself.

Our outstanding business settled, David complimented me on my "performance" at the meeting. Then, with Chiron obviously still on his mind, he lectured me on the importance of always being tolerant and courteous when dealing with drug companies or others important to YM's fortunes. While assuring him that I would take his advice to heart, I could not let the moment pass without pointing out that he hadn't exactly cornered the market on perfection. "Not perfect? ME?" he exclaimed dramatically as he put his hands across his chest, bursting into laughter. Vince and I joined him. At that moment, the truce was signed.[154] Peace was at hand. I would now have to work on the research funding, but that was for another day.

---

154 Did I forgive him? Yes. Would I forget what he did? Never!

CHAPTER SEVENTY-FOUR:

Eye On The Ball

My dad was an all-around athlete who loved golf. I remember him spending long summer evenings in our back yard, pitching wedge in hand, effortlessly lofting golf balls through the air with deadly accuracy. He kept trying to teach his oldest son the tricks of the trade. "You took your eye off the ball!" he would constantly admonish as I flubbed or sliced my shots over the white picket fence into our neighbor's flower garden. I never developed his talent for the game, but learned the valuable lesson that, in life as in golf, to succeed you have to keep your eye on the ball. Somebody forgot to do that at the startup of YM's new study.

It was very important to David Allan that the DPPE trial commence by "the end of the first quarter" of 2004. He had set that date in stone in all of the company's news releases. It was all about showing potential investors that YM could set goals and meet them. While the March investigators' meeting in Austria was the official trial launch for countries outside of North America, the regulatory agencies in most places were still assessing the protocol; no patients in a given country could be treated until a go-ahead was received from its regulators. In many cases, that would take a few more months. However, truth be told, countries varied widely in the stringency of their assessment. Possibly for that reason, Serbia had already given its approval to proceed.

On March 31, 2004, a press release appeared on the financial news wires: "*YM BioSciences Doses First Patient In Pivotal Breast Cancer Study.* 'We are very pleased to have commenced this important trial on time, and anticipate to have completed enrolment in approximately 18 months,' said Mr. David Allan, Chairman and CEO of YM BioSciences." So there it was. Serbia had helped him keep his promise. It didn't matter that no further recruits came aboard until several weeks later (as I said, regulatory approval often moves slowly). In business, appearances are everything. To be fair to David, it *was* an important milestone… no different than the milestone of that i.v. bag containing DPPE when I treated my first patient all those years ago. It's just that, whether for research or clinical trials, I was uncomfortable about setting "timelines and deliverables" to please investors.

Three months later, in June, I spoke with Vince. "You sound tired and harassed," I commented to my friend, noting the weary sound of his voice.

"Don't ask," he replied.

"What's the matter?"

"I've spent the last two weeks with almost no sleep. David didn't want this to get out, but I'm going to tell you anyway." He went on to explain that there had been a manufacturing error. Each vial of DPPE was supposed to contain five hundred milligrams of the drug, as stated on the label. After the first seven women had been entered into the study, Craig Binnie, YM's clinical products director, somehow discovered that the vials contained only four hundred and thirty milligrams. By that calculation, the first three or four patients randomized to the DPPE arm of the study had been underdosed by just under fifteen percent…not a huge amount, but a serious glitch nonetheless. As a result, the trial had screeched to a necessary halt until the problem was rectified.

According to Vince, the apoplectic David Allan immediately pointed the accusatory finger at everyone, finally settling on poor Craig (despite the fact that he had uncovered the error and brought it to everyone's attention) and Pharm-Olam, the trial's overseers. My take was that the Italian company that manufactured DPPE for the trial had taken *its* eye off the ball. They were the same contractor that had supplied the five hundred milligram vials of DPPE to Bristol-Myers Squibb.

"So was the DPPE dose also wrong in the MA.19 trial?" I inquired.

"No, we checked that. It's only this new batch where the potency is wrong. What can I tell you? *Nervous laugh.* I've been in touch with every site and all the regulators. We need to relabel all the vials and apply for a regulatory amendment in every country. This is probably going to delay us for at least two months." *I'll say it will!*

I decided to call David Allan. Although I was not surprised that he had failed to be more forthcoming, I was sympathetic to his plight. "Just be thankful that this was discovered very early on. After all, only a very few women[155] have received the underdose, and even there it can be corrected in subsequent cycles of treatment," I told him. While he agreed with my assessment, I could tell from the sound of his voice that he still had smoke coming out his ears. The delay while things were set straight would make his next "deliverable" difficult, if not impossible, to achieve: he had promised the financial community that, by the end of 2004, two hundred patients would be on the study.

Next, a nurse in Serbia took her eye off the ball. Actually, she may never have had it on the ball in the first place. "We have had our first SAE," Bruce Ross reported to me. By this, he meant "Serious Adverse Event". In any clinical trial, a non-critical side effect or mishap is referred to as an "AE" or "adverse event". Each

---

155 Because of the mistake, these patients would have to be assessed separately from the remainder of the women in the trial who received the correct dose of DPPE from the beginning.

is noted and recorded. If, for example, following a treatment a patient develops an itchy rash that lasts a few days, an AE is recorded and catalogued under "drug-related skin toxicity" or, perhaps, "drug-related allergic reaction", or both. If, two weeks after a treatment, a patient accidentally trips and falls while shopping at the supermarket, breaking an arm in the process, the event is still logged as an AE, even if the event is judged to be "non-drug-related".

An SAE is on a whole different level. After all, serious means *serious*. In this case, the nurse had mistakenly given a patient *ten times* the proper dose of DPPE!!

"Did she die?" I asked, holding my breath.

"No. But she had a convulsion from which she quickly recovered," Bruce replied. *Whew!!* There were no after-effects except in the nurse, who remained shaken and horribly upset by her potentially lethal mistake. "Just like those mice," I replied, telling Bruce the story about the famous trio of somersaulters. As a result of what had happened, he was now working on a stricter monitoring system whereby two people would have to check that a dose was properly calculated before any patient received a drug.

In August, I called Bruce to inform him that I had a potential candidate for the trial and to request an update on the "study numbers". Just back from Pharm-Olam's British office, he was delighted to hear the news and, as always, happy to share "non-classified" trial information, such as enrolment, with me. Despite the delay caused by the fiasco of the wrongly-labeled vials, the number of women in the study was now approaching twenty. With more and more centres coming on line in India, Russia and Eastern Europe, those numbers were set to improve dramatically. Despite this good news, I detected that Bruce's natural upbeat exuberance was wilted. I immediately asked why.

"To tell you the truth, Dr Brandes, I don't know if I'll be on this project much longer," he confessed, a sense of exasperation now clearly evident in his voice.

"Why do you say that, Bruce?" I asked, immediately worried by the thought that such a great guy would ever think of quitting.

"Dealing with YM is driving me to distraction," he replied. It turned out that Vince had been riding him hard, chastising him for his inability to sign up more U.S. and Canadian centres for the study.

Knowing how tirelessly Bruce had been working to recruit doctors, I felt this criticism to be totally unfair and told him so. Everyone knew from its inception that this trial would be mainly played out abroad. I also believed that, in turn, Vince was being pressured by David Allan to "get those numbers up".

"Vince is under a lot of stress and hasn't been himself lately," I explained.

"I suspect he tends to be a high-stress individual even when ordering dinner," Bruce drolly observed. I had to smile at that one. However, normally quick to return my calls or e-mails, I had not heard back from Vince for some weeks and was concerned about his silence.

"Oh, he's currently in Italy attending a christening and family wedding," Bruce reported.

I immediately e-mailed him, taking a light approach:

"Vince,

"I spoke with Bruce today about our first potential patient and he told me you had been with him in the U.K. and are now at the Vatican taking Cardinal lessons. Then he told me you were actually in Italy to be a godfather....or is it *The* Godfather? .... I also understand....that David Allan is up to his old tricks and giving everyone, especially you, a hard time. As they say in the Jewish section of Rome, 'Nil illegitimi carborundum.'[156] "Let's talk when you are back, whenever that is.

"Take care of yourself.

"LJB"

---

156 Latin for "Don't let the bastards wear you down".

I guess my attempt at humor was welcome. I soon heard back from him as he poured out his frustrations: "Lorne, I have to admit you put a smile on my face! Something that has been hard to do lately. There seems to be a total lack of understanding of the real drug development process and what it takes to do registration trials.[157] I am pushing myself and Pharm-Olam to the limit and it is still not good enough. The good news is that even after obvious reasons…beyond my control we are now back on track…I know that no one in the company has ever done this [or] realizes the effort necessary for success….unfortunately there [are] always such negative forces which are totally unnecessary from many individuals. Rest assured that this will be done with them or without them and I will continue to make sure we will be success-ful with the product you have created…

"Best regards,

"Vince".

Finally, when everything seemed to be settling down, a November e-mail from Paul Keane suggested to me that YM had taken *its* eye off the ball. In an attempt to improve recruitment of patients into the trial, the company now wanted to include women with "bone disease only". *WHAT???* I immediately suspected that the adherence to "timelines and deliverables" and the promise to accrue two hundred patients by the end of 2004 meant that the rules were about to be changed, and not in a good way. Now it was my turn to be driven to distraction, believing that such a move was poorly-conceived and could actually backfire.

Reaching for the phone, I called Vince at home on a Sunday evening. "I hear you are changing the protocol to include women whose only measurable disease is in bone."

"That's right. We hope that including them will help us with our accrual," he responded.

"Vince, since you pay me as a consultant, I assume you want my advice."

---

157 A registration trial is the final one that, if positive, usually leads to regu-latory approval of the drug.

"Of course, cuz," he answered.

"Okay, then. I want you to listen to me carefully. Patients with breast cancer that spreads *only* to the bones *live much longer* on average than patients whose cancer spreads to vital organs such as the lungs or liver. That is a well-known fact. If you don't believe me, check the medical literature. If YM wants an early resolution to the survival question, the *worst* possible thing is to include patients with bone disease only. That will likely *delay*, rather than expedite the very answer you are seeking. *So the bottom line is, don't do it.*"

Vociferously thanking me, Vince promised to discuss the matter with Paul first thing after the weekend. Taking no chances, I decided to e-mail Paul directly about my concerns. On Monday morning, he responded by forwarding replies that he had previously obtained from Kathy Pritchard, Lesley Seymour and Mark Vincent. None had a major objection to the issue of "bone-only" disease.

"Perhaps you could have discussed it with me before proposing this," I told him over the phone. Although very disturbed that I appeared to be the only one not consulted prior to this decision, I restrained myself as I quietly reiterated why I believed the others were wrong and the change was counter-productive. Paul did not appear moved by my argument.

"At the very least, are you planning to discuss this issue with the FDA?" I asked

"I don't think we need to," Paul replied.

"Now, I think that's a *big mistake!*" I countered. YM's study had been given Special Protocol Assessment status by the FDA and Paul did not feel the need to inform them of the change? It didn't take a rocket scientist to see the potential folly in this. In my opinion, changing the rules without consultation could cause problems for YM with the regulatory agency. Paul replied that he did not share my concern. "I guess you and I will have to agree to disagree," I stated for the record before hanging up.

What was it with these guys?? What they didn't know about oncology could fill text books. That aside, I couldn't understand why Kathy or Lesley hadn't given YM the same advice. It wasn't as if *they* didn't know the facts pertaining to survival and "bone-only" metastasis. Mark could be more easily forgiven. He was an oncologist, but did not treat breast cancer.

I decided to e-mail Kathy. After all, she was chairing the trial for North America.

"Are you okay with YM's proposal to include patients with bone disease only? Paul Keane tells me that they don't plan to discuss this with the FDA. You and I know that virtually no metastatic breast cancer study includes bone-only disease....we are measuring survival as the primary end point, but survival is significantly longer in bone-only patients. If they want an early answer on survival, that should work against them. I have told this to Paul, but he feels that they should include these...patients to speed up accrual. I look at this as quantity vs. quality and am unhappy. I would appreciate your candid opinion on this issue."

Her reply stunned me: "I think it will be okay. We can still measure time to progression ....as well as survival." *Time to progression? Could she not see the issue here?*

"But don't you think it needs to be passed by the FDA?" I e-mailed back, frantically hoping that the regulators, at least, would see the problem and nix the idea.

This time, my persistence paid off. "I think it might not be a bad idea," she replied.

A short time later, Kathy e-mailed Paul and his colleagues: "Do you think we should be running the bone lesion business by the FDA?"

The next morning, an e-mail arrived from Paul. The decision to include women with bone-only disease was revoked! Kathy's one-liner had apparently accomplished what my lengthy reasoned arguments could not. Although pleased with the about-face, I was ticked off by the lack of respect for my experience and knowledge. Why should Kathy's words carry more weight with YM than mine?

Dad: "Don't let it get to you, son. The important thing is that you kept your eye on the ball. That's what made the difference in the end."

Me: "Thanks, dad. I guess I was a better student of the game than you thought!"

CHAPTER SEVENTY-FIVE:

The Meeting

On December 2, 2004, I flew to Toronto for a meeting at the offices of YM BioSciences. A "scientific day" had been arranged for several investigators, including me, to present their latest laboratory findings. Things were heating up on the DPPE front in other labs as well as mine. I thought the idea of bringing everyone together at the same table was a good one, sure to foster new information, ideas and, hopefully, collaboration. According to Paul, in a change of business strategy for the company, YM would consider funding research.

Gary and I had spent the previous week putting together our data connecting DPPE to 12-S-HETE, the cancer-stimulating chemical related to the prostaglandins. Not only were the HETE levels in MCF-7 cancer cells affected by DPPE, increasing or decreasing depending on the concentration of drug added to the cell cultures, they were similarly altered in the blood of patients who received the drug with chemotherapy, an indicator of a potentially important biological effect. I was getting excited that, at long last, we were really onto something. A thorny issue with

YM had been our lack of publishable findings despite the infusion of funding over the previous three years. I could not argue that point, but was now optimistic that, after a lot of hard work, we had something of substance to put on the table.

My enthusiasm wasn't a solo act. Igor Sherman, YM's new director of clinical research and scientific affairs seemed genuinely impressed with the preliminary data I had sent him. Born and schooled in Ukraine, Igor immigrated to Canada, obtaining his PhD at the University of Toronto. Before joining YM, he had spent many years with big pharma, including AstraZeneca.

"Dear Lorne," he wrote, "… I think these are fantastic results and indeed may be the explanation of the mechanism of tesmilifene action…Furthermore, if your hypothesis is correct, which I suspect it is, it could form a basis of an invention and a patent, (e.g., selecting 12-HETE-overexpressing malignancies for therapy, expanding product claim to all tumors with elevated 12-lipoxygenase[158] levels, etc.); thus you should be careful with further disclosure. Best regards, Igor."

His effusive e-mail prompted me to reply:

"Thanks Igor.

"I agree with you that this may be an extremely important finding.…laboratory research can often be slow and plodding, with fallow periods when nothing seems to pan out. Then a spark ignites new excitement. This appears to be one of those times. I hope we can continue to pursue the 12-S-HETE story with YM's help."

Arriving at the Sheraton in mid-afternoon, the desk clerk informed me that the ever-generous Vince had reserved a deluxe room for me, complete with access to an executive suite down the hall that provided a tended bar and plenty of hors d'ouvres.

---

158 12-lipoxygenase is an enzyme that forms 12-S-HETE by removing a molecule of oxygen specifically at "the 12 position" of a fatty-acid (lipid) precursor; hence its name. 12-S-HETE also may be formed by a P450 enzyme called 4B1. We had never assessed the effect of DPPE and histamine on either 12-lipoxygenase or 4B1.

To top off the event's social calendar, David Allan had invited the participants and selected guests, including Kathy Pritchard; Mark Vincent; Igor; YM's European operations director, Dr. David Kennard; and prominent researcher and YM scientific advisor, Dr. Bob Kerbel, to dinner at his home that night. As David was reputed by Vince to be a good and attentive host, I was looking forward to the evening. "I rented a limo to take us," Vince announced as we headed out the hotel lobby. *Limo?*

Parked in front, doors swung open, was one of those outrageous black stretched "Elvis-mobiles". It had dark tinted glass, wrap-around leather seats, a side-bar stacked with cheap plastic champagne glasses, a ceiling-mounted stereo, a small TV with an unwatchable grainy picture and, studding the gaudy interior, scores of tiny lights that kept changing color. It was truly tacky, a brothel on wheels. The driver was so far forward, we couldn't see or hear him as he asked for directions. Glancing at the beaming Vince as he settled into the back seat next to me, I exclaimed, "You really *are* 'The Godfather'!"

Forty-five minutes later we arrived in Toronto's fashionable Rosedale district. Thousands of Christmas bulbs twinkled on homes and trees, lighting up the crisp late fall night. The joyous season was definitely upon us. Multimillion-dollar mansions, interspersed with more modest dwellings, lined the beautiful old streets; David, who lived in one of the former, greeted us as we walked through his large glassed front door into the gracious foyer. While his big mutt not-so-discreetly sniffed us, our host hung the coats in the closet. "My late wife had a great eye for color and design," he explained as we admired the eclectic mix of furnishings and warmly-painted walls on which hung expensive artwork. Two years earlier, her life had been tragically cut short by smoking-related lung cancer.[159]

As we sat in front of the burning logs in his fireplace, drinks in hand, Kathy came breezing into the living room. "Sorry I'm a bit

---

159 Ironically, her father had been chairman of the Canadian subsidiary of tobacco giant, Philip Morris.

late," she apologized breathlessly as everyone stood to greet her. "I agreed with you about the bone issue," she whispered in my ear as we exchanged a hug. I silently nodded my appreciation. She always tried to do the right thing.

"Dinner is served," David soon commanded, leading the way to the adjoining narrow dining room, its heavy long wooden table covered with starched linen and expertly set with beautiful china and expensive silverware. He had hired a small catering firm to prepare the food and wait on the guests. I was placed at the head of the table, to David's right and to Igor's left. Kathy perched at the opposite end, just in front of an impressive oversized antique armoire set against the wall. Wine flowed as we consumed the delicious fare. Through it all, David was the perfect host, warm and smiling with good stories to tell. "Such noise," he joked at one point, holding his ears as the volume of conversation and laughter rose by several decibels. There was no doubt about it; when at his best, he could be totally charming.

Perhaps his mellowness that night also reflected satisfaction with YM's increasing stature in the biotech world. Indeed, I believed David had good reason to be pleased with himself on several fronts. Although he would not meet his two hundred patient goal by the end of the month, if one also counted those who were going through the screening process, that mark had been achieved on a technicality.[160] In any event, two hundred women definitely would be on study by the end of January as new sites were activated. To add to his happiness, financial analyst David Martin had been impressed with "the DPPE story". I assumed that my four pages of answers to his questions helped him reach that conclusion. As a result, Dundee Securities initiated coverage of YM stock with a "Buy/Outperform" rating. "*A Solid Shot at Success*" was the title of the report. Dundee was not alone. Several other "Buy" endorsements by financial analysts in Canada, the U.S. and Britain soon followed, causing YM's stock to

---

160 Screened patients are those who are going through the tests required to determine their eligibility. Most end up going on the study

rise by almost fifty percent within a few months. David proudly kept all of the reports neatly bound in a folder on the table in the living room.

The icing on the cake came when Frost and Sullivan, a prestigious San Francisco-based industry consulting firm, named YM BioSciences "Breast Cancer Therapies Entrepreneurial Company of the Year (2004)"!

"Should I buy YM shares?" was a question I now frequently heard from friends and relatives as YM stock went up another notch.

"Only invest what you can afford to lose," was my standard reply. Me? I resisted the temptation.

There had been one other major coup for David. He had spent a great deal of time and effort lobbying Senator Christopher Dodd of Connecticut, among other U.S. officials, to change the law (the so-called Helms-Burton embargo) to allow his Cuban drugs into the United States, where they might benefit American citizens with cancer. However, even as Congress continued to balk, David successfully petitioned the FDA to grant so-called Orphan Drug Status[161] to TheraCIM, an Erbitux-like molecule that had been discovered at the University of Havana. TheraCIM had significantly fewer side effects than its rival[162] and was starting to look like a potential winner when combined with radiation in patients with serious cancers of the head and neck, or untreatable brain tumors.

---

161 The U.S. Orphan Drug Act grants seven years of exclusive marketing rights for effective drugs that treat diseases afflicting less than 200,000 people per year. Europe has a similar act that gives ten years exclusivity. By receiving this designation for TheraCIM, David had a shot at marketing the Cuban drug in the USA.

162 Like Erbitux, TheraCIM (generic name: nimotuzumab) is a specific antibody that targets the important EGF (epidermal growth factor) receptor, present on the outer membrane of certain cancer cells. However, while Erbitux and other EGF-blocking drugs often cause a severe skin rash on the face and body, TheraCIM appeared to be free of this unsightly side effect, a definite plus. Even if competing drugs are equally effective, the marketplace usually rules in favor of the one with the better safety profile.

YM had previously licensed it in Europe to a German company, called Oncoscience, but retained the North American rights.

Next, in a brilliant deal, David had turned over the drug's U.S. rights to a San Diego company, CancerVax Corporation. Together, he and CancerVax received an historic approval from the U.S. Treasury Department to develop TheraCIM for the American market. It marked the first time a U.S. company had been allowed to license a Cuban drug.

YM would receive milestone payments and royalties if TheraCIM succeeded. Suddenly, with DPPE and TheraCIM, YM had two chances to score big-time. I was impressed. Now realizing that Henry Friesen's earlier assessment about him being "brilliant and dynamic" was absolutely valid, I went further. Whatever else he might be, David Allan was an outstanding tactician in the tricky world of biotechnology.

The following morning, we all gathered in a conference room in a building across the parking lot from YM's small offices. Following a few words of welcome from Vince and David, and an overview of DPPE by Mark Vincent, Peter Ferguson, one of Mark's research colleagues at the University of Western Ontario, held everyone's attention as he presented some riveting data. This is what he found: as I had originally observed, DPPE alone was often stimulatory to cancer cell growth in the test tube. When added to chemotherapy drugs such as doxorubicin and Taxol, DPPE only enhanced their killing of "nasty" cell-types, the ones that were MDR+ (multiple drug resistant) and contained all those P-gp pumps.

The exciting part of this was that, in Peter's experiments, the effect occurred at low concentrations of DPPE that could be achieved in patients receiving the drug. Since the Bristol-Myers lab previously showed that DPPE only blocked the pumps at much higher concentrations, it was now abundantly clear from Peter's experiments that drug resistance was being circumvented by some other mechanism, just as Rob Warrington had concluded almost ten years earlier!

Peter's data also lent great support to our already-held notion that DPPE selectively helped chemotherapy target aggressive cancers, the ones that were most likely to have large numbers of MDR+ cells. *Now the story was really starting to come together. At last, there was corroborating laboratory evidence to back up the ability of DPPE to potentiate chemotherapy and increase survival.* David Allan smiled while the rest of us nodded our approval at the significance of what had just been presented.

Next, one of Kathy's colleagues, University of Toronto researcher Eldad Zackesenhaus, presented an overview of his laboratory program. His interest was focused on a small population of so-called tumor stem cells, primitive precursors of the billions of cells that form a breast cancer. These stem cells have drug-resistant properties and likely have the potential to mutate the tumor into an aggressive, metastasizing form. He thought that the DPPE/chemotherapy treatments might specifically hone in on them, preventing the emergence of resistant disease and improving survival. If true, use of DPPE with chemotherapy early on, in the adjuvant setting, might take them out all together and be predicted to save countless lives. It was what I had been saying intuitively for years. Now there appeared to be an elegant high-tech lab approach to test this concept. *More smiles and nods around the table.*

Finally it was my turn to present the data that had so excited Igor Sherman just two weeks earlier, linking DPPE treatment to changes in the level of 12-S-HETE. Saving the most enticing findings for last, I showed the effect of DPPE to alter blood levels of 12-S-HETE in four patients with breast cancer who were receiving the drug in combination with chemotherapy: very high blood levels of 12-S-HETE dropped precipitously sixty minutes into the DPPE treatment in a lady with spread of her breast cancer to the lungs; a repeat measurement three weeks later showed the same result. On the other hand, in three patients with lower blood levels of 12-S-HETE, DPPE treatment caused a considerable *rise* in two.

Since those two, and the first lady, all seemed to be responding to the treatment, it was possible that the "up" or "down" effect of DPPE on blood levels of 12-S-HETE was an indicator of disease response. Indeed, one group of researchers had recently proposed that 12-S-HETE from tumors gets into the blood and might be monitored as a "tumor marker" in patients on treatment for active breast cancer.

To explain the variable effect of DPPE on 12-S-HETE levels in patients, I hypothesized that, because cancers are almost always made up of mixed populations of cells, perhaps how DPPE affected the 12-S-HETE level overall was determined by the proportion of aggressive cells, with their higher HETE levels, to less-aggressive cells, with their lower HETE levels. In mainly high-grade tumors, DPPE might drastically lower 12-S-HETE, whereas in lower-grade tumors, the opposite might result. "Whatever is going on here, it appears to be important," I concluded, making a pitch for badly-needed money to allow us to continue our promising work.

The presentations now ended, I glanced over at the previously-enthusiastic Igor. He was expressionless, totally silent. "We now have some tough decisions to make," Paul concluded. *Why were alarm bells going off in my head??*

CHAPTER SEVENTY-SIX:

Upsandowns

When our children were growing up, we spent every July at Wasagaming, on Clear Lake, in Riding Mountain National Park, the site of my 1994 histamine meeting. The kids loved it so much that, as adults, they made the trek with us back to the old cabin we always rented. Amazingly, it hasn't aged much over the decades. I wish I could say the same for us.

Just beyond town, the lakeside road undulates over a small hill where hundreds of rocks are embedded in the berm next to the sidewalk. A little known fact is that this "wall of stones" was a make-work project for German POWs during World War II.[163] Near the top of the hill stands an inverted V-shaped cottage signpost on which is etched "Upsandowns", a phrase that aptly described life in the first three months following the meeting.

---

163 Following capture by the Allies in North Africa, some German soldiers were shipped over the ocean to Manitoba to be interred in the park. They appear to have had it a lot easier than any of our boys who were captured by their side. Then again, the long cold prairie winter was punishment in itself, guaranteeing that anyone trying to escape should think twice about risking hypothermia and being eaten by the wolves.

A week after returning from Toronto, I called Jennifer Seibert, who had recently moved from Chicago to manage YM's intellectual properties. In addition to the fact that her ancestors sailed to America with William Penn, who founded Pennsylvania and established the Quaker faith there, I was impressed by her grasp of the issues at the scientific presentations the week before. Moreover, she appeared to be very sympathetic to my need for research funds to follow up our findings on 12-S-HETE.

"Do you think YM will fund me?" I inquired.

"I have been asked by Craig Binnie to sit on the committee[164] and hope to come up with a 'creative' way to make that happen," she assured me. While I was happy with her response, I also recognized that the word "creative" implied that she might be my only ally. After all, somebody obviously had told the previously-supportive Igor Sherman to clam up. Why? I didn't know. "I need an answer by February. My money runs out by the end of March," I told her. That was no exaggeration. Once again the gas tank was heading towards empty.

"I think we should definitely have things worked out by then," she replied. I hoped so.

Christmas/Anniversary dinner at the Russells two weeks later was, as always, wonderful. Once again the angels turned rapidly on their thin pedestal as the candle flames licked at their wings. To add to the happiness, Jason, wife Kathryn and granddaughter Lily breezed into town over the holiday. Much to our pleasure, Kathryn had recently learned that she was three months pregnant. On January 4th, the four and one-third of us celebrated Jill's birthday at La Vieille Gare (The Old Train Station), a longtime favorite restaurant in St. Boniface. Knowing that we were coming, owner Irene Kirouac was there to greet us. Many years earlier, as Lyonel's resident-in-training, I had helped care for her handsome

---

164 The committee's chairman was YM product development manager Craig Binnie, a PhD and former researcher in the field of bacterial gene cloning. He had worked for Pfizer in the U.K and, then, Cangene, a Canadian company, before joining YM.

teenaged son when he was hospitalized with acute leukemia. A bone marrow transplant failed and he succumbed to the disease. Nonetheless, she remained forever grateful for our efforts.

Two days later, Jill and I jetted to Fort Lauderdale for our annual January in Pompano Beach. Jason, Kathryn and Lily had flown home the preceding day. It was exactly one year since the double-funeral for my parents had cast a pall on our trip. This time, we were looking forward to a more relaxing and carefree vacation. It was not to be.

Arriving at our Florida destination in the early evening, we stocked up at the local Publix store and then grabbed a hamburger at a nearby restaurant. As we unlocked the door of our condo, bags of groceries and a six-pack of beer in hand, the phone was ringing. It was Carolyn. "Call Jason right away," was all she could say. We did. Sobbing as he recounted the news, our shaken son told us that his thirty-two year old wife had awakened that morning with bleeding. They had rushed to the hospital where an ultrasound examination confirmed that she had a miscarriage. It also showed a totally unexpected and serious problem in her right kidney.

"She has an appointment with a urologist tomorrow. The doctors at the hospital found a large tumor. They told us it could be cancer. We're really, really scared," Jason tearfully reported. So were we. *It's one thing to lose a baby. On top of that you learn that "you may have cancer"?* As luck would have it, the young urologist to whom they were referred was wonderfully kind, spending over an hour going over the findings and answering all of their anxious questions. When Jason told him I was an oncologist, he immediately called me.

"It looks quite suspicious for renal cell,"[165] he confided. Once CT scans were performed, he would call back. Two days later the phone rang. "The bad news is that the CT confirms the ultrasound findings. The tumor is the size of a small orange, about three inches in diameter. Unfortunately, because of its central location,

---

165 "Renal cell carcinoma" is the medical term for the usual type of cancer that affects the kidney.

we will probably have to remove the entire kidney. The good news is that it appears contained. No other abnormalities are detected on the scan." I let out a sigh of relief. Kathryn's survival depended to a major degree on the absence of spread to the major blood vessels of the kidney or beyond. Only complete surgical removal of the tumor could guarantee a shot at a cure.

Despite the sunny warm Florida days, a dark cloud hung over our heads as we waited for Kathryn's surgery. When it finally came, all went well. There were no surprises. Now we had to wait for the pathologist to examine the tissue and give a final verdict. We finally learned the news when, on our way home to Winnipeg, we stopped in Toronto to visit our daughter-in-law at the hospital. A copy of the pathology report had been left for me by her doctor. It was a low-grade malignancy with no sign of spread. "That little baby must have been sent from heaven to save my life," a tearful Kathryn proclaimed. I had to agree.

Back home, I had my own medical appointment to keep. Two years earlier I had noticed a "hole", right above the centre of vision in my right eye. After a couple of false starts, the problem was diagnosed as glaucoma, probably inherited from dad. My ocular pressures were not astronomical, only two or three millimeters higher than they should be. Nonetheless, damage had been done to the right optic nerve. Eye drops and laser treatments were prescribed in quick succession as my ophthalmologist kept a close watch on the "upsansdowns" of my eye pressures. I was a very compliant patient and did exactly as he instructed, never missing a drop. The phrase "I'll be seeing you" took on a whole new meaning.

"I'm very worried about your right eye," he reported in late December. Despite the fact that my ocular pressure, now fourteen, was well within the normal range, I had lost a bit more peripheral vision. Persistent small hemorrhages on the optic nerve indicated that, despite the lowered pressure, the process was not under good control.

Now it was my turn to be scared. "What do we do now?" I asked.

"I've done as much as I can. I want to refer you to a colleague. I think you need surgery[166] to drop the pressure in that eye," he responded glumly.

I was shocked. "What about trying different drops?" I suggested. I had read that a combination of two eye fluid-reducing substances in one drop seemed to be more effective in many patients. Dad had been prescribed the combo drops for years.

He just shook his head. "No drops will get you down to where you need to be," he replied matter-of-factly.

"And where, exactly, do I need to be?" I countered.

"Seven, eight, ten.....who knows?" he shrugged. *That's a big help!*

"I think you had better come with me to my appointment," I told Jill. I needn't have said anything. She would have been there whether or not I asked her. We found my new, much younger doctor to be both high-tech and more upbeat in her approach. "Your retinal scan shows the damage is mainly along the lower border of the right optic nerve. The left optic nerve looks pretty good," she reassured me, pointing out the areas in the colored picture so that I could see them for myself. Then, using a hand-held gun-like device to painlessly "zap" my eyes, she measured the thickness of my corneas. Finally, she gently lifted my upper lids to measure my eye pressures. As she did so, I was struck by the subtle smell of lovely perfume emanating from her hands...a nice touch.

After a few minutes of peering at my retinas, she sat back. "I don't want to operate except as a last resort. *Whew!!* The procedure can cause complications. *Ouch!!* Your pressure is really quite

---

166 The procedure is called "trabeculectomy", literally the creation of a tube to channel fluid from inside the eye to the outer surface, where it drains into a little "valve" of tissue created under the sclera (white of the eye), just out of sight under the upper eyelid. Sometimes, as a result of excessive drainage, the pressure drops too low and the eye then has to be "pumped up" with saline. Sounds scary? I thought so, too.

good now, at fourteen, and since your corneas are actually on the thick side of normal, the pressure in your eye could actually be a bit lower than what I measure. Let's see if we can't get it down further by switching to a combination drop twice a day. That's in addition to the other one you take at night. I have found this approach helpful in many patients." I didn't need convincing. After all, hadn't I made the same suggestion myself? Three weeks later she rechecked my pressures, her hands smelling as lovely as ever. "Four points lower! I couldn't do much better with surgery," she reported with a big smile. Mine was even bigger. I could have kissed her. Although she would have to follow me with additional tests and pressure checks, I was now more optimistic. Hopefully, if we could maintain this level, all would be well. In this case, the "down" was an "up"!

Life's "upsandowns" continued when, quite unexpectedly, Frank LaBella re-entered the scene. The "up" his return afforded me was, unfortunately, at the expense of a "down" for him. Why had he come back to Winnipeg? Although happy in Gainesville, and despite being an American citizen, it turned out that Frank's long absence from his homeland made him ineligible for Medicare coverage, a fact that, uncharacteristically, he had overlooked during his careful analysis prior to making the move south. His inability to obtain affordable private health coverage soon become a major issue, so much so that he, Arlyne and their horse made the long journey home to the Manitoba prairie only two years after leaving.

Happily, Frank was given back his old pharmacology department office where, when not napping on the lumpy red sofa, he could continue to read *Science* and *Nature*, contemplate the universe and write learned papers. "So what's happening with DPPE?" he asked on the day I resumed taking my "Frank" walk.

"I'll tell you what. I'm in the process of writing a book about it. Why not read what I've written to bring you up to date?" I answered.

"Sure," he replied.

"Just as long as you understand that I have written candidly about everything, including our relationship," I quickly added. Frank nodded.

"Aren't you nervous about letting Frank read your book, especially the part about his refusing to have his picture taken for the *U.S. News and World Report* story?" Jill asked when I told her.

"Nope. He knows it's all true," I replied. Frank never ran away from the truth.

A week later, I again visited him. "I've read the book as far as it goes," he commented dryly.

"So, what do you think?"

"An engaging read," he agreed. "However, I take exception to being described as a boring lecturer and, even worse, your criticism of my singing."

"Okay. Fine. But is it just possible that I could be correct?"

"I must admit that when Arlyne can't fall asleep she asks me to stand up and give a lecture, but I *don't* sing off-key!" he insisted.

"Frank, a person never hears himself as others do," I countered.

Five minutes later the two volatile ethnics were still going at it, picking up where we had left off two years earlier!

CHAPTER SEVENTY-SEVEN:

Beware The Ides Of March

Julius Caesar was assassinated on March 15, 44 BC (the middle of the month was called the Ides in the Roman calendar). History records that he was betrayed by a group of conspirators led by Brutus, the son of one of his lovers, Servilia. As Shakespeare told the story, the Emperor was on his way to a meeting of the Senate when a soothsayer warned, "Beware the ides of March," to which Caesar replied, "He is a dreamer; let us leave him. Pass." Compared to what befell poor Caesar, March, 2005, was only slightly less disastrous for me. It all revolved around a broken promise.

The month actually began on a positive note. The clinical trial was accruing ever more patients. YM was now increasingly confident that it would be able to meet its goal of seven hundred patients by the end of September, 2005. "As of today we have 270 patients randomized and 332 screened in the study," Vince reported in a February 28th e-mail. Ten days later the numbers were even higher. "The study is cooking along nicely. As of five minutes ago screenings were 347 and randomizations 290!" Bruce Ross e-mailed. "I am doing OK, could be better but overall

OK. Same old stuff (YMB, YMB, and YMB)," he added. It was obvious that there were some persisting frictions.

"Vince is a drama queen," Bruce complained a few days later, his frustrations boiling over. Vince had a more matter-of-fact perspective. Earlier, he had elevated Bruce to be international project manager for the trial, but had to relieve him of that responsibility[167] after only four months because "he didn't have people skills". That this had occurred was unfortunate because, in addition to liking both men, I believed each to be talented and highly committed to my drug. Working tirelessly, traveling the world to make the trial a success, Vince was not one to stop and smell the roses. From time to time, he probably vented on Bruce, among others, in the Pharm-Olam organization. If anything, Vince could be hardest on himself. I frankly told him that if he didn't quit being so antsy, given his weight problem he could be a prime candidate for a heart attack or stroke.

That said, Vince wasn't the only one who was antsy. I still had not received any word about funding for my research. Time and money were about to run out. Three months earlier, I had submitted a detailed proposal to YM, clearly defining the experiments needed to confirm the 12-S-HETE data that I had presented at the December meeting. Naturally, I included a budget to cover Gary Queen's salary and the cost of all the supplies needed to do the experiments. Finally, in early February, I received an e-mail from Craig Binnie.

After reviewing our data, his committee had concerns that the test we were using to measure the levels of 12-S-HETE was not giving consistent results. Nonetheless, they remained interested in a possible effect of DPPE on the substance. Money would be provided to work out any bugs.

"...We are very interested in the hypothesis that DPPE acts at least in part via the 12 - lipoxygenase pathway. If we can together

---

167 Laura Downing, in Pharm-Olam's Reading, U.K. office, took over as project manager for the duration of the study. Vince spoke very highly of her abilities.

provide the quality data needed to establish the relationship between these two then we will have increased confidence in being able to present this in the more critical scientific arenas. I also reiterate our previous point that we are prepared to fund the assay development work which should allow you to satisfy our needs and to retain the services of your technician for the immediate future. His experience will be invaluable," he wrote.

In a followup conference call to discuss various issues surrounding the test, Paul Keane, who was very familiar with the type of commercial kit we were using to perform our measurements, had some suggestions for experiments to make sure that the results were reproducible. Gary, who was with me on the phone, spent a half-hour going over the technical details of his methods. "That's fine," Paul replied after Gary agreed to send him the raw data to examine. "We definitely want to fund this," Paul said at the end of the call. I looked at Gary, giving him the high sign.

After we hung up the phone, I told him, "Paul sounds very positive. It looks like we're going to be okay. Your job seems secure. Now let's do exactly what they want. Once everyone is happy with the reproducibility of the test, we can move forward with our experiments." After going over the material we had faxed him, Paul e-mailed, "Let me know the financial implications." I called him with a 12-month estimate. He said he would pass it on to Craig Binnie. I was hopeful that a cheque would soon follow.

For the next four weeks, Gary made good headway in reducing the "background noise" of the test. There remained one serious problem....I still had not received any money from YM. Sweat poured down my forehead as I counted the remaining morsels in my grant. I was now at the point of no return. Subtracting the vacation money owed to Gary in the event of a severance, I would be in "Chapter Eleven" by the end of March. "I wish I could help, but it's up to the committee," Paul Keane replied in response to my desperate e-mail.

I immediately called Craig, but he was "out of the office". I quickly shot off an e-mail to him. "Craig, I will be obligated to give

Gary Queen notice…if his contract is not going to be renewed….
It all comes down to whether we will be funded by YM for our
work on 12-S-HETE. I would appreciate knowing when you plan
on making your decision. I am sure you understand the importance of this request." He did not reply. *What was going on here???*
I called Vince on his cell phone, leaving him a message to call me
as soon as possible. The next afternoon, Vince returned the call
from his home. He had just had some minor eye surgery and took
a few days off to recover.

"I need the money right now or it's all over," I pleaded.

"The committee just met this morning. I'm afraid they turned
down your proposal," he replied. *I don't believe this!!!* Now I
understood why Craig Binnie had not answered my e-mail. I
could only hope that one day he would find his missing pieces of
male anatomy. As I was in the middle of my clinic, it was not a
good time or place for further discussion. We agreed that I would
call Vince that evening. "You don't look very happy," observed
Michelle Powder, my always-attentive clerk. She was right. I had a
headache for the rest of the afternoon.

Driving from work that night, the world never looked darker.
No money and it was all over. In the good old days, I could turn to
Lyonel or Peg Sellers for a life preserver. Now, both were gone.[168]
I had been out of the grants competitions for several years. That,
plus my perennial lack of success with the panels meant that a
new application to a national funding agency had about as much
of a chance as Winnipeg's temperature hitting ninety in January.
In any event, I didn't have the luxury of time it would require for
a national grant review. My money was all but gone. I was on the
precipice, about to fall into the abyss.

*Judge: "Dr. Brandes, you have been found guilty of trying to
determine whether there is a link between DPPE and 12-S-HETE."*

Me: "Yes, your honor."

---

168 Peg died of cancer in the mid-1990's. I took care of her in her final illness.
    Most of her original advisors are gone as well. Lyonel and I resigned
    from the Sellers committee a few years earlier to let in "new blood".

Judge: "For that egregious act, this court hereby sentences you to life without research. Guards, take him away!!"

As I mixed myself a stiff martini at home, the recent discussions and e-mails kept going around in my head: "...*we definitely want to fund this...let me know the financial implications...I also reiterate our previous point that we are prepared to fund the assay development work...".* Had my brain played tricks on me? Did I hear only what I wanted to hear? There was certainly one way to find out. While any conversations would have to remain "my side of the story", the written missives could be easily retrieved from my laptop. They would contain the real evidence.

After wolfing down yet another of Jill's always wonderful dinners, I turned on the computer. The e-mails were there all right, the statements just as I had remembered them.

I picked up the phone and called Vince. "My issue is that we have been promised money to validate the test and that promise has been broken."

"All I know is that the committee was unanimous in recommending not to fund you," he replied sympathetically. I knew it was now make or break time.

"Vince, I am going to e-mail you something important that may have escaped your attention. Maybe after you have read it, you will get back to me." With that, I forwarded him Craig's "...*we are prepared to fund the assay development work...*" statement.

A short time later, a chastened Vince called back. "It's pretty clear, isn't it?" I said.

"Yes, it certainly is," he replied soberly. Then: "He had no authority to put that in writing." Although floored by his remark, I remained adamant. "Whether or not he had the authority, I believe YM has a moral obligation to fund me," I replied evenly.

"I'll speak with David and get back to you," Vince promised.

Two days later, I received word from Vince that David Allan had approved just under thirty thousand dollars for us to continue our work. I immediately e-mailed YM's CEO a short note of thanks. He did not reply.

This whole sordid affair caused me to reflect on my relationship with the company to which we had licensed DPPE. Promises had been made and then broken. Were Paul and Craig overruled by someone? Who and why?[169] But, hey, hadn't YM made everything "right" in the end? Yes....but for the wrong reason: my possession of an "unauthorized" e-mail!

Now, the flame remained lit but was flickering precariously. Would we be successful in keeping the research alive? The next ninety days would tell. Or would they?

---

169 In a subsequent e-mail, Jennifer Seibert gave this explanation of events: "In January, we [YM] learned that the FDA...required us to repeat all of the animal toxicity data. This was a largely unplanned and major expense. We all had to work hard to get the support and resources in place. The most unfortunate outcome of the Dec 3rd scientific advisory committee (from my perspective) is that each and every scientist left that room thinking there was a huge pot of money that they were entitled to. The reality is that every penny of that money is needed to fund the clinical development of DPPE." Referring specifically to my concerns over how YM had treated me, she wrote: "The most difficult aspect of seeing a technology move into a company for commercial development is the feeling of loss of control. As the product matures, the number of people involved and required to support the product also grows. This is a natural process. Each and every inventor gets totally p——d off at some point with the company and becomes insulted at their lack of involvement. To a certain extent, commercializing a product is much like raising an infant. Sometimes you have to just let go and take pride in seeing your technology walk across the floor. You have a whole company of people working every day for the success of DPPE. You have investors all over the world equally interested in the success of this product. You have achieved what many inventors can only dream about. There is no intent to treat you badly. There is no plan to exclude you from anything. Please be patient with us. We are running across the floor."

CHAPTER   SEVENTY-EIGHT:

The Horoscope

"How are things?" Mark Vincent asked in an e-mail two months later.

"I'm fine," I lied, adding, "for the second time in my life, I await the fate of DPPE." *That was certainly true.* To help guard my sanity this go-around, I had started taking piano lessons, something I had always wanted to do but somehow never found the time. "Piano lessons? I see a performing duo in the future: I sing, you accompany. Let's face it, the Italian has it by genetic design," Frank wrote after learning the news. He was right. I would never be an Ernie Ramsey let alone a Vladimir Horowitz, but that was okay.

"Hey, mister, is your kid in there?" a twelve-year-old hot-shot, guitar in tow, had inquired when I appeared for my first lesson several months earlier. Before I could answer, the studio door suddenly burst open as a four-year-old prodigy skipped out to find her mother. "No, *I'm* in there," I told the amazed youth as I got up from the chair to meet my new twenty-something music teacher.

My musical flashback was soon interrupted by Jill. "I think you should hear what your horoscope says about you today," she exclaimed, wide-eyed, over coffee that morning. Despite my total disdain for such things, I indulged my dear wife as she imparted what the stars and planets had in store for Scorpio: "... *Ever since 1999, you know you've been building to your 'moment', which...let's face it...is virtually imminent. The next few years ahead are your time of harvest!*"

While Jill was amazed at the precision of the wording, certain that the horoscope was an important "sign" portending success, I was far less sure that it could be trusted. After all, there were countless Scorpios out there. How could the same prediction apply to each and every one of them? Moreover, how could I have been "building to my moment" since 1999, the year of DPPE's great disaster? Not until 2001, a full eighteen months later when the survival data matured, had its "resurrection" occurred. Yet, in truth, DPPE had always remained alive, even if that fact was not appreciated for a time. Rumors of its demise had been, as they say, "premature".

All right, then. The notion of 1999 was not totally outra-geous. What was the *"moment"* to which the horoscope referred? I assumed it could be the outcome of the new trial. Although the exact meaning of *virtually imminent* could be argued, with the number of patients having now climbed to well over four hundred, and the study taking dead aim at full accrual of seven hundred women by September, 2005, the answer conceivably could come within twelve months, by mid-2006. That possibility soon appeared more likely when Bruce Ross e-mailed: "...rumor has it that approximately 100 deaths have occurred; of course nobody but the [Data Safety Monitoring] group[170] know which death is which." In the grand scheme of the universe, a year, or even two, *was* fairly imminent. And if the survival advantage

---

170 Except for an external three-member Data Safety Monitoring Board, absolutely no one was privy to information about differences between the two treatment arms. If, in fact, there were already 100 deaths by May, 2005, the first analysis, when 192 deaths occurred, likely would take place by late spring or summer 2006.

again strongly favored women receiving DPPE, I had to agree that it definitely would be harvest time. *Suddenly, I was more impressed with the potential accuracy of my horoscope!* Soon there were other signs confirming my favorable heavenly alignment. "Your pressure is staying down beautifully, your vision is stable and the hemorrhage in the right optic nerve has gone away," my lovely new ophthalmologist reported with a smile. She had just rewarded me for spending thirty agonizing minutes gazing straight ahead at a small screen, first with one eye, then the other, afraid to blink for fear that I would miss pressing a hand-held button whenever I detected a faint flash of light generated by that infernal visual fields machine. The test was nothing short of sheer torture.

The next day, one full month before the deadline, Gary and I put the finishing touches on our laboratory report for YM BioSciences. There was absolutely no doubt that we had done everything asked of us and had fine-tuned the assay for 12-S-HETE. The results of our tests looked very good. But would that lead Craig Binnie and "the committee" to recommend more funding? Somehow, given their track record, I remained very pessimistic....that is, until there suddenly occurred a major jolt in the celestial bodies that governed my fate. Out of the blue, Craig announced his departure to join a rival biotech company.

Scrutiny of the data now fell to Paul Keane who soon contacted me to say that he was very satisfied with the new test results. This was followed by an e-mail: "...as agreed would you proceed with experiments looking at the effects of tesmilifene on 12-S-HETE production in MDR+ cell lines? If you would be kind enough to submit an outline of experimental work and budget that would be great." *Ah, to be a Scorpio with my planets perfectly aligned!*

Paul's approval could not have come at a more opportune time. As fate (or the stars) would have it, that very morning a major breakthrough had been announced at the annual ASCO meeting: a four-year followup of women with aggressive early-stage breast cancer showed that, when combined with adjuvant chemotherapy,

Herceptin (known generically as trastuzumab),[171] a targeted antibody that locks on to a cell membrane receptor called "HER-2"[172], significantly decreased the chance of the tumor coming back or spreading. Previously, chemotherapy and Herceptin combinations had been shown to be effective in boosting survival in late (metastasized) breast cancer.[173] Did this news carry with it a certain familiar ring? I certainly thought so.

From the reaction of the oncology community to the new findings, there was no doubt that, in newly-diagnosed cases of HER-2-positive breast cancer, the paradigm had shifted and the rules of the game changed. But there were drawbacks. At most, twenty percent of women with aggressive tumors had the high levels of HER-2 needed to respond to Herceptin. Moreover, the drug could weaken the heart in some women, an effect significantly magnified when it was combined with doxorubicin. DPPE also increased survival in MA.19 but, in contrast to Herceptin, did not increase heart toxicity when combined with doxorubicin, did not seem to require high levels of HER-2 in breast tumors to be effective and, in the phase two studies, appeared to work in prostate and other non-HER-2-expressing cancers to boot.

---

171 Generic names, doled out by officials of the United States Adopted Names (USAN) Panel, can be real tongue-twisters. In the case of trastuzumab, the suffix "-zumab" means "humanized monoclonal antibody", indicative of the fact that the drug is a type of vaccine, while "-tu-" indicates activity against a tumor. As for "tras-", who knows??? The tradename, Herceptin, is a clever play on the HER-2 receptor.

172 HER-2 stands for "human epidermal growth receptor, type 2". Natural protein substances, called epidermal growth factors (EGFs), fuel breast cancer cells that have large numbers of receptors for them on their membranes. By specifically attaching to the HER-2 receptor, associated with some aggressive breast cancers, trastuzumab blocks EGF, prevents cell division and also helps chemotherapy to kill the cells.

173 The 25% relative increase in survival observed in patients with Her-2-positive metastatic breast cancer who, in clinical trials, received Herceptin plus chemotherapy, appeared to pale in comparison to the 50% relative increase in all 150 patients, and an absolute 143 % increase in the subgroup of 100 patients with aggressive breast cancer, who received DPPE and doxorubicin in the MA.19 trial.

That said, I still wondered whether DPPE could be acting in a "Herceptin-like" way with the additional benefit of increasing survival in *all* women with aggressive breast cancer, not just the minority with high levels of HER-2. "To be, or not to be, like Herceptin. *That is the question!*" I shamelessly soliloquized. The possible answer was that DPPE might be acting "downstream" from HER-2, rather than at the receptor itself. In other words, DPPE and Herceptin might be affecting the same chemical pathway that increases the sensitivity of cancer cells to chemotherapy, but at different locations along the road. If so, HER-2, vital for Herceptin's effectiveness, might be irrelevant to the ability of DPPE to help chemotherapy kill aggressive cells. Fueling my excitement about this possibility was a published paper that linked overactivity of the HER-2 receptor to the stimulation of 12-lipoxygenase, *the very enzyme that forms 12-S-HETE.*

Now, more than ever, we needed an answer to what DPPE was doing to levels of that substance in cancer cells and in the bloodstream! With another six months' funding now guaranteed, I could only pray that my astrology would remain favorable long enough for Gary and me to find out. Not to worry. I soon learned that our solar system's largest planet was hurtling my way. "Jupiter enters your sign in late October where it stays for a year, bringing you good fortune and luck. It doesn't get much better than this," the horoscope in that weekend's newspaper assured me. *Scorpio rules!!!*

CHAPTER SEVENTY-NINE:

The Little Engine That Could

Sure enough, as Jupiter and I came within a month of our rendezvous, Vince Salvatori stood poised to keep his longstanding promise to me. "I was in Houston this weekend giving a pep talk to the country managers to get 700 patients by [the] end of this month. We are at 662 today," he had dutifully reported in a September 12th e-mail. The pep talk must have worked, as just three days later YM's website posted an impressive mid-month total of 672!

Then, with but one week remaining until, in David Allan's parlance, "the end of Q3", came the latest update: "690 patients today - 10 more to go," Vince wrote. I could not conceal my awe at the rapid pace. "That's really fantastic," I replied, asking him to let me know personally when the magic number was reached. "Expect a call by the end of next week, cuz!" he shot back, confident that it was now just a matter of days. Pharm-Olam, which was equally sure, faxed everyone the following announcement: "*Re: YMB 1002-02. Pleased be advised that recruitment for the above study*

*will stop on 30th September 2005. All patients must be in screening
and registered by this date."*

The jangling of the phone woke me shortly after seven o'clock
the following Wednesday morning. "We're there!" Vince stated
simply. I could tell that he was talking through a very wide smile.
Now wide awake, so was I. He had placed the first call to David
Allan and was now letting me in on the good news. "David must
be very happy," I observed.

"Happy? Try ecstatic," Vince replied. Shortly after noon, a
company press release appeared on the financial newswires.[174]

> YM BioSciences completes enrolment of pivotal
> trial for tesmilifene
>
> Wednesday September 28, 1:12 pm ET
>
> First interim analysis planned for mid-2006
> could lead to approval
>
> MISSISSAUGA, CANADA, Sept. 28 /CNW/ -
> YM BioSciences Inc. (AMEX:YMI, TSX:YM,
> AIM:YMBA), the cancer product development
> company, today announced that it has completed
> enrolment in its 700 patient[175] pivotal trial of
> tesmilifene for the treatment of metastatic and
> recurrent breast cancer.
>
> "We anticipate that the first planned interim
> analysis of data from this pivotal trial will
> occur in mid calendar 2006," said Dr. Vincent
> A. Salvatori, Executive Vice President of YM
> Biosciences. "If survival results are similar to
> those in the first tesmilifene Phase III trial then,

---

174 YM's stock finished the day down five cents on the news. Oh, well.....

175 Vince decided to allow woman who were still undergoing screening at
the time the trial closed to enter the study if they were found to be
eligible. The final total was 723 patients.

through a Special Protocol Assessment agreed to with the FDA, the data could be sufficient to seek regulatory approval."

"Enrolment for our 700 patient pivotal trial was achieved on schedule in just 18 months, demonstrating the quality of the clinical group we have assembled at YM," said David Allan, Chairman and CEO. "We are committed to maintaining this momentum as we progress the trial towards completion and look forward to the results of several planned interim analyses, any of which could produce data suitable to submit the drug for approval. The first analysis will occur following 192 events and subsequent analyses, if required, will occur every 64 events which we expect on approximately a quarterly basis. The threshold for success at each interim analysis decreases."

Reflecting on the story behind the story, I couldn't help but think of YM as the corporate "little engine that could". Finishing a study this size in only eighteen months would be the envy of any multinational pharmaceutical giant employing thousands, let alone a small Canadian biotech company consisting of a dozen or so people!

Indeed, in an interview that he had given a year earlier, David Allan proudly explained how his tiny organization was capable of such a feat: "Skill and talent as well as serendipity. We are a very small company. We are in fact 15 people, and I don't really know any other 15-person company that has initiated a Phase III registration trial. So, I think the answer is in our corporate structure. Ten years ago, when we founded the company, we created it as a management company and outsourced the majority of the work, the toxicology studies, the stability studies, the manufacturing was outsourced, our statistical analyses were outsourced, and in fact, our drugs were outsourced because we are an in-licensing company that avoids original research.

"Our job as we see it is development through clinical research. Ten years ago, when we created this model, people would say to us that [it] was not a real company. Well, I think it's the very leanness of the organization that is designed to rely on external skills, talents, and resources to be able to advance drugs at a very, very small internal overhead. To give you the numbers, our corporate overheads - salaries, rents and so on - are about $3 million a year for a company that has three drugs in development, and one of them in a registration trial. But, it really is all a function of the structure and style of the company that we've put together."

I decided to call David on his cell phone. He was in New York for the day, probably meeting with financial types. After we exchanged mutual congratulations, he turned philosophically droll: "Lorne, at the end of the day, you will be regarded either as the Prince of Light, or doomed to spend your remaining days in the darkness of the dungeon." *Roar of laughter from David.* We quickly agreed that it would be much better both for us if it were the former.

The discussion then turned serious. "What do you think about this hair-growth business?" he asked, referring to recent reports from trial investigators in Russia and Georgia that although, as expected, everyone's hair fell out initially, there appeared to be signs of regrowth after the first few chemotherapy treatments in patients on the DPPE arm of the study. "If true, it suggests a certain degree of hair follicle protection by DPPE," I replied, adding hopefully, "maybe it also means that increased survival will follow."

David then revived a pet peeve. While appreciating the role the University of Manitoba and province had played in the early years, he felt that little interest or enthusiasm from either had come his, or YM's, way subsequent to the halcyon days of Bristol-Myers. Early on, he had written eloquent letters to them, asking for their support, and felt that he was ignored. In this, he was not wrong.

Indeed, I often sensed the same thing myself and pondered why. Perhaps there was a degree of residual "shell-shock" after the hope and hoopla of 1996 ended in the crash of 1999, resulting in a certain timidity to re-associate too publicly with the up-and-down fortunes of the drug. Or perhaps it was the old "*Yes, but what have you done for us lately?*" routine.

Then there was the time element. The passing of five years had taken with it many of my most ardent supporters. Lyonel, Georgie and Ernie were gone. Gary Filmon's days as premier had long passed. Terry Hogan had stepped down; his replacement, Dr. Joanne Keselman, seemed supportive of my efforts, but had a disturbing knack for not returning my calls. Marion-Vaisey Genser and Janet Scholz were also absent the scene, the former long-retired and now ill, the latter having recently moved to Calgary where she set up her own consulting practice. Finally, Brent Schacter's successor as CEO of what is now called CancerCare Manitoba, tended to steep himself in bureaucracy, seldom straying from his fourth-floor office. Although aware of DPPE and its potential importance, he had not asked me about its status for almost two years! Dismayed, I decided that I wouldn't add to his already heavy administrative burden with news of our progress.

No excuse offered would pass muster with David, however. He simply could not understand why, in light of the now-finished trial, "those people in Manitoba" continued to show, as he put it for the umpteenth time, "not the slightest interest in DPPE". Indeed, in true David Allan fashion, he had recently taken on some of "those people" over the issue. "Frankly, his behavior has been off-putting for all," Garold (Gary) Breit, the University of Manitoba's new head of technology transfer had e-mailed me after an unpleasant encounter with Allan at an international biotech trade show in Philadelphia two months earlier.

According to Breit, not only had YM's CEO vociferously accosted Joanne Keselman at the trade show ("getting in her face", as Gary put it), but then, at a reception, took on Manitoba's then-Premier, Gary Doer, for several minutes before being gently sidetracked by the premier's security detail. The general feeling among those present was that David was overly aggressive and had shot himself in the foot. Despite that, his tactic was not totally without effect, as a "letter of support" from the premier[176], co-ordinated through Breit's office, soon found its way to Allan's desk!

Words of support from Gary Breit also came my way. On hearing that the trial had finished, he left me a warm message: "Dr Brandes, I wanted to call and say congratulations to you on this DPPE trial. You know, this is an important day [for] the drug and, frankly, for patients...we're happy for you...incidentally, I have advised folks in the University and the province...we're all excited....give me a call....kudos to you." I reached Gary at home that night and had a heart-to-heart with him. "You know, it wouldn't hurt for people here to e-mail or write David Allan the same kind of message you left me this morning. Like him or not, he really deserves recognition for what he has done. Stroking his ego also might do wonders for any future collaboration and business dealings." Breit readily agreed with the wisdom of my words, saying he would "speak to the others".

Now, with the trial closed, what was there to do besides wait? The answer depended on whether you were me or YM BioSciences. As I quickly learned, the company had a whole lot to do. "I can't believe it. Here they were in a pivotal trial with DPPE and they did practically nothing that was required. What was going through their minds?" an exasperated Vince asked soon after during a phone call. He was referring to Bristol-Myers. YM was having to spend additional millions, working day and night to plug the gaping regulatory holes the drug giant had failed to fill in.[177]

---

176 "It was a pleasure meeting you at the Canadian reception in Philadelphia during BIO 2005," the premier stated in his opening sentence. Don't you love politicians?

177 I posed Vince's question to Jeff Usakewicz. "I think that being such a huge company with all the needed resources, Bristol-Myers' management probably felt that they could quickly ramp things up to obtain the required data once MA.19 was positive.

The long and short of it was that, without a complete dossier on drug manufacture, product stability, additional animal toxicity studies and human pharmacokinetics, a New Drug Application could not be submitted to the FDA, even if the trial was successful. Data that had been sufficient for Agnes Klein to allow me to begin my clinical studies years earlier was totally inadequate to bring the drug to commercial fruition. Ironically, Vince had just hired Scott Bentham from the Canadian branch of Bristol-Myers (!!) to oversee product development and make sure that nothing in the DPPE file was overlooked.

As opposed to YM's frantic agenda, with the exception of my research effort, I was in a "mark time" mode, about to reprise my role in *Groundhog Day*. The only difference this time around was that, instead of waking up to the clock radio at the same time each morning, wondering about the verdict of Bristol-Myers and the NCIC, my thoughts would be focused on the three-member Data Safety Monitoring Board (DSMB) appointed by YM BioSciences: Dr. Joyce O'Shaughnessy, a widely-known breast cancer specialist; Dr. John Crown, professor of oncology and holder of the cancer research chair at Dublin's St. Vincent's University Hospital; and Dr. Lee-Jen Wei, professor of biostatistics at Harvard.

Reviewing the C.V. of each, I immediately suspected that we and DPPE were in good hands. A *cum laude* Yale Medical School grad, Dr. O'Shaughnessy had been a special assistant to the director of the NCI in the late 1980's, co-ordinating the agency's development of approval guidelines for new cancer drugs with the FDA. She eventually left government service and moved to the Baylor-Sammons Cancer Center in Dallas, affiliating herself with U.S. Oncology, a private sector cancer treatment and research healthcare network. I noted that one of her stated interests was in making drugs like doxorubicin and epirubicin more effective in breast cancer therapy....a perfect fit for her involvement in the DPPE study.

I had a similar feeling about Professor Crown, especially on learning that he, too, had taken a laboratory discovery from the bench to the clinic. In an incredible parallel to my own story, his research had uncovered a possible DPPE-like effect of a widely-used anti-inflammatory drug, known by the tradename, Sulindac, to potentiate chemotherapy in resistant tumor cells overexpressing a cell membrane-associated protein pump called "MRP1", different in form, but similar in function, to our old friend the Pg-P. Like me with DPPE, Crown had taken his baby into phase 1 and 2 clinical trials, combining it with epirubicin! Obviously, he and I had much in common.

Finally, there was Lee-Jen Wei, a widely-cited heavyweight in the field of clinical trial design who was especially interested in statistical methods of interim analyses and survival assessment.[178] For this reason, I was somewhat disconcerted to learn from Vince in the back of a limo (where else?) on our way to Toronto's airport, that Professor Wei had expressed some early skepticism about certain aspects of Dr. Whitehead's method of planned sequential analysis. A quickly-arranged trans-Atlantic flight and face-to-face meeting between the two in Whitehead's University of Reading office apparently smoothed out the wrinkles.

During the ride, Vince also told me that he had briefly talked with the members of the DSMB at the yearly ASCO meeting in Orlando the previous May, after their first deliberation a few months into the trial. "They were all smiles when they came out of that room," Vince observed.

"Which means?" I asked my friend.

"Which means…I think….we're going to have a positive trial," he opined.

"Why do you say that?"

"Lee-Jen is a tough sell. He wouldn't have gone out of his way to smile broadly and tell me that 'things are going very well' unless they are," Vince reasoned.

---

178 Princeton-based Advanced Biomedical Research, a contract research organization specializing in analysis of clinical trials, was actually responsible for "crunching the numbers" of the study. Their findings then went to the DSMB for its appraisal.

I was not as impressed as my friend that any specific conclusion could be drawn from Wei's comment or demeanor. "I guess we always tend to read into things what we wish. Maybe he was simply indicating that the study was progressing very well and that no major concerns about DPPE, safety or otherwise, had been identified," I argued. *Once bitten, twice shy.* With that, Vince appeared less sure of himself, agreeing that his interpretation was purely speculative. "Of course, I hope that you are right," I quickly added, nudging him back into a smile. All would be revealed eventually, maybe as soon as the following spring.

CHAPTER EIGHTY:

Hopes And Wishes

My family celebrates every new year twice: first, during the Jewish festival of Rosh Hashanah, usually in September, and second… well, we all know about that one. Although totally secular, I always attend synagogue on the annual High Holidays, sitting quietly as I listen to the age-old chanting of the cantor and reflect on my life. Of course, it doesn't hurt that, for years, Jill was the lead soprano in the choir. "Have a sweet year," my late mother would say on Rosh Hashanah as she served us traditional apple slices dipped in honey.

In recent times, with DPPE on our minds, Jill would make a wish that "this will be *our* year". Don't get me wrong. Life for us had always been a full plate, never *only* about my drug. But, to be perfectly truthful, we often thought about DPPE. How could we not? Now, with only a matter of months to go before the verdict was in on the YM BioSciences trial, we both realized that, one way or the other, 2006 likely would be "it"….the make or break year.

Suspecting the same, others with whom I kept in touch conveyed their hopes and best wishes. "Lorne, here's to success!!!" the always supportive Agnes Klein e-mailed. Ditto for Greg Burke, who wrote: "I have been watching the DPPE story. I hope it pans out."

"I will try to remember to breathe while waiting [for] the results," Lee Schacter, now a private pharmaceutical consultant, replied when told that the trial had finished. "Looking forward to early 2006," enthused Jeff Usakewicz. "Wouldn't a good-news story be wonderful!" exclaimed CTV-medical reporter Avis Favaro, while Susan Brink, now at the Los Angeles Times, wrote, "I'm really hoping this works for you—and for women." *Me, too!*

So how *really* confident was I that this would be "our year"? Hope and horoscopes aside, in my opinion the chance of success at the end of the day was fifty-fifty, no more, no less. Irrespective of the highly encouraging survival increase in MA.19, there were enough examples of one-hundred and eighty degree differences in results in major clinical trials that one could never be totally confident in the reproducibility of robust findings. That, in a nutshell, is why regulatory agencies almost always insist on two positive phase three studies before granting approval to a new drug or therapy.

Yet, on the "glass-half-full" side of the equation, compared to 1999 we had much more going for us this time around. First, this was a fully-completed trial, not aborted when an early endpoint did not meet a drug company's expectations. At the time the MA.19 study was stopped, all women receiving DPPE were immediately crossed over to the doxorubicin-alone arm. How much better might the survival data have been if this had not occurred? Second, the new trial was over twice the size of MA.19, decreasing the likelihood that there would be statistical ambiguity in the results. Finally, the YM BioSciences trial was designed to capitalize on the subgroup analysis of MA.19, enrolling only those high-risk women most likely to benefit from the addition of DPPE to chemotherapy. Of one thing I was certain: we gave this trial our best shot. If it came up negative, so be it. I would not have any lingering doubts or concerns that DPPE was tested incorrectly or given the bum's rush out the door.

Then there were the promising results on the prostate cancer front to tweak our optimism. Even as we awaited the verdict on the breast cancer trial, a phase three DPPE study in advanced prostate cancer was in the design stage, driven forward by the ever-enthusiastic Derek Raghavan, and given impetus by the just-published results of the phase two study that he and I had originally started under Bristol-Myers and completed under YM BioSciences. The announcement from YM, carried on the financial wires, was accompanied by the usual ruffles and flourishes:

"YM BioSciences…today announced the publication of a research paper in the November 2005 issue of the *Journal of Urology* that reports results from a Phase II trial of tesmilifene plus mitoxantrone/prednisone for the treatment of hormone-refractory prostate cancer. The paper reported that….the 2-year survival rate of 21%[179] mandates further assessment in a Phase III trial.

" 'The high proportion of patients experiencing a…PSA decrease, and dramatic amelioration of pain suggests that this novel regimen may be more effective than mitoxantrone/prednisone alone, especially when the characteristics of advanced age and extensive bony metastases are considered…,' noted Dr. Derek Raghavan, lead author of the paper …

"The South West Oncology Group, a U.S. National Cancer Institute cooperative group, has proposed to sponsor a Phase III trial, which is currently in design and will compare tesmilifene plus mitoxantrone/prednisone against mitoxantrone/prednisone in hormone-refractory prostate cancer patients…..

" 'This publication further establishes that tesmilifene has the potential to enhance the positive effects of a variety of

---

179 Hormone-refractory prostate cancer patients typically have a median survival of less than 12 months and a 2-year survival of only up to 10% in most studies.

chemotherapies and can be applied across a range of tumor types,' said David Allan, Chairman and CEO.'"

Aside from the clinical developments, a recent spate of supportive laboratory evidence also raised hope that we were truly on to something. Corroborating the earlier findings of Peter Ferguson, Laurentian University's Dr. Amadeo Parissenti found that low concentrations of DPPE could significantly decrease resistance to doxorubicin and Taxol in cancer cells growing in the lab. Unlike Peter, who employed established MDR+ cell lines, Amadeo had adopted a widely-used method for inducing high levels of multiple drug resistance in sensitive cancer cells by exposing them over many weeks to increasing concentrations of chemotherapy drugs. This Darwinian process eliminated the sensitive cells, selecting out survivors that could withstand fifty, or even one hundred times, the usual amount of drug. However, despite reducing the degree of chemotherapy resistance in these almost bunker-proof cells, DPPE did not completely reverse the problem.

Yet, where there is smoke, there is fire, and I thought I spotted the fire. "Do you remember the old adage, 'An ounce of prevention is worth a pound of cure?'" I asked Amadeo. It all went back to my analysis of MA.19 and the hypothesis that DPPE was preventing the emergence of drug resistance so that, over time, doxorubicin remained effective to kill aggressive cells. *Preventing resistance in the first place, rather than decreasing it after the fact, might be the answer to how DPPE worked.*

Now, with Amadeo's laboratory technique firmly established, the hypothesis could be definitively tested by adding DPPE to the cell cultures at the same time as they were being treated with increasing concentrations of chemotherapy drugs to make them resistant. If the cells still retained much, or all, of their original sensitivity despite weeks of exposure, *voilà*!! The minute I said it, a light went on in Amadeo's eyes. It was the obvious next experiment. I could hardly wait for the results.

And what about the provocative suggestion that DPPE might be targeting tumor stem cells? Coincident with Dr. Zacksenhaus and his colleagues gearing up for the start of their experiments, I attended a Winnipeg dinner meeting where oncologist and molecular biologist, Dr. John Mackey of Edmonton's prestigious W.W. Cross Cancer Institute, presented an overview of the treatment of metastatic breast cancer. "Chemotherapy is only palliative in late breast cancer because most of the tumor cells we currently target with antineoplastic drugs are at the end of their life-cycle," he stated.

John's point was well-taken. The common notion that all cancer cells divide in perpetuity is incorrect; killing off most late-stage cancer cells that no longer multiply may shrink tumors but has little biological effect on the cancer's capacity for new growth or spread. To succeed in controlling metastatic spread and thereby prolong life, he believed we must turn our attack on the more primitive "seeds", the tumor stem-cells that had the ongoing capacity to make new clones of dividing cells. But could it be done?

To my surprise and delight, John then put up a slide of the survival curve from the MA.19 trial. Looking my way, he commented, "Based on the magnitude of difference in survival in the two arms of this published study, I believe that Lorne's drug, DPPE, may be the first example of an agent that can accomplish this." As he said this, my colleagues smiled, toasting the possibility by raising their now largely-empty glasses. I nodded my thanks to the group and to John for his comments, explaining that a research project to look at this very possibility was being initiated.

There was more. Exciting news arrived from the laboratory of my colleague, Andras Falus, a professor at Budapest's Semelweis University. At my request, Maria Deli, a researcher in his department, had carried out experiments to determine whether DPPE

might increase the permeability[180] of blood vessels in experimental brain tumors in rats. For decades, doctors and scientists
have grappled with the "blood-brain barrier", a term to describe
the fact that, as compared to the cells lining blood vessels in the
rest of the body, those feeding the brain are cemented tightly
together, greatly reducing the number of microscopic "openings"
whereby chemotherapy drugs and other substances can exit the
blood stream and penetrate into the surrounding tissue. Not
only that, it turns out that the brain's blood vessel cells are a rich
repository for the drug-busting P-glycoprotein pump! As a result,
the central nervous system is often a sanctuary for cancer cells,
and a common site of relapse in diseases such as acute leukemia,
where chemotherapy kills malignant blood cells everywhere but
in the brain.[181]

Now, Maria had shown that DPPE treatment in rats significantly breached the blood-brain barrier, especially in the blood
vessels feeding brain tumors, making them much more "leaky".
The implication was huge, suggesting that DPPE might improve
the ability of chemotherapy drugs to treat brain tumors and leukemia. One thing was becoming increasingly clear: DPPE had
impressive biological activity at multiple levels that might improve
the outcome in patients with cancer.

As to our own progress on the 12-S-HETE front, we now had
evidence that, in eight of eleven patients with breast cancer, including five of six with high grade tumors, DPPE caused a significant
change, either up or down, in serum levels of the substance.

But suddenly there was a question. "Have you tested to see
whether any of the 12-S-HETE may be coming from the platelets

---

180 Permeability refers to the ability of a substance such as a liquid to pass
     through openings, for example, through a membrane. Since stimulat-
     ing the formation of certain prostaglandins and HETEs can affect this
     process, I thought DPPE might increase blood vessel permeability, espe-
     cially in vascular tumors.

181 For that reason, it is standard practice in the treatment of acute leuke-
     mia to prophylactically inject a chemotherapy drug called methotrexate
     directly into the spinal fluid, bypassing the blood vessels.

in the blood?" Paul Keane had asked. In my blind enthusiasm that the tumor was the major source of the chemical, I had over-looked an obvious source…platelets, those same little "corks" that make new histamine when they clump, had long been known to produce HETE substances as well.[182]

There was an easy way to find the answer. I had Gary collect an additional blood sample in a tube containing an anticoagulant to prevent it from from clotting and then remove the unclumped platelets by spinning the sample in a centrifuge. With the platelets gone, the specimen retained but a fraction of the 12-S-HETE that we had seen previously. My hypothesis about the tumor being the main source of the substance in the blood lay in tatters!

Clearly, we now needed to see what effect DPPE had on the residual, non-platelet-related, level of 12-S-HETE in the blood and to focus more of our attention on what the drug might do to levels of the chemical in MDR+ tumor cells in culture dishes. As I made a wish that the research program, and Gary with it, survive past January 1st, I allowed a little optimism to creep in. After all, the positive findings of multiple colleagues could not be ignored.

---

182 The production of both histamine and 12-S-HETE by platelets during aggregation seemed to me to be an important clue that two substances might also work closely together to stimulate tumor growth.

CHAPTER EIGHTY-ONE:

The Rehearsal

With Christmas, Hannukah and our 39th wedding anniversary now about to converge, my thoughts turned once more to angels…. specifically, the angels on the Russell's infamous candle holder. Would they revolve during our annual dinner feast? *I'm not kidding. I was really concerned.* After all, in the months following December 25, 1998, the one and only time the angels failed me, DPPE was prematurely declared a loser in the MA.19 trial and jettisoned by Bristol-Myers. Despite Jupiter's favorable position in my "house" this time around, I just couldn't take the chance that a repetition of that bad omen might nix the outcome of the YM BioSciences study. Ergo, the angels *must* spin on December 25, 2005! Anything less and I would be sleepless for much of 2006.

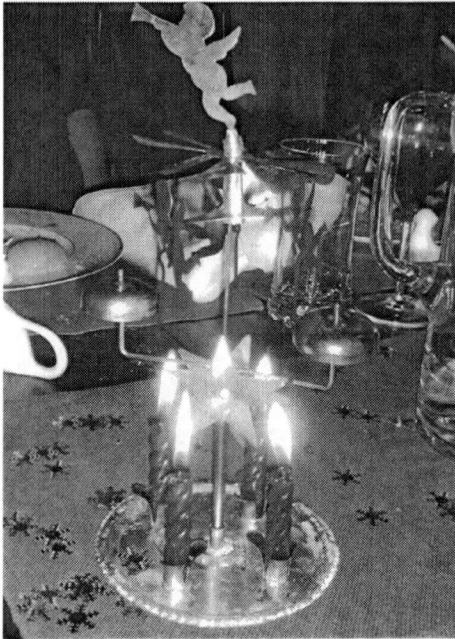

The Angels candleholder (Personal photo collection)

My worry progressed to the point that, on December 22nd, I left the following message on the Russell's answering machine: prior to the "big night", they should have a dry run, a dress rehearsal if you will, to ensure that the angels were in ship-shape. "If there looks to be any problem at all, just leave the candle holder off the table this year," I solemnly instructed before hanging up. On hearing this, would they think I was nuts? Yes....with the exception that Tony had added YM's stock to his portfolio the year before. It would be to his advantage that the angels spin; otherwise, his investment might suffer accordingly!

Yet, not all good news was dependent on the angels. A week earlier, a gift arrived from YM BioSciences in the form of an e-mail from Jennifer Seibert. My research funding was being renewed for another six months! "Hi Cuz, This is my holiday present to you...," Vince Salvatori wrote soon after.

To be absolutely truthful, the money did not come as a complete surprise. Two weeks before, Paul Keane had called to ask me if I would be willing to put our 12-S-HETE study on hold. He wanted me to consider going back to the C-3 fibrosarcoma model that we had originally used to demonstrate the ability of DPPE and doxorubicin to cure early tumors and increase survival in mice. This time around, he wanted us to determine whether DPPE could prevent these tumors from developing drug resistance to doxorubicin, equivalent to what I hypothesized may have occurred in humans treated with the drug in the clinical trial.

"But what about Amadeo Parissenti's cell-culture experiments?" I inquired. It turned out that Amadeo had run into trouble when the human cancer cells he employed suddenly died off during an elaborate experiment to test this hypothesis in the test tube. It was now back to the drawing board to determine what had gone wrong and how to fix it before he could carry out new studies. *Oh, the trials and tribulations of research!* In the meantime, Paul hoped that we might obtain more direct proof of the concept by using mice.

Given the apparent link between 12-S-HETE and aggressive breast cancer, I wasn't crazy about abandoning this line of research. Yet, I recognized the wisdom of Paul's request. One aspect of our results that continued to be problematical was the variable "up-down" effect of DPPE on serum levels of the substance. Even after removing the platelets, DPPE treatment dramatically increased 12-S-HETE in some patients' blood but decreased it in others. Why?

Even if an answer to that question could be found, would the change in the level reflect what was happening in the tumors themselves? At this point, I was far less sure than when we began this line of investigation. On the other hand, experiments looking directly at whether DPPE could prevent the emergence of resistance to doxorubicin might lead us across the finish line. *All right then. As they say on New Year's Eve, out with the old and in with the new.* "I don't see any problem in changing direction and carry-ing out the experiments you propose," I told Paul.

Based on our previous work, the testing should be reasonably straightforward. A small amount of solution containing the C-3 tumor cells would be injected into the shaved skin of the hind quarters of sixteen mice. After two or three weeks, each mouse would be expected to develop a sarcoma tumor, measuring about five millimeters in diameter. The mice would then be divided into two groups. The first group would receive six weekly injections of saline followed by a low (subtherapeutic) dose of doxorubicin; the second group would receive six weekly injections of a human-equivalent dose of DPPE (fifty milligrams per kilogram in the mouse) followed by the same low dose of doxorubicin.

Why give a non-cancer-killing dose of doxorubicin over several weeks? Just as with cancer cells in the test tube, chroni-cally exposing the cancer cells in the mice to a low dose should "prime" the tumor to overproduce those P-glycoprotein pumps and become drug-resistant.

Our aim was to determine whether, as compared to the mice receiving saline plus doxorubicin, formation of the P-gp pumps would be hindered in the mice receiving DPPE plus doxoru-bicin. The answer would be obtained by cutting out the tumors at the end of the several weeks of treatment and carrying out a test, called a "western blot",[183] to measure the level of the specific protein that comprises the P-gp pump.

However, getting started immediately would be a challenge. Times had forever changed when it came to obtaining permis-sion to carry out animal-based experiments. Our 1990 tumor studies in rodents had been conducted in "prehistoric" days, when

---

183 The "western blot", a common test for separating and identifying pro-teins, is so-called because of its technical similarity to the "southern blot" (named after its inventor, the British biologist M.E. Southern) for locating a particular sequence of DNA in cells or tissues. A related technique for locating a sequence of RNA has been named (tongue-in-cheek) the "northern blot". Who says there isn't humor in science?

completing a standard two-page questionnaire was the norm for research applications involving mice or rats. Approval to proceed usually came within days or, at most, two or three weeks. Not so in 2005. The form, now in excess of twenty pages, had hoop after hoop to traverse, including the requirement to take an animal ethics course and pass a test. The average application now took two to three months and several revisions to be approved, if at all. Indeed, the research bureaucracy had become so top-heavy, the paperwork and review process so onerous, that investigators had been known to throw up their hands in despair.

As an example, Frank LaBella told me the following story that he swore was true: a neurosurgeon conducting research wanted to study how magnetic fields affect the ability of spiders to spin their webs,[184] but his application was rejected by the Animal Care Committee. The reason? Spiders need to feed on live insects, taking "little nips" at a time from their entangled victims; some committee members were concerned that the insects might suffer undue pain as they were slowly being eaten! *Oy vay!* According to Frank, the committee finally relented when the idiocy of this criticism was pointedly rebutted.[185]

"This may have to wait until I return from my January holiday in Florida," I told Paul. He assured me he understood. Although our experiments would be delayed until we received the go-ahead to use the mice, the money would flow from YM. In addition to guiding the animal protocol through its review, during my

---

184 Physical and chemical agents can be tested for central nervous system toxicity by measuring their effect on the spider's ability to spin its web. For example, marijuana makes spiders lose concentration and stop spinning before the web is finished. Benzedrine ("speed") causes them to spin their webs rapidly, resulting in large holes, while caffeine makes them unable to spin anything more than a few randomly-strung threads.

185 Like every major university, Manitoba has had its share of threats by animal rights activists to disrupt research. While they may be misguided, their tactics have succeeded in raising the level of awareness that animals used for research must be treated as humanely as possible. That said, the pendulum may have swung too far left, as exemplified by the case Frank mentioned.

absence Gary could spend his time setting up the western blot test. With that settled, we closed up the lab to spend time at home with friends and family.

"Merry Christmas. Happy Hannukah. Happy Anniversary," the Russell family exclaimed in unison at their front door on Christmas Day evening, or "angels, do your stuff" time as I had come to regard it. "That was quite a message you left us, Dr. Brandes," clucked Susan Russell once we had removed our outerwear and gone into the large family room. For emphasis, she played back my words, still on the telephone answering machine, for all to hear. "This is serious business, Mrs. Russell," I assured her, all the while nervously peering through the dining room door at the beautifully-set table. At its centre sat *the* candle holder.

"I sure hope you had the rehearsal, Mr. Russell," I confided to Tony over a cold glass of Corona and hot spring rolls. He just smiled. A half-hour later, my host disappeared into the dining room for several minutes and then called me to come in. As I entered, my eyes opened wide. *The candles had been freshly lit and already the angels were slowly spinning!* Was I relieved, or what? With that, dinner was formally announced and everyone took their seat around the table. "Just look at those angels!" I crowed as we pulled on the ends of the "crackers" and put on the paper crowns that fell out.

By the time our goblets were topped up with red wine, and the turkey, stuffing and cranberry sauce served, a high-pitched ringing of chimes filled the air as the thin length of brass that hung from the now rapidly-revolving heavenly figurines struck the two bells perched below. Their constant *ping, ping, ping* was such music to my ear that I crooned back, "We meet and the angels sing. The angels sing the sweetest song I ever heard…."[186].

"Don't you think we've heard enough of that tune?" Jill asked with a tone of exasperation after I sang it a second time. *Did she not understand the significance of what was happening here?*

---

186 *And The Angels Sing.* Ziggy Elman and Johnny Mercer. © 1939. WB Music Corp

Unrepentant, I continued *sotto voce*. Come dessert, as I savored my favorite Figgie pudding, the candles finally started to flicker. Undaunted, the angels stubbornly continued their circular journey, coming to a standstill only when the flames finally died out as the last sip of coffee went down. *If this wasn't a good sign, nothing was!*

After dinner, I warmly complimented Tony for making sure that the evening's performance was flawless. With that, he confessed that there had been no rehearsal. *What?? Surely an explanation was in order*! And so it was given: after discussing my request, the Russell's daughter, Carolyn, a graduate engineer, had carried out a top-to-bottom inspection. The red candles were of uniform height, had good wicks, and fit straight and secure into their respective holders. The rotating platter on which the angels were mounted spun evenly atop the thin needle-tipped rod arising from the base. The heat vanes were freshly polished and correctly aligned. Carolyn's conclusion: everything was in good working order; my concern notwithstanding, a "dry run" was not necessary.

"In the end, we decided it would be best to leave up to fate whether the angels turned," my friend told me. After slowly digesting this shocking information, I decided he was right. After all, hadn't Jupiter made sure that everything turned out just fine?

CHAPTER EIGHTY-TWO:
Billion Dollar Drug?

Paul Keane had encouraging news to tell me on my return from
Pompano Beach. After seemingly endless talks, he and his YM
colleagues had succeeded in gaining the agreement of Sanofi-
Aventis, the world's third-largest drug firm[187] after Pfizer and
GlaxoSmithKline, to test DPPE with the company's taxane deriva-
tive, docetaxel (Taxotere).[188] The pharmacokinetics of the two

187 Here we go again. As with other major drug companies, Sanofi-Aventis
is the current iteration resulting from a long series of complex industry mergers. In 2004, Sanofi-Synthélabo (Paris-based, with a strong
U.S. presence), took over French rival, Aventis (formed in 1999 when
Rhône-Poulenc merged with Hoechst Marion Roussel, itself the product
of a 1995 merger of Germany's Hoechst with France's Roussel-Uclaf and
U.S.-based Marion Merrell Dow, the latter resulting from a 1989 takeover, by Kansas City's Marion Pharmaceuticals, of Merrell Dow, the 1980
offspring of Dow Chemical's buyout of Richardson-Merrell). The Sanofi
empire includes vaccine-makers Pasteur and Toronto's Connaught laboratories (both incorporated as Sanofi Pasteur).

188 Like Bristol Myers' Taxol, Sanofi-Aventis' Taxotere is widely used in
breast cancer treatment. Taxotere has the advantage of requiring only
one hour to administer, compared to three hours for Taxol.

drugs in combination would be assessed as part of a collaborative phase two study of safety and efficacy in women with aggressive metastatic breast cancer. Sanofi-Aventis would supply the docetaxel, worth about one thousand dollars a dose!

It was a small commitment, perhaps, but to my mind a seemingly important one, the first positive signal from a drug company since the fizzled Pharmacia deal. Vince concurred with that assessment. "No question, they are interested or they would not have agreed to give us Taxotere for the study," he told me. S-o-o-o, if DPPE produced a survival advantage in YM's soon-to-be analyzed trial, this company *might* be the one to license it at the end of the day.

As I had already tested DPPE and Taxotere on patients in Winnipeg, I was confident the trial would confirm my findings that the treatment was well tolerated and highly active. Moreover, as I had repeatedly observed with other chemotherapy drugs in combination with DPPE, troublesome chronic side effects associated with Taxotere, such as damage to the nerve endings in the hands and feet (called peripheral neuropathy), seemed to be substantially reduced.

YM's deal with Sanofi-Aventis did not escape Wall Street's notice. A short blurb, rather hopefully titled "*YM BioSciences' Cancer Drugs Are Working*", soon appeared on the financial newswires.[189]

> "Another tiny biotech, YM BioSciences (YMI), trading on the Amex, may also have a winner: tesmilifene for metastatic breast cancer. Now in phase III trials, tesmilifene has been shown to improve the effectiveness of commonly-used chemotherapies in prolonging life. In January, YM signed a pact with Sanofi-Aventis (SNY) to

---

189 I suspect the story may have resulted from a business writer attending a presentation in New York by the ever-traveling David Allan. As David might say, "Good on him!"

investigate the effect of combining tesmilifene
with Sanofi's docetaxel to treat fast-growing
tumors. The study will test whether using tesmilifene together with docetaxel enhances the
survival of seriously ill patients without increasing toxicity. Initial research will be conducted
in Europe and the U.S....Mitchell Kaye of
XmarkCapital Partners, the lead investor, with
10%, says tesmilifene could generate annual sales
of $1 billion. Now at 3.53 [U.S.] a share, YM could
hit 15 [dollars] in a year, Kaye figures...."

Predictably, the magic phrase "annual sales of $1 billion" caused
an almost immediate run on YM shares, pushing up their price
by leaps and bounds. To add to investor excitement, there quickly
followed this announcement:

YM BioSciences cancer drug wins fast U.S. review

Mon Feb 13, 2006 11:18 AM ET (Reuters)

"Shares of YM BioSciences Inc. jumped to a
52-week high....after the biopharmaceutical
company said U.S. regulators agreed to a 'fast-
track' review of its lead breast cancer treatment
drug....The fast-track program expedites the
review of new therapeutics intended to treat
serious or life-threatening diseases and address
unmet medical needs."[190]

While it was tempting to dismiss all of this as just the latest
example of market hype causing a bunch of neophytes to part
with their hard-earned money in the hope of snagging a big profit,
there was no denying the billion dollar potential of a successful
DPPE. Future royalties aside, based on recent precedents it was

---

190 Fast-tracking would only occur if the trial result was positive. I'm not
    sure that most investors understood this nuance.

likely that YM could demand hundreds of millions of dollars up front as its share of the deal; any number of major pharmaceutical companies would willingly pay such a large sum for a proven drug sure to gain rapid regulatory approval, especially if they perceived the potential to generate ten-figure profits for years to come.

Fully realizing that fact, YM was moving full steam ahead. Not one second was to be wasted in the event of the study's success. "Dear Cuz," Vince Salvatori wrote in early February, "...[I am] putting together a very aggressive plan to submit the NDA [to the FDA] by the end of the year. I am sure you are aware, this is an enormous undertaking for any company! But we do the impossible - so was recruiting 723 patients in 18 months."

One fact seemed indisputable: whoever turned out to be YM's ultimate partner would have spent no money, i.e. taken no risk (also referred to as "good business" in corporate boardrooms) on DPPE's development.[191] Given that fact, would the drug, costing mere pennies to make, be reasonably priced when it hit the shelves? Not likely! For starters, the payment to YM would be roughly equivalent to what the company would have spent had it taken the drug from discovery to approval; that money would have to be recouped. Next, they would be faced with very expensive new costs for post-marketing (so-called phase four) development. This would take the form of new clinical trials, both in the adjuvant (early) breast cancer setting and in other forms of cancer. Not to carry out such studies would be extremely short-sighted, since success in even one or two new areas would pay back in spades the money spent, ensuring ever greater corporate profits (and, possibly, new use patents). Moreover, number crunchers would undoubtedly factor in such costs when recommending a price for DPPE.

Then, like all new drugs, the cost per dose of DPPE would be calculated to amortize maximal profit over the remaining life of its patents, before the lower-cost generic drug makers moved in

---

191 Assuming that, heaven forbid, Bristol-Myers Squibb did not make a successful offer.

for the kill (there are only five to seven years left on most drug patents by the time of approval). And oh yes, add to the equation the multi-millions of dollars that would be spent on an aggressive "awareness" campaign, possibly including those TV, newspaper and magazine ads targeting the public: *"Ask your doctor if tesmilifene is right for you."* Critics of drug advertising contend that such costs are always passed on to the consumer.

Finally, I suspected that a premium would be imposed for DPPE's potential to greatly increase survival. For example, life-prolonging Herceptin, expensive to manufacture, is priced at approximately six dollars per milligram. Depending on the weight of the patient, this translates into a cost of *two to three thousand dollars every three weeks*. With this as a guide, any pharmaceutical company marketing department likely would argue that, although cheap to produce, if DPPE increased survival significantly more than Herceptin, and was potentially active in *any* woman with aggressive breast cancer rather than just the twenty percent whose tumors over-expressed the HER-2 protein, it should cost at least as much per dose as the latter, perhaps significantly more.

Let's face it. The oncology drug genie has been long out of the bottle. DPPE…a potential billion dollar drug? *What about a multi-billion dollar drug?* Easily, based on current big pharma economics.

Since I was to share in the profits, I should have been thrilled by that prospect, yes? Okay, yes…but only up to a point. There was a serious moral dilemma here. As a practicing oncologist, I knew all too well that everywhere in the world, whether the medical care system was public, private, or a mix of the two, the exorbitant price of new cancer therapies was becoming a major impediment to their use. Each new drug was a potential budget-buster. As a result, lack of funding often delayed entry into the clinic, sometimes for years, let alone months. Consequently, thousands, perhaps tens of thousands, of deserving souls missed benefiting from the very advances intended to improve their outcome. What could be more inhumane to patients (and counter-productive to drug company profits)?

With this in mind, I vowed I would lobby whoever licensed DPPE to price the drug significantly below current industry "standards". My pitch to company executives would be as follows: "Ladies and gentlemen, why are there hundreds of Toyotas for every BMW on the road? To me, the answer seems obvious. The average working person's budget may accommodate the monthly payment for a Toyota whereas usually only the well-heeled have the cash for a BMW. Now, why not apply that thinking to DPPE? Price it like a Toyota rather than a BMW and what you initially lose in profit per unit eventually will be gained back in sales volume as a result of public and private health-care payers being more able to absorb the cost. Delay in making the treatment widely available to patients with cancer will be substantially cut and everyone, *including you*, will win."

Was I optimistic that such a "radical" argument would win the day? Remember Richard Kaplan's words to me that day at the NCI? "I pray every day for world peace, but so far....."

CHAPTER EIGHTY-THREE:

The Numbers Game

I have always loved Franz Schubert's Eighth Symphony, named the *Unfinished* because it ends after only two movements, leaving the listener to wonder what might have followed. How ironic that in early March, while awaiting an end to that other unfinished symphony, DPPE, I toiled at the piano to learn the theme from the first movement of Schubert's masterpiece! Oh, how I struggled. Why couldn't I get through it just once without making mistakes? *Help me, Ernie!* But, frustration with my musicianship aside, practicing for two hours every night continued to be a calming influence, a great distraction, my remedy against the *Sturm und Drang* of that which I could not change.

To the best of my knowledge, David Allan did not play the piano. For the man whose favorite musical instrument was probably the bell that opened and closed each trading day on the stock exchange, the wait was becoming agonizing. After YM's share price almost doubled in three weeks, I called to congratulate him. "You must be very happy with your stock flying so high," I exclaimed when he picked up the phone. His sombre answer was not quite what I expected: "Lorne, the only thing that will make me [expletive] happy is when we get the result of the [expletive] trial and learn that your [expletive] drug has worked." Although he then laughed, possibly to mitigate his vulgar choice of epithet, there was now no doubting what was first and foremost on his mind.

Yet, whether he cared to admit it or not, I knew that the "street's" valuation of YM was of overriding importance to him. Ten months earlier, when the company's shares tanked on low volume, languishing at well under three dollars for a couple of months, shades of "Mr. Hyde" reappeared during a phone call. "Absolutely nobody believes your story," he told me. The cause of his black mood? Try as he might, he still could not get big pharma to show any real interest in DPPE. Oh sure, there were plenty of "let's wait and see" responses, but nothing more substantive. The almost accusatory tone of his voice left me more depressed than angry. After all, I knew he was risking the future of his company on the successful development of my drug.

"David really appears to be down on DPPE," I remarked to Paul Keane a few days later.

"Oh, I think it's less about that and more about money," Paul replied.

"Has his bad disposition anything to do with the low market value of the stock?" I inquired.

"No question," Paul answered. "When the shares drop, I think David becomes terrified that YM could be ripe for a hostile take-over and he would be out. It could well happen, you know. At its current price, the company really is very undervalued. Our investors could be easily persuaded to accept an attractive buyout."

"Well, let's sincerely hope that doesn't come to pass," I replied, a flashback to the takeover of Pharmacia by Pfizer quickly coming to mind. *Good grief!*

There was no doubting Paul's words. Although YM had yet to earn a cent of profit, its portfolio *was* greatly undervalued. DPPE aside, the company's Cuban-discovered drug, TheraCIM, was moving forward nicely in clinical trials in both head and neck and brain cancer, still free of the nasty skin rash, diarrhea and other side effects that plagued its already-marketed competitors.[192] David had also recently acquired Delex, a Toronto company with a promising phase two drug called AeroLEF, a unique inhaled form of the potent narcotic, fentanyl, intended for the treatment of severe cancer-related pain. This was all well and good, but without a fresh infusion of cash, additional clinical trials required for continued development of his drug pipeline, including DPPE, would be stalled.

Now, in March, 2006, stock analysts were finally paying attention to YM's portfolio. I knew that for a fact. Suddenly there was a demand for my participation in conference calls with financial types. "How do you explain the increase in survival when there was no difference in the response rate or time to progression?" was the usual first question, invariably followed by, "So how does tesmilifene work?" *Is everyone reading from the same notes?*

Whether because of, or despite, my answers, David was soon able to raise the additional forty million dollars he so desperately needed. This was accomplished through an "off-the- shelf" issuance of nine and one-half million shares of YM stock, priced at U.S. $4.25, to "major healthcare institutional investors", as they were described in a press release. U.S. and Canadian brokerage firms S.G. Cowen, Dundee Securities and Canaccord Capital handled the transaction. Despite a temporary drop resulting from a dilution effect and the discounted price, within days the stock took off again. A favorable report from C. E. Unterberg, Towbin, a "specialty" Wall Street firm that advised clients on investing in up-and-coming drug and biotech companies was the likely reason.

"We are initiating coverage of YM BioSciences, an emerging late-stage development biotechnology company focused in the area of oncology, with a Buy rating," Katherine Kim, a senior

---

192 Although, if successful, it had the potential to rake in substantial profit, a major question mark continued to be its marketability in the United States. Only the U.S. Treasury Department could determine that, but so far it wasn't commenting.

analyst and VP with the firm wrote, adding " ...we do not believe the value of tesmilifene is reflected in YM's current stock price.... positive clinical trials will bring significant visibility to this drug among both the financial and medical communities...A large 700-patient confirmatory Phase III trial in aggressive metastatic breast cancer is underway with the first of 3 interim analyses expected to occur around mid-year 2006. We believe that tesmilifene has a reasonable shot of hitting its pre-specified primary endpoint of at least a 33% difference in overall survival. Assuming success, we expect an NDA filing in early 2007 with potential approval in late 2007." *Yes!!*

"You know, we may have our answer very soon. I'm even talking March. How scary is that?" a noticeably happier David asked me in a subsequent call.

"Why do you say March? I thought we were looking at May or June at the earliest," I replied. Recently, Vince had written me that his best guess was the latter two months.

"I think we can predict from MA.19," David responded confidently. "Look, consider this: over 300 women in the current trial were entered by the end of March, 2005. We are now a year beyond that, in March, 2006. Okay. Half of those women, approximately 150 or so, would have been randomized to receive chemotherapy alone and the other half to DPPE plus chemotherapy. Now, what was the median survival for the 100-odd patients with aggressive disease on the chemo arm in the MA.19 trial? *Just over twelve months.* Right? So, based on that, it's likely that most of those first 150 patients on the chemo arm of this trial have died. Now, depending on the number of deaths in the first 150 DPPE-treated women which, hopefully, will be much lower, the 192 "events" needed to trigger the first survival analysis could be reached *any day now.*"

One thing was certainly clear: if David could not sleep at night, he counted patients instead of sheep! Realizing that there were some major holes in his reasoning, I refrained from commenting and changed the topic, leaving him mildly deflated that his brilliant deduction did not seem to catch my fancy.

A few days later, I decided to put my own perspective on the record. "...I suggest that we shouldn't rely too heavily on the 'numbers' from MA.19 to predict when we may reach... 192 events in the current study," I wrote, reminding him that while the MA.19 study employed a single chemotherapy drug (doxorubicin), the YM trial used two drugs (epirubicin and cyclophosphamide). Since combinations of chemotherapy drugs are often more effective than single drugs to treat breast cancer, the time to death might be longer on average in the new study. Furthermore, while a maximum of six cycles of treatment was given in the first trial, patients in the YM study were treated for up to ten cycles, a difference that once again could result in an increased survival time. The bottom line? Beware of comparing smaller apples with larger apples.

There were two additional problems with David's equation. First, as compared to the late 1990's when the MA.19 trial was in progress, several new treatment options might improve the subsequent outlook in women whose tumors progressed on the 2005 YM study. Second, while he was correct that the *median survival* of women with aggressive breast cancer treated with doxorubicin alone in the MA.19 trial was just over twelve months, his calculation did not seem to take fully into account the implication of the term.

It is easiest to think of the median as "*the number (or numbers) in the middle*", above and below which the rest of the numbers fall. Consider the example of 4, 6, 7, 7, 9, 12, 12, 14, 20, 21, 21 and 23. Each number, twelve in all, represents the survival, in months, of a single patient with breast cancer. The number(s) in the middle, or median, is 12. This means that, while the median survival was 12 months, five women died under that time, surviving between 4 and 9 months, while the remaining five lived longer, ranging from 14 months to just under 2 years! Therefore, it would be incorrect for anyone to assume that, because the *median* survival of women with aggressive breast cancer in MA.19 was twelve months, all, or most, died within that time, or that the same held true for the first 150 women in the current trial.

"Actually, I think that to have to wait *longer* for the first analysis could be a good sign that DPPE is working," Igor Sherman suggested just a day after my conversation with David. By this he meant that if patients in the arm receiving DPPE plus chemotherapy survived much longer than patients in the control arm, this might significantly increase the time taken to reach the required 192 deaths. Perhaps Igor had a good point there. Then again, maybe he didn't. It was all just a mental exercise, conjecture, or as I termed it, "maybe, could be, possibly…". Finally, even YM's CEO agreed on the futility of engaging in idle speculation. "It'll be what it'll be," he conceded a couple of days later in an e-mail.

In the end, playing the "numbers game" had one unintended consequence. Soon after, while continuing to hammer away at the *Unfinished*, I strayed from the notes to look at the page number in my music book. It was twenty-six. "What page will I be on when we finally learn the result?[193] Thirty-two? Forty-eight? Sixty-seven…?" I suddenly heard myself asking. *Did I really say that?* Rolling my eyes, I went back to practicing Schubert.

---

193 In reality, it could take many additional months before an answer emerged. After assessing the results following the first 192 deaths, the Data Safety Monitoring Board likely would make one of three recommendations: stop the trial for success (and file with the FDA); stop the trial for futility (meaning the end of the road!!); or continue the study (without further comment) and perform subsequent planned analyses.

CHAPTER EIGHTY-FOUR:

Hurry Up And Wait

There is an old saying: "Living is what you do while you wait for something to happen". Of the "somethings" that did happen over the next two months, the first interim analysis was not among them. April and May came and went without a peep from the trial's Data Safety Monitoring Board. For whatever reason, David now took to publicly speculating that August loomed large for an answer. Why couldn't he just be quiet and let it happen when it happened? Come on. It wasn't in his genes to do so.

His intense focus on "when" was all the more unwise because, with the data still immature and follow-up time relatively short, the first analysis had a high chance of *not* yielding a conclusive result. This possibility was not lost on savvy financial analysts like Philippa Flint of Canada's RBC Dominion Securities. While optimistic for DPPE's long-term success, she advised her clients that the required minimum of fifty percent survival improvement needed on the first go-around was a high hurdle, unlikely to be achieved. Yet, in reality, nobody could predict anything with assurance. We would all learn together... whenever. I quietly suspected that, with the three members of the DSMB likely to convene in Atlanta during the ASCO meeting, "whenever" or, at least, a signal as to "whenever", could come in early June.

And while we waited, life *did* go on. In April, twenty-five faculty members, myself included, were honored by the University for patenting our innovations. Jennifer Seibert flew to Winnipeg to represent YM. Prior to the late-afternoon awards ceremony, Jennifer and I spent some time in the lab with Gary Queen, reviewing his latest experiments. The western blot test was up and running. Gary could now detect the level of P-gp in various cancer cells. Over the next few weeks he would be treating our first batch of mice, then testing their tumors to see if DPPE could prevent doxorubicin from increasing the level of the pumps.

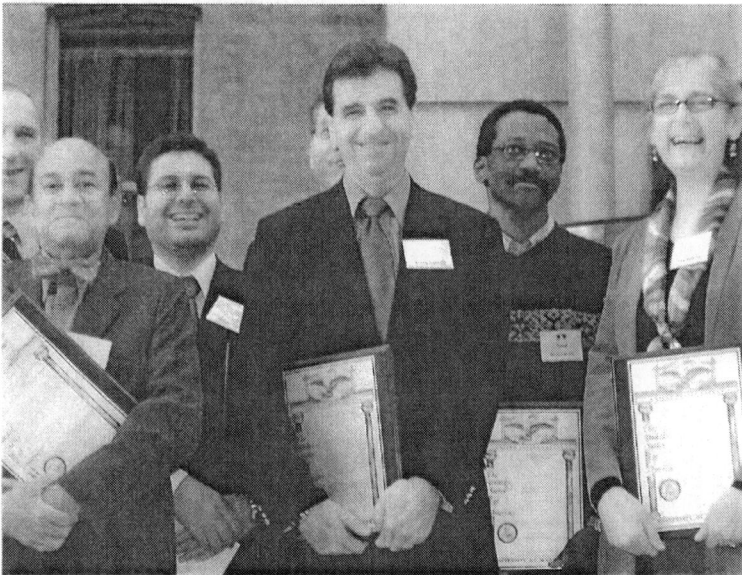

Faculty, including me (centre) being honored for patenting our innovations
(Personal photo collection)

Jennifer seemed pleased with our progress. "Have you looked for P-gp in the cultured C-3 fibrosarcoma cells...you know, before you inject them into the mice?" she asked. Why had we not thought of the obvious? Thanking her profusely, I promised to make it our next order of business. Gary nodded in agreement. It would turn out to be a key suggestion.

Early May arrived with the surprise announcement that, after months of deliberation, YM's board had approved the acquisition of a small Pennsylvania-based oncology drug firm called Eximias[194], now freshly renamed YM BioSciences USA. In exchange for its stock, YM gained almost thirty million dollars in cash, a sorely-needed base of operations in the United States and, as David Allan observed, "a seasoned oncology management team". The former president and CEO of Eximias, Gail Schulze, who had twenty-five years of late-stage drug development under her belt, would now be president of YM BioSciences and CEO of the U.S. subsidiary, while David would remain in full command as overall chairman and CEO of the combined company.

"This [transaction] will ensure YM is well positioned for the prospect of the clinical and regulatory success of tesmilifene without necessarily having to rely solely on a partner for commercialization," read one eyebrow-raising statement in the press release. Was David signaling that YM might now go it alone in bringing a successful DPPE to market? "I think that's unlikely," Paul Keane replied to my nervous query. But make no mistake about it, he, Jennifer and Igor Sherman were delighted by this new development. They were impressed by Gail and the new YM, formerly Eximias, VPs including Dr. Lisa Deluca (regulatory affairs), John Bennett (corporate development), Scott Jackson (marketing) and Gary Floyd (operations). "David can now just concentrate on raising money and let people with real know-how lead us forward in developing our portfolio," Jennifer succinctly concluded.

---

194 Backed by major U.S. and Canadian venture capital firms and pension plans since its inception in 1998, the company recently had a chemotherapy drug, called nolatrexed, fail in a phase 3 trial in liver cancer. With nowhere to go, and the blessing of its backers, it agreed to the buyout by YM.

But where did this leave YM's Canadian staff, especially the two senior veterans, Paul and Vince? Despite David Allan's reassurances that they were safe, having seen first-hand the fallout after Pfizer took over Pharmacia, I believed that here, too, there were likely to be casualties. In Paul's case, the Eximias acquisition likely posed no major threat. Now past seventy, he had often told me of his plan to retire on his own terms, possibly once the future of DPPE was known for certain. Having been successfully treated for early prostate cancer two years previously, and with his finances in good shape, he confided that he looked forward to more golf, travel with his wife and, of course, "time with the grandkids".

But I was less sure what lay in store for the much younger and less sanguine Vince. Although he was to remain YM's executive VP, now fully responsible for the "Cuban portfolio", I suspected that the influx of highly-experienced Eximias people might seriously diminish his influence within the company. For example, while "Cuz" would continue to oversee the "DEC" trial, Gail Schulze had been tapped by David Allan to be DPPE's prime mover on all other fronts. A proud man, Vince could not have been pleased about this.

Increasing my worry, his responses to my recent e-mails once again had been both infrequent and vague, usually just a one-liner saying that he was traveling and would call when he had a moment. Invariably, that moment never came. Knowing him well enough to believe he was unhappy, stressed out, or both, I decided to take the bull by the horns, writing, "I am wondering if everything really is OK with you. Does the recent takeover of Eximias and integration of its team into YM affect your situation with the company? If so, I hope it's strictly in a positive direction. But without any word from you, how would I know? Hope you feel free to respond."

His reply was anything but direct: "Exceptional on your part! I am doing the impossible - will give you what I promised! Your cuz, Vince." *Exceptional on my part?* I assumed by this he was referring to my insight in asking the question. But beyond the usual "yadayada" about keeping his commitment to me, I feared his silence spoke volumes. *Was the YM door about to revolve?* I prodded a bit more: "If I understand your cryptic response, I would just ask that you let me know if and when you decide to change paths."

This time he leveled with me: "Thank you Lorne. A very sincere message and do appreciate your concern. At this point I do not plan to go anywhere but it truly is difficult times for me. That is the reason I have not made any contact - it is always best not to say anything. My main priority is to get the DEC study done and let's hope there is a better future for me." Saddened that my intuition had been correct, I tried to buck up his spirits, writing back, "I just want you to know that whatever the outcome of the DEC trial, I will always be grateful for your very hard work. And remember, sometimes the sky is darkest before that rainbow appears." I hoped he took my words to heart and would remain with YM.

Given the reality that the "DPPE torch" was being passed to Gail Schulze, I had already placed a get-to-know-you call to her Berwyn, PA, office.

"I'm very pleased to make your acquaintance," she responded when I introduced myself.

"So how are you getting along with David?" I asked. *No use beating around the bush.*

Gail's answer was direct and to the point. Having been grilled by David during several pre-acquisition meetings, she had already clashed with him. Her firm tone of voice as we talked about this and other matters made it abundantly clear that she had tough executive skin. I believed it unlikely that she would brook nonsense from anyone, including David Allan.[195]

"I should fly up to Winnipeg to meet you," she suggested at the end of the call.

"Name a time and day, and I'll be here," I told her. I sure liked her style!

---

195 She'll add a dose of reality to the place," YM board member, Henry Friesen, commented to me.

The end of May brought an illuminating discovery. "Have a look at these western blots," Gary Queen suggested as he handed me several pages of data from his first analysis of the cultured C-3 sarcoma cells. His finger pointed to a horizontal dark line located at just the spot where one would expect to find the P-gp. If this was as it appeared, the implication was enormous: by chance, the tumor cells that Arnold Greenberg gave me all those years ago may have been MDR+ as a result of overproducing P-gp pumps. Given what we now knew, had they *not* been drug-resistant, DPPE might have had no effect to help doxorubicin cure mice injected with them. *And, if DPPE had no effect in the mice, history would have been totally different. Could there be a more random event than that???*

"Any news on the trial?" a colleague asked as she poked her head through my office door late one afternoon in early June. Believing in my work, she had recently invested a few dollars in YM. "Still awaiting you-know-what," I replied, preferring buzz-words to describe the limbo in which I found myself. As we spoke, I glanced over at the calendar. It was Monday, June 5. The ASCO meeting would end the next day. "Actually, it could come quite soon. I'll let you know when I hear something," I assured her.

True to those words, I awoke the next day to find an e-mail from Vince. "Reached 212 events but the DSMB needs 2-3 more weeks to analyze. Message was 'continue as planned'. I am at ASCO now and difficult to call. Best regards..." So, the Data Safety Monitoring Board *had* convened during the ASCO meeting. But what, exactly, was their decision? I quickly e-mailed Vince: "I'm a little confused. Does 'continue as planned' mean that 50% was not achieved and we go to the next analysis, or that the committee hasn't finished the first analysis to make that determination?" His reply still left room for doubt: "They asked for a full analysis and they will review within a month."

Perplexed, I decided to call Paul Keane. He was holding the fort at YM while the rest of his colleagues attended the ASCO meeting. Paul had also just heard the "news" but, not sure himself as to what was going on, awaited a call from Vince to discuss the situation. He promised to get back to me once he knew more.

"Apparently the DSMB has requested information on the estrogen receptor status of a small subset of patients," Paul explained when he called back a few hours later. "In addition, instead of 192 'events', it appears that by the time the DSMB convened, the number of deaths was actually 215; the statisticians were not prepared for that many, but have now agreed to include the extra patients. They have told us it will take three or four weeks to review the additional data and complete the analysis. Until then, in the absence of any safety issues, they have advised us to carry on with the study as planned."

My ears pricked up at his use of the phrase "complete the analysis". Did this imply that the DSMB already knew where the numbers stood with the first 192 patients? If so, why would they now need weeks instead of days to complete their assessment of 215? To me, the overall equation appeared relatively straight-forward. Of the 215 deaths so far, "X" had occurred in the DPPE plus chemotherapy arm and "Y" in the chemotherapy-alone arm. Since the time from first treatment to death was known for every patient, it should not take long to calculate the number of months each woman lived, construct an overall survival curve for the subjects in each arm of the trial and apply the appropriate statistical test, called a "hazard ratio (HR)",[196] to assess any difference between the two.

"Paul, what is your take on all of this?" I asked.

"I think we can treat this generally as good news," he replied. "They haven't told us to stop the study for futility, *something they are absolutely obligated to do*. This suggests there is probably a trend favoring DPPE. The one thing they *have* told us for sure is that there are no safety issues. Apparently, there is to be a press release tomorrow with all the information." *Press release?*

---

196 The HR was the number of deaths in the DPPE group divided by the chemotherapy-alone group.

"Why would there be a press release when there has been no decision? I don't see that it serves any useful purpose at this point," I replied.

Paul shared my opinion. "I agree, but you know David. I understand that since the meeting with the DSMB, he has been madly running around the place like a whirling dervish."

"Why?"

"Because, dear boy, as a result of this he is no longer in C-O-N-T-R-O-L and he *needs* to be in control. So he puts out a news release where he can say what he wants, whether he needs to or not."[197] I instantly understood. It was time to say goodbye, hang up and wait for the announcement that would come early the next morning.

> YM BioSciences announces update on tesmilifene pivotal trial.

> Wednesday June 7, 7:00 am ET

> "MISSISSAUGA, ON, June 7 /CNW/ - YM BioSciences Inc. (AMEX:YMI, TSX:YM, AIM:YMBA) advises that the milestone of 192 events required for the first interim analysis in its pivotal Phase III trial of tesmilifene in metastatic and recurrent breast cancer has occurred.

> "The Data Safety Monitoring Board (DSMB), at its meeting conducted during ASCO on June 5th, 2006 required further clarification of the data in respect of a small number of patients. When this is received it will permit the DSMB to complete a formal statistical analysis. YM anticipates that this should occur within the next four weeks.

---

197 I later learned from Paul Keane that the chairman of the DSMB told David that it was not necessary to make a public statement at that time and advised against it.

"The DSMB advised YM that there were no safety concerns and that the trial should continue as planned.

" 'We look forward to learning the outcome of this first interim analysis in several weeks,' said David Allan, Chairman and CEO of YM BioSciences. 'The reporting of no major safety concerns provides additional confirmation of the safety of tesmilifene observed in earlier clinical trials'...."

As Igor Sherman had been in Atlanta with the others, I sought his version of events. Igor's long experience with drug trials aside, I found him to be very level-headed, not given to letting his emotions override rational thought. "Lorne, we did not expect this. It was quite bizarre, actually," he told me, going on to describe the meeting with the DSMB as "a somewhat tense" affair. "They were quite stone-faced, giving nothing away," he added.

"How did David react?"

"Quite well during the meeting but, you know, once he left the room, he really didn't know what to make of it."

"What did *you* make of it, Igor?"

"I think....actually, I believe...they saw the data before our meeting and that we may be very close to a positive result. Otherwise, I cannot understand why they would ask for all the additional time and for the estrogen receptor information...which, by the way, I think is not really that important. I think they are nervous not to give a premature decision, especially since this is the first time that the FDA has allowed this type of analysis in a cancer trial. So they are being very conservative."

"Then I take it from your comments you are optimistic DPPE will succeed at some point?"

"I think so, yes," my friend responded.

"How can you be so sure?" I inquired.

Igor then stunned me with a statement that, for him, bordered on the emotional: "Lorne, I don't just *believe* your drug works. I *know* your drug works."

He went on to recount his visits to Russia and Georgia (the now-independent former Soviet state), inspecting the various sites participating in the trial and speaking with the doctors treating the patients. Many had been involved in the previous NCIC MA.19 study of DPPE and doxorubicin and, as a result, had been eager to participate in the YM trial. "I have learned from them that some of their patients treated with tesmilifene and doxorubicin on MA.19 are still alive all these years later."

"What about women treated with doxorubicin alone? I assume a few of them are also still alive?" I held my breath awaiting his answer.

"No." I slowly exhaled. *Amazing!*

"Well, let's hope that the same result applies to the current trial," I exclaimed.

"I believe it does. At every site I have visited, some treating twenty or thirty women, there were always more deaths in the patients who have *not* received tesmilifene." I could only hope that Igor's observations portended eventual success.

Time almost stood still as day after day went by without further word from the DSMB. Once again I tried to distract myself at the piano, practicing *Toreador Song* from Bizet's opera *Carmen*, all the time wondering whether, in the end, DPPE might suffer a fate similar to that of the doomed gypsy temptress.

The answer finally came in an e-mail from Vince late on Friday, June 23rd. The DSMB had simply advised YM to "continue as planned". Apparently a fifty percent or greater difference in survival had not been achieved at this early point in time. Although not what YM and I had hoped, the recommendation was still a far cry from the "stop the trial" order from Bristol-Myers almost exactly seven years previously. The announcement of the decision was made at the end of market trading the following Monday:

YM BioSciences announces independent Data Safety Monitoring Board recommends tesmilifene pivotal trial continue as planned

Monday June 26, 5:00 pm ET

"MISSISSAUGA, ON, June 26 /CNW/ - YM BioSciences Inc. (AMEX:YMI, TSX:YM, AIM:YMBA) today announced that the independent Data Safety Monitoring Board (DSMB) for the pivotal Phase III trial of tesmilifene in metastatic and recurrent breast cancer has completed its first planned interim safety and efficacy analysis and concluded that the trial continue as planned. The interim analysis was based on 215 events (deaths) which occurred as of June 8th. The second of three planned interim analyses is designed to occur after 256 events and is expected to occur in the calendar third quarter of 2006. YM remains blinded to the study data.

" 'The next interim analysis for our trial is expected to occur shortly and, as per the statistical plan and design of the trial, at each subsequent analysis the level of survival improvement tesmilifene must demonstrate is lowered. Thus the probability of success improves with each interim analysis,' said David Allan, Chairman and CEO of YM BioSciences. 'We are pleased that tesmilifene continues to display a good safety profile and remain optimistic based on the efficacy results tesmilifene produced in its first Phase III trial....' "

The markets took the news in stride. YM's falling stock stabilized and even recovered a bit. Like Igor, financial analysts and investors remained optimistic DPPE would eventually succeed.

David, too, was upbeat in a message he left on my voice mail: "Lorne…no worries. We are not anxious in the least. In fact, our modeling[198] of the situation suggests that it very well may have been extremely close or even positive….the first time around… ….so don't you worry about it. I'm pretty sure there is no way that one gets those data from your first trial without seeing [positive] data on the second trial."

Mirroring David's optimism, a series of e-mails soon arrived: "Hang in there …I sense this is all good… As Mick Jagger once crooned, 'Time is on your side'," Jeff Usakewicz wrote.

"Since the BMS study showed a survival advantage, it might just take longer to reach than expected," Lee Schacter added.

"I think this is actually pretty encouraging for a cancer drug," agreed my University of Chicago colleague, Dr. Jon Moss.

"Still looking good. I want one of us to be rich and famous for a humanitarian contribution," Frank LaBella remarked.

"Remember that anything positive at this point is pure gravy! No need to be depressed if the trial actually has to go to completion. Most trials do!" Nic Stiernholm counseled.

Yet, given that I had "been there" once before, the consensus that a positive outcome was just a matter of time did not mitigate my more sober assessment: the hard truth was that the first pitch had just been thrown, swung on, and missed. Although it continued to ride the up escalator, nobody could predict whether DPPE would eventually hit the home run needed to win the game or, like the mythical Casey, strike out. Would there be joy in Mudville? Until that answer came, the never-ending visit to the dentist continued.

---

198 According to Paul Keane, David and Mark Vincent remained absolutely obsessed by the numbers, spending hours with pen and paper constructing estimates on how DPPE might have fared. It was pure speculation on their part. Only the DSMB knew the truth. If, as David suggested, the result was positive the first time around, I believe the DSMB would have declared that the trial be stopped for success then and there.

CHAPTER EIGHTY-FIVE:

Continue As Planned

As Gary continued to toil away in the lab, I tried to distract myself by attending to my patients and enjoying the warm summer weekends with Jill and my family. July brought the promised visit from YM's new president, Gail Schulze, accompanied by Paul Keane. Table talk at dinner that night at an upscale restaurant in beautiful Assiniboine Park was somewhat muted. "There is no use in discussing future plans until we know the outcome of the trial," Gail observed matter-of-factly. Paul soberly nodded in agreement. Of one thing both were certain: given the rapidity of patient accrual, the second interim analysis was likely to take place much sooner than later. Silence followed as we reflected on this fact.

A few minutes later, our waiter came over to the table to find out how we were enjoying the meal. "Excellent. Would you mind taking our picture?" I asked, hoping to lighten the mood.

"Of course," he answered.

With that I kneeled down between my two seated visitors and put my outstretched arms around their shoulders .

"Here's to the success of DPPE," I said as the three of us smiled for the camera.

Sure enough, the second interim analysis occurred a mere six weeks later. Unfortunately, it did not result in the definitive success that we were hoping for.

> YM BioSciences announces independent Data Safety Monitoring Board recommends tesmilifene pivotal trial continue as planned.

> "MISSISSAUGA, ON, Aug. 22 /CNW/ - YM BioSciences Inc. (AMEX:YMI, TSX:YM, AIM:YMBA).....today announced that the independent Data Safety Monitoring Board (DSMB) for the pivotal Phase III trial of tesmilifene in metastatic and recurrent breast cancer has completed its second planned safety and efficacy analysis following 256 events and concluded that the trial should continue as planned.

> "We are encouraged by the DSMB's conclusion that our pivotal Phase III trial should proceed," said David Allan, Chairman and CEO of YM BioSciences. "Based on the study design, we believe the trial continues to have the prospect to yield a positive outcome. Further, this analysis also confirms that tesmilifene continues to demonstrate a good safety profile."

Was I getting nervous? You bet I was. Any survival benefit afforded by DPPE was clearly shrinking with each interim analysis. Agnes Klein's words to me at that 1997 NCIC meeting now rang ever louder in my ears: "Just remember, there's a rule of thumb that drugs usually perform better in phase two than in phase three," she had said.

Yet, if David Allan shared my nervousness, he did a good job of hiding it. When I called to get his take on the situation, he answered my query with a question of his own: "How many cancer drugs in phase 3 trials have survived two interim analyses, let alone one?" Without waiting for my response, he replied with a flourish, "Only tesmilifene!"

Was it just bravado on his part? Perhaps. But he had good company at YM. They all seemed to think that something positive was happening in favor of DPPE. How else to explain the recommendation to continue the trial after the second analysis? Even if it was less robust than MA.19, the survival curve in the DPPE arm must be pulling away from the control arm. After all, if the difference wasn't starting to become apparent by now, the DSMB was obligated to say so and stop the study.

It's amazing how we play mind games at such times. I was no exception. One moment I thought of Agnes' admonishment and the next I dwelled on the enthusiastic doctors in Russia and Georgia telling Igor about the increased survival in their patients who received DPPE. Yes, but didn't Igor also describe the meeting with the DSMB members at ASCO, where they requested more data prior to completing the first interim analysis, as "a somewhat tense" affair? Why were they tense if things were going well? "Put it to rest," I told myself.

A few days later, Gary Queen came to my office. "Can we talk?" he asked from the doorway.

"Of course. Come in and close the door."

Gary, who kept his eye out for news of the trial, had just read the latest YM press release.

"Are you concerned?" he asked after sitting down.

"Let's just say that we haven't been told to stop. YM is hopeful that something positive is brewing. But the short answer to your question is that I would have preferred an answer by now," I replied.

"When do you think the final analysis will occur?"

"At the rate we are going, we should have a 'yes' or 'no' by December." Then, remembering how everything grinds to a halt over Christmas and New Years, I added, "January at the latest."

"If it's 'yes', do you think they will continue to fund us?"

"I think so, because at that point YM will have renewed confidence in my research and will definitely want us to determine whether DPPE is overcoming drug resistance in our animal models. I also wouldn't be surprised if they sponsored us for an Industry/University grant," I answered.

Always the realist, Gary then told me that while he would be happy to keep working if the research continued, I shouldn't worry if, for any reason, things didn't pan out and I had to let him go. Having turned sixty, he and his wife had increasingly talked about retirement; their savings and pensions would see them through. I was glad he shared that with me. The one thing I always dreaded was having to cut my loyal technicians loose for lack of funding. Sadly, in that arena I had a lot of previous experience. Although both of us hoped for a happy outcome, Gary had just taken a load off my mind.

CHAPTER EIGHTY-SIX:

Unanswered Calls

The leaves of summer quickly turned brown and fell off the trees by the middle of October. As snowy December began, there was still no word from the DSMB. Since Vince was always my best source of information at YM, I called him. "Hi cuz," he greeted me, sounding very upbeat.

"Shouldn't we be hearing something very soon?" I asked.

"Any day now," he replied.

"When you hear, call me, okay?"

"Absolutely," he promised.

But Christmas came and went without a word from Vince. Another yearly feast was consumed at the Russells. And, oh yes, the angels did their stuff perfectly.

As our annual January pilgrimage to warm, sunny Pompano Beach was just days away, I checked in with Vince. "Hi cuz. Nothing to report yet, *b-u-u-t* our sources tell us that we should have the answer any day now."

"Is everyone at YM on tenterhooks?"

"Actually, everyone at YM is very optimistic. We are convinced that we have a positive outcome. Everyone from David on down thinks it will be a winner."

"I hope you are right. Now, Vince, Jill and I will be in Florida until the end of January. I want you to promise me again that as soon as you get any news…any news at all….you will call me immediately."

"You have my word," he replied as I gave him my cell number and then asked him to repeat it back to me to be sure he had heard correctly.

Two weeks later my phone rang as I sat reading under an umbrella by the pool.

"Hi cuz. We just heard from the DSMB. We have reached the required three hundred and twenty deaths to trigger the final analysis but they want us to make sure that there are no outstanding data before they proceed."

I was puzzled. "At this point I don't see how any outstanding data will change the survival curves…*unless we are on the borderline between a positive or negative trial.*"

If he was unnerved by that possibility, Vince didn't let on. "I guess they just need to dot all their i's and cross all their t's before issuing their findings. I'll phone you the minute I know."

Not surprisingly, Vince's call was quickly followed by a David Allan press release:

> YM BioSciences provides update on tesmilifene pivotal trial
>
> "MISSISSAUGA, ON, Jan. 15 /PRNewswire-FirstCall/ - YM BioSciences Inc. (AMEX: YMI, TSX:YM, AIM:YMBA)…today announced that the independent Data Safety Monitoring Board (DSMB) for the pivotal Phase III trial of tesmilifene in patients with metastatic or recurrent breast cancer has notified the Company that the milestone of 320 events required for the

third interim analysis in its pivotal Phase III trial has occurred.

"Since the last 'data sweep' was completed in November 2006, the DSMB advised the Company to conduct a further data sweep to bring the survival data current prior to performing the third interim analysis. This data sweep is ongoing and the Company expects this work to be completed and to have a formal recommendation from the DSMB in February 2007. A data sweep is conducted on a periodic basis prior to each interim analysis.

"Although we are eager to learn the outcome of this third interim analysis, a meticulous review by the DSMB of any new data is entirely in keeping with the rigor of this trial," said David Allan, Chairman and CEO of YM BioSciences. "Because of the interest in this third analysis and expectations that it might occur this month, we decided to confirm that the threshold number of events has been reached. We have no additional information from this trial at this time."

After reading the announcement, I assumed that we could now enjoy our remaining two weeks in Florida unencumbered by any further news. "The answer won't come until early February after we are home," I told Jill.

As it turned out, that was wrong. Out of the blue, Vince called back ten days later, on Friday, January 26th. "Hang on to your hat, cuz. The DSMB has finished the analysis. We have scheduled a Monday morning conference call with them. I will call you as soon as we know," adding, "We are all very excited. Everyone is expecting a celebration."

Requesting that Vince convey my best wishes for success to everyone at YM, I hung up and told Jill that YM was confident of the outcome and that our long wait would be over on Monday.

The following day, one of south Florida's periodic cold waves, the result of an Arctic air mass swooping down from Canada (where else?), sent the temperatures "plummeting" into the mid-sixties, with expectations that by Monday morning it would be in the fifties. As usual during cold snaps, the streets of Pompano Beach emptied out except, that is, for the hardy Canadians! After all, however cool it may get in south Florida in January, it is still miles ahead of the weather north of the border. "No matter the temperature, we Winnipeggers always get our money's worth," I would say to shivering Floridians.

To help keep our minds off DPPE, we spent the weekend with longtime condo friends Mark (Skip) and Elaine Pitkow, shopping at CityPlace in luxurious Palm Beach on Saturday, and attending a movie matinée on Sunday.

True to the weatherman's prediction, Monday, a.k.a "D-day", dawned with the temperature in the low fifties. As the Pitkows had packed up and checked out of their condo pending a late afternoon flight home, the four of us decided to have lunch at an ocean-side restaurant in nearby Deerfield Beach. "I expect my phone to ring at any time," I told my friends. They were both well aware of the situation and as anxious as Jill and I to know the outcome. All during lunch I kept looking down at the phone, checking to make sure that the signal indicator on the screen remained strong. The last thing I wanted was to be out of range of a cell tower when that call was made!

However, even though we took our time, finally finishing dessert and coffee at one-thirty, the phone remained silent. *What was going on? The conference call should have been over hours ago!*

"I would be lying if I told you I was not extremely nervous," I admitted. As Jill and I traded worried looks, Skip gave me a supportive pat on the shoulder and suggested we stroll down the sidewalk next to the beach. "Good idea," I agreed. After all, a watched pot never boils.

We walked up and down for the next hour. No call. Finally it came time to drive our friends back to their car at the condo. After we said our goodbyes and they drove away, Jill and I went upstairs to our unit. It was now 3:30. "It had to be bad news, otherwise we would have heard long before now," I reasoned. Jill eased herself down into the large easy chair facing the TV. She just looked into space, her eyes filled with tears.

All that hard work, and this tortured silence was our reward.

I decided then and there that if they weren't calling me, I would call them. First, I tried Vince, but for once, his Blackberry just rang and rang until a generic voice announced, "The cellular customer you have dialed is not available. Please leave a message at the tone or hang up." I hung up.

Next I called Paul on his office line; he hated cell phones and did not use one. But once again the phone rang and rang without a pickup. Ditto for David Allan. Over the next hour, I went through this useless exercise three more times. Finally, in desperation I called Paul's home; his wife answered. "I'm sorry but Paul isn't here yet. I'm not sure when to expect him," she said. I left her my number and asked her to have him call me as soon as he arrived.

I looked over at Jill and shook my head in defeat. "I think I'll sit on the balcony. Do you want to come?"

"No," she replied. "At this moment I just want to go home." She started to cry. I bent down and kissed her.

"Is it okay if I go outside by myself?"

She nodded and I stepped out the door into the sunlight.

The weather was finally starting to warm up in the late afternoon sun; it was now pleasant enough that I didn't need my jacket. I spent the next several minutes looking out over the intracoastal waterway, deep in thought.

Suddenly I remembered that there was one person I had not yet called. I looked up Gail Schulze's number in my cell phone contacts and pressed the keys. After two rings she picked up.

"Hello?" Her voice sounded distant and strained. I wasn't sure it was her.

"Gail, is that you?"

"Yes." I now detected a distinct quaver.

"It's Lorne calling." *Silence.* At that moment I instinctively knew that she was sorry she had answered. After what seemed like an eternity, she finally said, "I'm in a meeting. I can't talk now."

"Gail, I just want to know one thing. Was the trial successful?"

"*No….*I'm sorry but I have to go."

Click.

After a few minutes spent in stunned silence, I went back inside to tell Jill.

"It's over darling. We lost."

"I know," she responded softly.

We hugged each other for a very long time.

CHAPTER EIGHTY-SEVEN:

Absolutely No Difference

Early the next morning, the phone rang. It was Paul. He began with an apology for the way I had learned the bad news. Following the conference call, David decreed that no one was to call out or answer their phone until YM responded publicly to the bad news. Apparently, Gail had forgotten to turn off her cell phone; when it rang she inadvertently answered it and became rattled when she heard my voice.

Yes, his wife had given him my message. He had left the office early and was actually at home when I called but was completely drained and too emotional to talk. He had needed a good night's rest. I then listened quietly as he recapped the events of the preceding day.

"We all went into our boardroom quite confident...a bit nervous, yes...but everyone had high hopes. I even wore my green tie for good luck.

"When we were told on the conference call that the trial was completely negative we were thunderstruck. I don't have to tell you that the mood in the room instantly changed to one of shock and sadness…Vince, Igor, Gail, David…everyone.

"We learned from Dr. O'Shaughnessy that when the first interim analysis showed absolutely no difference in the survival curves, the DSMB members were taken aback… given the MA.19 results they hadn't expected this."

"Maybe that's why they asked for additional time to review estrogen receptor data on some of the patients…to make sure that there wasn't some explanation for the negative finding," I interjected.

"Perhaps. I don't know," Paul replied. "In any event, mindful of what had happened when Bristol-Myers prematurely stopped MA.19, they didn't want history to repeat itself. Since there were no safety concerns about DPPE, they unanimously agreed to let the trial continue.

"But when the second interim analysis was identical to the first, there was a lot of discussion as to whether they should declare futility. Still, because the trial had accrued so rapidly, and only a little over 28 months had passed since the first patient was entered, absent any concerns over side effects or inferiority of the tesmilifene arm, they again decided to let the trial continue to give the data more time to mature.

"Finally, when we reached 320 patient deaths earlier this month and there was still absolutely no difference in the survival curves, the DSMB called it quits."

With that, there was little for me to say, except that I, too, was shocked by the absolutely negative outcome. How could the results of MA.19 and the DEC trial be so different? We spent the next few minutes fruitlessly speculating over possible scenarios, and then turned to whether YM itself would survive this catastrophe. Our discussion finally at an end, he promised to send me all the trial data as soon as he received them. I thanked him for everything and wished him well.

Later that afternoon the bad news was made public:

YM BioSciences announces termination of the tesmilifene Phase III pivotal trial in advanced breast cancer

—- The Data Safety Monitoring Board advises the trial is very unlikely to demonstrate a survival benefit for the tesmilifene arm —-

"MISSISSAUGA, ON, Jan. 30 /CNW/ - YM BioSciences Inc. (AMEX:YMI, TSX:YM, AIM:YMBA)…today announced that the independent Data Safety Monitoring Board (DSMB) for the pivotal Phase III trial of tesmilifene in patients with metastatic or recurrent breast cancer has completed its third planned safety and efficacy analysis. The DSMB advised the Company to stop the trial based on an interim analysis of 351 events, indicating it is very unlikely significant differences in overall survival will be shown between treatment arms as the data mature. The trial was not stopped due to safety concerns relating to the product. The Company plans to submit data from this trial to an appropriate medical meeting after it completes its review.

"Dr. Joyce A. O'Shaughnessy, a leading breast cancer researcher, oncologist and the designated Safety Officer of the DSMB, and Professor Lee-Jen Wei, Chair and Statistician of the DEC Trial Data Safety Monitoring Board stated that, 'We extend high praise to YM BioSciences. The DSMB is of the opinion that the trial was well-conducted and well-executed.'

" 'We are very disappointed by this outcome and will be evaluating the data to understand why tesmilifene did not add a clinical benefit in this trial,' said David Allan, Chairman and CEO of YM BioSciences. 'Upon completing the review of the Phase III data, the Company will consider its options relating to tesmilifene.' "

****

The following day, Jill and I flew home to pick up the pieces and begin our lives anew. Now there would be one less "family member" to worry about. DPPE had finally come to the end of the road. There would be no further options to explore. There would be no next time.

EPILOGUE

I suppose it is somewhat unusual to almost complete a book and then not finish it for eight years. When DPPE failed so abruptly in January, 2007, I shelved the manuscript on the assumption that nobody would be interested in reading about an unsuccessful drug. And, to be honest, in the aftermath I regarded myself as a failed scientist. But that was not the view of my family and colleagues, who felt that single-handedly taking a drug from discovery to clinical trials was a singular accomplishment of which I should be proud, and that such a unique and interesting story was, and remains, worth telling, no matter how it turned out.

As a result, I finally decided to revisit DPPE. And so, for the first time in eight years, I read my yet-to-be-completed manuscript. Call me biased, but I found that what I had chronicled remained compelling, if not entertaining. It was time to finish the book.

Now that the remaining chapters have been completed, I want to address three questions that I am most frequently asked, and update (when possible) what has happened to the key players in the story.

"Which result should we believe? MA.19 or the YM (DEC) trial?" While nobody will ever have the answer, the fact remains that, despite taking advantage of the subgroup analysis of MA.19 showing that DPPE plus doxorubicin was most effective in increasing the survival of women with aggressive breast cancer, a theory buttressed by independent researchers who found that DPPE increased the ability of chemotherapy drugs to kill aggressive multiple-drug-resistant (MDR+) cancer cells in the lab, YM's pivotal study (with the notable exception of DPPE-treated patients in Georgia) failed to confirm the robust survival advantage seen in MA.19. It is not the first time, nor will it be the last, that clinical studies contradict one another.

"Shouldn't they have repeated the trial?" Given the complete negativity of the DEC study, there was no interest by YM or anyone else in going one more round. I certainly understood that and accepted it.

"Were human epidemiological studies ever carried out to determine whether antidepressants stimulate cancer growth?" In fact, several studies were subsequently published. Some said "yes", some said "maybe" and others said "no". But, as I feared, none tested the question our rodent studies raised (the stimulation of existing cancer), with one possible indirect exception: a large Danish study of over 30,000 antidepressant drug users found a 40% increase in cancer of all types in the first year after filling a prescription (403 cases were observed; 283 were expected). Cancer rates then decreased to normal over the next seven years except for a continued increase in non-Hodgkin's lymphoma in chronic users of tricyclic antidepressants.[199] Yet, the Danish investigators dismissed the increase in the first year, reasoning that the inclusion of these "early" (i.e. first-year) cancers "assumes a biologically-implausible induction time of zero." That might be true if the drugs *caused* cancer, but not if they *stimulated* subclinical cancer.

---

199 Dalton SO, Johansen C, Mellemkjaer L, Sorensen HT, McLaughlin JK, Olsen J, and Olsen JH. Antidepressant medications and risk for cancer. Epidemiology 2000; 11: 171-176.

While one might also argue that the excess of cancer cases in the first year might have been more apparent than real, and due to the prescribing of drugs for depression following a recent diagnosis of cancer, the reported incidence of depression in patients with cancer is 14%,[200] considerably lower than the 40% increase in cancers observed in the first year of the Danish study.

Moreover, there is an eerily similar counterpart in a New York study published almost fifty years ago,[201] at a time when phenothiazine-type antipsychotic drugs, now known to be associated with an increased incidence of breast cancer in rats, and whose chemical structures overlap the tricyclic antidepressants (e.g., amitriptyline), had recently come into widespread clinical use. As compared to the general population of New York state, deaths due to cancer were "much higher" among patients in the state's psychiatric hospitals in the first one to four years after hospitalization. Mortality rates then declined over the ensuing years; indeed, patients hospitalized for over ten years had lower cancer mortality than the general population.

Therefore, a plausible explanation for the excess of all cancers in the first year in both studies is that some people who were prescribed antidepressant or antipsychotic drugs had early (undiagnosed) cancer. Stimulation of growth of subclinical cancers by the drugs could have resulted in the rapid development of clinically-evident tumors, especially within the first twelve months (in other words, the human equivalent of our rodent studies). Over time, this "early provocation" selected for people without cancer, resulting in rates that eventually became equivalent to, or even lower than, the general population.

---

200 Akechi T1, Nakano T, Okamura H, Ueda S, Akizuki N, Nakanishi T, Yoshikawa E, Matsuki H, Hirabayashi E, and Uchitomi Y. Psychiatric disorders in cancer patients: descriptive analysis of 1721 psychiatric referrals at two Japanese cancer center hospitals. Jpn J Clin Oncol. 2001; 5:188-94.

201 Katz J, Kunofsky S, Patton RE, and Allaway NC. Cancer mortality among patients in New York mental hospitals. Cancer 1967; 12: 2194-2199.

And what about those biphasic/bell-shaped curves of tumor stimulation, such as the ones I found in fluoxetine (Prozac)-treated mice and rats, that the FDA's Dr. Temple refused to accept?

In a 2005 paper entitled, *"Hormesis: a revolution in toxicology, risk assessment and medicine"*, University of Massachusetts Professor of Environmental Health Sciences, Dr. Ed Calabrese, took up the fight, making a strong case for bell-shaped or biphasic dose responses. He applied the term "hormesis" (from the Greek verb, *hormao*, meaning "to rouse or set in motion") to this phenomenon. Moreover, he believed hormetic dose responses to be the rule, not the exception. One notable quote from his paper: "The consequences [of the hormetic response] for human health are serious. As the concentration of a drug in the human body decreases over time, the agent against which the drug is targeted could enter *a growth-stimulating zone*, a condition that could be good for a microbe or a tumor but bad for the patient."[202] Subsequently, after an exhaustive review of the scientific literature, Calabrese reported that over 120 different agents, including prescription drugs, caused biphasic responses of tumor growth in 136 tumor lines comprising over 30 tissue types.[203]

So were our rodent studies, and the "bell-shaped" curves for antidepressants and antihistamines to stimulate cancer growth a non-reproducible phenomenon? Had we "created a stir where a stir should not have been created"? Not in my opinion, unless, of course, one chooses to ignore Dr. Calabrese's findings and the two epidemiological studies I have reviewed.

Now for a follow-up on the people and companies in my story:

Despite the failure of DPPE in 2007, YM BioSciences did not go under, although one by one the key players left the company: Paul Keane retired; Vince "Cuz" Salvatori was replaced by Dr.

---

202 Calabrese EJ. Hormesis: a revolution in toxicology, risk assessment and medicine *EMBO Rep.* 2004; Spec No: S37-40.

203 Calabrese EJ. Cancer biology and hormesis: human tumor cell lines commonly display hormetic (biphasic) dose responses. Crit Rev Toxicol. 2005; 35: 463-582.

Nick Glover; Gail Schulze and Jennifer Seibert pursued other opportunities in the pharmaceutical industry; and Igor Sherman started his own biotech company.

True to form, David Allan continued to wheel and deal. After selling off YM's Cuban drug, TheraCIM (nimotuzumab), to a company in Singapore for $2 million, he bought an Australian company, called Cytopia, for $10 million to acquire their portfolio. One of their drugs, called CYT387, was showing promising results in early-stage trials to treat a chronic and often fatal blood condition called myelofibrosis. When followup studies were positive, he raised $70 million on the street to finance a phase 3 trial; in doing so, he caught the eye of Gilead, a major California-based pharmaceutical company.

Suddenly, in late December, 2012, Gilead took the financial world by surprise when it announced that it had successfully concluded negotiations to buy YM BioSciences for $515 million in a straight cash deal. As a result, YM ceased to exist in early 2013. David Allan undoubtedly profited handsomely and exited a winner.

Since leaving YM in 2002, Nic Stiernholm has had a brilliant career in the Canadian biotech industry. He is CEO of Trillium Therapeutics.

Sadly, David Harper, who had been responsible for gaining my interest in licensing DPPE to YM, died in 2009, yet another victim of pancreatic cancer; he was only fifty-five.

At Eli Lilly, Bernie Abbott left the company some years ago. When contacted during the writing of this book, he seemed pleased to hear from me, but politely declined to discuss his years at Lilly.

At Bristol-Myers Squibb, Renzo Canetta continues on as oncology VP. After several lean years and depressed stock prices, the company is once again at the forefront of cancer therapy, having in-licensed monoclonal antibodies that powerfully stimulate the immune system to shrink advanced melanoma and lung cancer.

After departing BMS, Lee Schacter held several positions in the pharmaceutical industry. He is currently the executive medical director (oncology) at Clinipace Worldwide, a consulting company that designs clinical trials.

Bill Slichenmyer, who first headed the DPPE project at BMS and then disappointed me when he was oncology VP at Pfizer, left the company after it was reorganized following Hank McKinnell's departure in 2006; after stints as chief medical officer at AVEO Oncology and Merrimack Pharmaceuticals, he recently joined Alacrita, a medical consulting firm.

David Lebwohl, Bill's replacement at BMS during the MA.19 trial, has been with Novartis for more than a decade, having risen to be a senior VP and head of oncology clinical development. I would not have predicted it, but good for him!

After leaving BMS, Jeff Usakewicz finished out his career at AstraZeneca and is now happily retired.

At Health Canada, now well into her seventies, Agnes Klein, who guided DPPE through the regulatory process all those years ago, is the director of the Centre for Evaluation of Radiopharmaceuticals and Biotherapeutics. What a lady!

At the FDA, Greg Burke who, while head of the oncology/pulmonary drug division, shared with me his concern about liver tumors in rodent toxicology studies of antihistamines, and supported the concept of biphasic/bell-shaped curves, retired several years ago after a post-FDA career at Novartis. Private by nature, it appears he then dropped out of sight; hopefully, he is enjoying himself wherever he may be.

At the University of Saskatchewan, Rob Warrington, whose seminal work on L-histidinol led me to combine DPPE with chemotherapy, and whose lab collaborated on the tumor growth-stimulation studies of antidepressants and antihistamines, recently retired, leaving behind an outstanding career in research and teaching.

At the University of Manitoba, after moving to Phoenix, Arnold Portigal, our master negotiator responsible for licensing

DPPE to BMS, was appointed treasurer of the board of trustees of the American Cancer Society (ACS) Foundation, a post he held until early 2002 when he stepped down after experiencing signs of early Alzheimer's disease. Despite his slow decline, we kept in touch for several years; he died just recently. Arnold was a real *mensch.* I will miss him.

Janet Scholz, who helped me protect DPPE before filing a use patent, now resides in Nelson BC where she runs her own consulting company.

Marion Vaisey-Genser, whose decision to underwrite the early patents for DPPE opened the door to all that followed, died of lung cancer in 2005. I will always be in her debt.

Terry Hogan, Marion's successor, died in 2007, two years after stepping down as research VP. Carl (Kris Kringle) Pinsky and Clive Greenway, two of the staunchest supporters of my histamine hypothesis, followed soon after, in 2008.

Henry Friesen, who advised me to invest in radiolabeled DPPE, went on to head Canada's Medical Research Council, reorganizing it into the Canadian Institutes for Health Research (CIHR). He was also the founder and first chair of Genome Canada; I doubt that Henry will ever fully retire, although I understand he now spends winters in Florida....a good start.

Leigh Murphy who, along with Robert Sutherland, was responsible for stimulating my interest in the nature of the AEBS, still leads an active research program at the recently renamed Research Institute in Oncology and Hematology, focusing on the estrogen receptor. She has encouraged me for years to finish this book.

Ed Kroeger, who showed that DPPE and tamoxifen were weak H_1 antihistamines, continues in his role as U of M's assistant dean of graduate studies.

Gary Glavin, who linked prostaglandins to the ulcer-preventing action of DPPE, also left research to become a U of M administrator.

To everyone's surprise, Jon Gerrard, whose lab definitively showed that intracellular histamine acts as a second messenger in blood platelets, left academia at the height of his career for a life in federal, and then provincial, politics.

Frank LaBella, who greatly broadened my horizons in pharmacology and had the brilliant insight that the "intracellular receptor" to which histamine binds is on cytochrome P450, is an emeritus professor in the pharmacology department where he continues his research; we often bump into one another at the gym and rehash old times in the locker room. Now an octogenarian, he still rides his horse and keeps current on the latest developments in science.

As for me, shortly after the demise of DPPE, I closed up shop in the lab; after 35 years devoted to basic research it was time to hang up my skates and focus all my efforts on the practice of oncology and other academic endeavours. Was I sorry to leave behind the frustration of rejected grant applications? What do you think?

And what about Professor Kahlson's intracellular histamine as a driver of cell growth? After Frank and I left the field, interest dwindled although review papers on the subject often cite our studies on the AEBS and histamine binding to P450. Maybe in the future another young researcher will read our publications and have a "Eureka" moment that will once again propel the story forward.

I end with this observation: the development and early human testing of DPPE by a single investigator at a single centre was entirely a product of 1990's culture. I do not believe that it could happen in today's world. If tons of paperwork, countless presentations, and the need for approval by layer after bureaucratic layer, and committee after endless committee, doesn't prevent a similar discovery from getting off the ground, the institution's risk-averse lawyers almost certainly will. C'est la vie.

Lorne J. Brandes, MD, FRCPC
Winnipeg, MB
November, 2015.

ABOUT THE AUTHOR

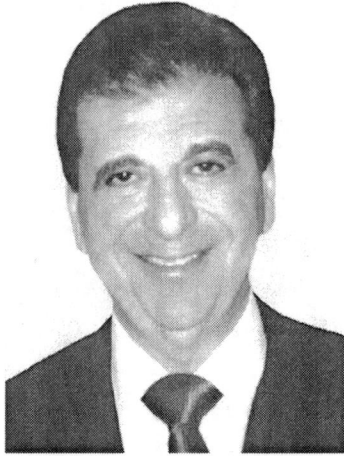

Dr. Lorne Brandes

A former senior oncologist at CancerCare Manitoba, Dr. Brandes received his MD (cum laude) from the University of Western Ontario in 1968, and his Fellowship in Internal Medicine from the Royal College of Physicians and Surgeons of Canada.

Following his internship and first year of residency at Western, he was privileged to spend 1970-71 with chemotherapy pioneers, Drs. David Galton and Eve Wiltshaw, at the Royal Marsden Hospital (London). He then completed his training in hematology/

oncology at the University of Manitoba under Dr. Lyonel Israels, one of Canada's foremost hematologists and medical researchers. Dr. Brandes joined the Faculty of Medicine at U. of M. in 1975, where he was a professor in the Department of Medicine until his retirement in September, 2015 after forty years of service.

Dr. Brandes was also affiliated with CancerCare Manitoba's Institute of Cell Biology (now renamed the Research Institute in Oncology and Hematology) where, for 35 years, he conducted a successful research program. During that time, he made a drug discovery at the laboratory bench that he took into human clinical cancer trials.

Over the years, he treated most types of cancer but, subsequently, limited his practice to breast and prostate cancer. He greatly enjoyed teaching the art and science of oncology to the many students and post-graduate physicians who rotated through his clinic at CancerCare Manitoba.

An avid reader and lover of the arts, he enjoys playing classical piano, keeping up to date on medical science and, until 2012, wrote health blogs for CTV.ca. He and his wife, Jill, have two children and four grandchildren, all in Winnipeg.

CPSIA information can be obtained
at www.ICGtesting.com
Printed in the USA
LVOW11*0252180917
549085LV00002B/27/P